Minimally Invasive Approaches in Endodontic Practice

Gianluca Plotino
Editor

Minimally Invasive Approaches in Endodontic Practice

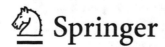 Springer

Editor
Gianluca Plotino
Studio di Odontoiatria
Grande Plotino Torsello
Rome
Italy

ISBN 978-3-030-45868-3   ISBN 978-3-030-45866-9   (eBook)
https://doi.org/10.1007/978-3-030-45866-9

This Springer imprint is published by the registered company Springer Nature Switzerland AG
The registered company address is: Gewerbestrasse 11, 6330 Cham, Switzerland

This book represents the evolution of my thoughts of the last 18 years of clinical and scientific work, since I was graduated in 2002. I met on my personal journey several people, colleagues and friends who have deeply influenced my life and my way of thinking, both privately and on the working field.

First of all, I want to express a special thanks to my family and the beloved ones, who always support me in everything I do and give me the strength to keep going beyond myself.

I want to thank Nick and Ferr, partners, brotherly friends and indispensable support in my activity.

A special thought to Vinio, Enzo and Gaetano, the people who has more influenced my vision in dentistry and endodontics, helping me to think out of the box and consolidate a lateral thinking and to the teachers that I found during my pre-graduate and post-graduate education: Francesco and Gianluca.

Finally, I am grateful to all my authors and co-authors for their efforts to create such fantastic book!

Gianluca Plotino

Preface

The minimally invasive approach represents a hot topic of the moment in dentistry. Since the technologies, the materials and the techniques are evolving so fast in the dental world, all the disciplines in dentistry advocated for minimal intervention and maximum respect of the healthy natural structures.

"The less is more" concept is a philosophy of living, based on the principles of minimalism and simplicity: very often people confuse "simple" with "simplistic". The objectives of *minimally invasive dentistry* must not have to be misinterpreted by assuming that they are interested only in simplistic procedures. Instead, this philosophy is interested in promoting optimum, minimally invasive treatment for patients in all areas and specialties of dentistry.

"Minimally invasive dentistry" is a philosophy based on evolution of the instruments, materials and techniques, which permits the clinicians to overcome some myths and dogmas deep-rooted in the field and embrace the paradigm shift concept. It represents a fundamental change in the basic concepts and experimental practices of a scientific discipline. Paradigm shifts, which characterize a scientific revolution, arise when the dominant paradigm under which normal science operates is rendered incompatible with new phenomena, facilitating the adoption of a new theory or paradigm.

Minimally invasive concepts easily involved the endodontic world, which is one of the most prone field of dentistry to evolve and overcome old concepts in favour of most actual ones.

In fact, in the last 20 years, endodontists faced a continuous (r)evolution of the field, embracing, very fast, new technologies, materials, instruments, device and concepts in the day-by-day practice. Embracing the concept of minimally invasive endodontics and implementing it in practice represents the perfect example how some paradigms of the field were substituted by new ones based on new phenomena.

The scientific world has now the mission to validate these new concepts and promote evidence-based protocols for clinicians.

The journey that I have tried to trace in the present book aims to give the reader a balanced view on the *minimally invasive* approaches in endodontic practice, describing the most advanced clinical procedures, supported by the most updated scientific data.

I would like to underline here a concept that is very important for me: everything in dentistry, and specially in endodontics, must be based on and guided by the anatomy.

It is the anatomy that dictates every single step of our treatments and procedures embraced to reach a predictable long-lasting clinical result. This is the reason why I would like to conclude this preface stating that the term *minimally* must be seen as a synonymous of *anatomically*, so that I always like to call it: **Anatomically Invasive Endodontics**.

Rome, Italy   Gianluca Plotino

Contents

The Role of Modern Technologies for Dentin Preservation in Root Canal Treatment

1

Carlos Bóveda and Anil Kishen

Contents

1.1 Introduction

Conventional root canal treatment relies on 2-dimension (2D) radiographic images and clinical assessments to comprehend root morphology and root canal anatomy. Despite several technological advances, abiding to typical conventions and/or attempting exploration at the expense of dentin tissue to reveal anatomical variation is still a common practice in root canal treatment (Fig. 1.1). The cause of conventional root canal treatment failure may be attributed to multiple variables. Although conventional practices in root canal treatment display a clinical success of 68–85% [1], among others, missing root canal anatomy, leading to residual intracanal infection [1], and compromised mechanical integrity, leading to fracture [2], have been considered as important causes of endodontic treatment failure.

Bacteria residing in missing canals can contribute to signs and symptoms of failure in endodontically treated teeth [1]. In a study that examined 5616 endodontically treated/retreated maxillary first/second molars, failure to locate

C. Bóveda (✉)
Cátedra de Endodoncia, Facultad de Odontología,
Universidad Central de Venezuela,
Caracas, Distrito Capital, Venezuela
e-mail: carlosboveda@carlosboveda.com

A. Kishen
Graduate Education, Faculty of Dentistry, University
of Toronto, Toronto, ON, Canada
e-mail: anil.kishen@dentistry.utoronto.ca

© Springer Nature Switzerland AG 2021
G. Plotino (ed.), *Minimally Invasive Approaches in Endodontic Practice*,
https://doi.org/10.1007/978-3-030-45866-9_1

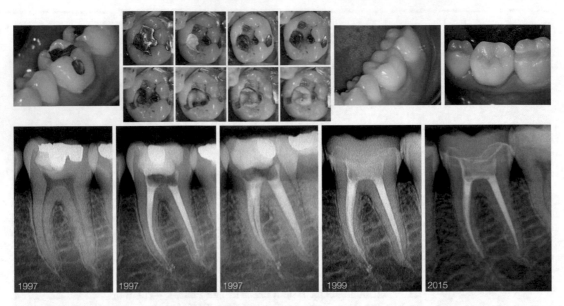

Fig. 1.1 Conventional root canal treatment. This protocol is based on the clinician interpretation of 2D radiographic images with complete unroofing of the pulp chamber space and straight-line access to the roots and canals at radicular level, arbitrary determination of the taper of the preparation as well as clinical inspection for possible anatomical variations detectable with visualization. The restorative procedure for this approach includes a cuspal protective restoration to increase the long-term success. Follow-up on this case is 18 years. Restoration by Dr. Edward De Veer, Caracas, Venezuela

MB2 canal resulted in a significant decrease in the long-term prognosis of endodontic treatment [3]. In another prospective study [4], the incidence of missed canals were reported to be 42% of all the 1100 endodontically failing teeth. Along the same line, it is also suggested that an optimum root canal enlargement coronally and apically is essential for adequate root canal irrigation and subsequent antimicrobial efficacy [5]. Thus, locating all root canals, adequately enlarging the canals, and irrigating the canals with antimicrobial irrigant are major objectives in root canal treatment (Fig. 1.2).

Compromised structural integrity contributes to cracks and fractures in root-filled teeth. Residual dentin thickness plays a key role in teeth survivability after dentin structure loss through iatrogenic and non-iatrogenic reasons [2]. Excessive removal of dentin during coronal enlargement and post space preparation have been reported as contributing factors for vertical root canal fractures [6–8]. The preexisting root morphology and root canal anatomy will influence the degree of dentin removed and residual dentin thickness post root canal instrumentation [9]. Correspondingly, oval-shaped canals become considerably affected when round preparations are created. This results in considerably less remaining dentin thickness, eccentrically in cross-section of the root [6, 10] (Fig. 1.3). The pericervical dentin (PCD) denotes the dentin situated 4 mm coronal and 4 mm apical to crestal bone [11]. It has been demonstrated that the PCD would influence the bending resistance and stress/strain distribution pattern in the root. Increased bending and stress/strain distribution would increase the propensity of vertical root fracture in tooth with reduced PCD [7]. Balancing (a) the degree of root canal enlargement with the requirements of irrigation methods to achieve optimum disinfection and (b) the goal of preserving root dentin during instrumentation so as to maintain the mechanical integrity of the root can be a real conundrum in endodontic practice. The current technological advances have been focusing towards optimizing these goals in root canal treatment.

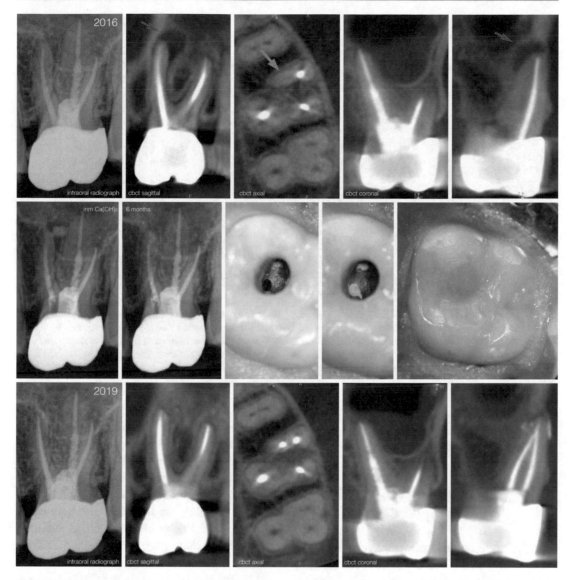

Fig. 1.2 Missing anatomy (untreated canals) is one major failure etiology in root canal treatment. Intraoral radiographs are occasionally able to point out aspects related to this situation (i.e., periradicular pathoses). CBCT slices show them consistently and detailedly. This information (clear visualization of cause and effect) leads to a more precise diagnose and to an appropriate procedure. This particular case was solved with a selective root canal retreatment, the solely reintervention to treat the missed MB2 in two appointments with the use of intracanal medication. 3 years follow-up

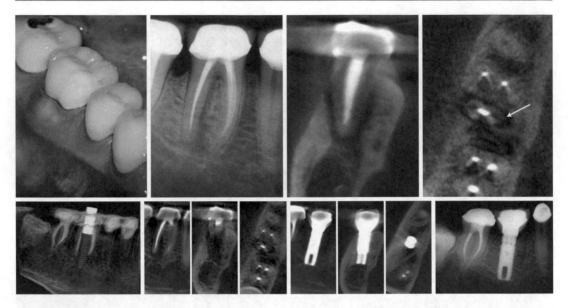

Fig. 1.3 Even though conventional root canal treatment has been reported quite successful (68–85%), cases still fail, including those where despite the fact that accepted protocols have been applied, the structural response is compromised and/or some anatomy may be missed. Presented case is failing after 10 years of endodontic and restorative procedures due to vertical root fracture of the distal root. Classic indication for an osseointegrated dental implant retained crown. Case solved by Dr. Maria del Pilar Rios C (Caracas, Venezuela)

1.2 Technologies for Dentin Preservation: Phase 1—Planning

1.2.1 Cone-Beam Computed Tomography (CBCT) Imaging

Conventional dental radiographs offer a 2D transparency of a 3D object. It has been the standard of practice in dentistry for decades. In endodontics, due to the anatomical and morphological challenges posed by the intricate root canals in the core of the tooth structure, radiological approach has been an invaluable tool to obtain essential information of the anatomical landmarks and morphological characteristics of the pulp chamber/root canals to achieve the established standard of care in root canal therapy. However, the interpretation of dental 2D radiographic images can be challenging due to its inherent limitations such as superimposition of teeth and surrounding dento-alveolar structures, as well as the inability to reveal the true 3D con-figuration of the dento-alveolar structure [12]. The 2D radiographic interpretations may also be highly subjective and would be influenced by different parameters, such as X-ray beam angulation [13]. The cone-beam computed tomography (CBCT) imaging, on the other hand, provides high-quality 3D views of the tooth and surrounding structures, with interrelation images in three orthogonal planes [14] (Fig. 1.4).

Limited Field of View (FOV) CBCT has been successfully employed in endodontics for a long time now. The current CBCT applications in endodontics includes (a) a variety of clinical situations when intraoral radiographs present inconsistent results, (b) display complex anatomies, for initial treatment of teeth with potential for additional canals, (c) when complex morphology of root/root canal is suspected, (d) for the identification/localization of calcified canals, (e) when intraoral radiographs are inconclusive for the detection of root fractures, (f) in cases of nonhealing treatments, (g) in cases of endodontic complications, (h) certain traumatic injuries, (i)

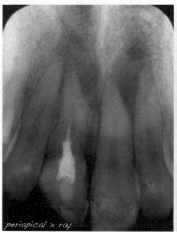
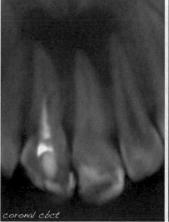
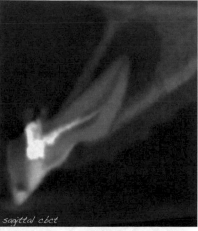

Fig. 1.4 The 2D transparency of a 3D object reveals only what may be observed from such position. In clinical endodontics this means that relevant information for the understanding of the situation might be hidden due to the limitations of a superimposed image. Actual case shows an unusual deviation on the axis from the crown to the root on a maxillary central incisor, not detectable from a conventional buccal X-ray. A lateral view is needed to fully appreciate this condition, as this one provided by a sagittal CBCT slice

in the presence of resorptive defects, and (j) for the outcome assessment in cases when signs and symptoms are present or (k) when FOV CBCT was the imaging modality of choice at the time of treatment [15]. Question arises if any clinical situation is suspected based on the conventional 2D radiographs. Resorptive defects are not always detectable via intraoral radiographs (Fig. 1.5). Even when intraoral radiograph shows a concern, valuable additional information of the concern may be hidden (Fig. 1.6). The potential of extra canals is such an issue. In such cases, without certainty in the knowledge of root canal anatomy, there is always a need to explore for what might be a possibility in the tooth, and this exploration without preexisting knowledge can be at the undesirable expense of dentin tissue.

CBCT scans contain valuable data for less invasive root canal treatments (Fig. 1.7). A detailed evaluation of the preoperatory volume should offer the following information, not clinically presented by other radiographic methods:

- Detection of periradicular lesions
- Determination of the point of entry for root canal treatment
- Assessing anatomical details

- Size and position of the pulp chamber
- Number of roots and canals
- Root canal configuration
- Root curvatures
- Working length determination (root length)
- Canal splitting
- Horizontal root bulk and canal dimension at pericervical region

1.2.1.1 Detection of Periradicular Lesions

Bender and Seltzer [16, 17] investigated the limitations of intraoral radiography for the detection of periapical lesions. Their study revealed that in order for a lesion to be visible radiographically, the cortical plate of the supporting jaw bone must be engaged. Thus, it turns out that intraoral X-rays are capable of showing some periapical lesions, but in many instances they do not reveal it when present, while CBCT shows periapical lesions consistently [18]. With the use of CBCT, any radiolucent changes at the root apex, related to periapical disease, can be detected earlier than with conventional intraoral periapical radiographs [19]. CBCT slices identified 62% more periapical radiolucent areas on individual roots of posterior mandibular and maxillary teeth,

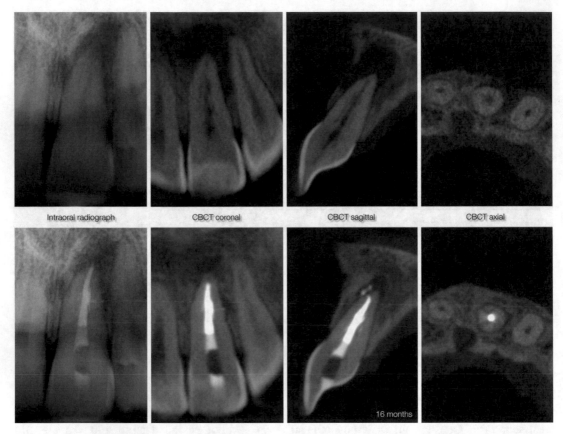

Intraoral radiograph   CBCT coronal   CBCT sagittal   CBCT axial

16 months

Fig. 1.5 Intraoral radiographs are not always capable to show or suggest the presence of dental resorption clearly, nor show the real condition of supportive structures around an endodontically compromised tooth. This affects the perspective whether a CBCT study is indicated or not when following restrictive indications for the use of such resource. Having the appropriate information ends up affecting the diagnostic impression and the decision-making process regarding the procedures suggested for any condition. Case presented shows an internal resorptive defect not clearly seen in the initial intraoral X-ray. The panorama revealed on the CBCT slices guides the diagnose and the therapy selected. Having proceeded without this knowledge increases failure possibilities. Follow-up on completed endodontic therapy is 16 months. It shows advanced repair, but not complete yet. The tooth remains asymptomatic, later follow-up is guaranteed

compared with intraoral periapical radiographs [12]. Please note that when treated early, the outcome of root canal treatment is more successful [20]. This information is crucial when the presence of a radiolucency is considered determinant in the decision of the number of treatment appointments [21] (Fig. 1.8).

1.2.1.2 Determination of the Point of Entry for Root Canal Treatment

The point of entry is defined as the most convenient location to initiate the preparation of access cavity for endodontic treatment. The most coronal projection of pulp chamber should be considered as an important location for this purpose. Conventionally, the point of entry for root canal treatments is determined generically, without individual considerations. Not considering individual information could affect the selection of point of entry in cases. Trying to obtain this information from intraoral radiographs may lead to incorrect decisions, since conventional radiographs show projection distortions that could create inaccurate suggestions (Fig. 1.9). This landmark may be accurately determined with the use of appropriate CBCT slices. CBCT has proved valuable as a tool for exploring root canal

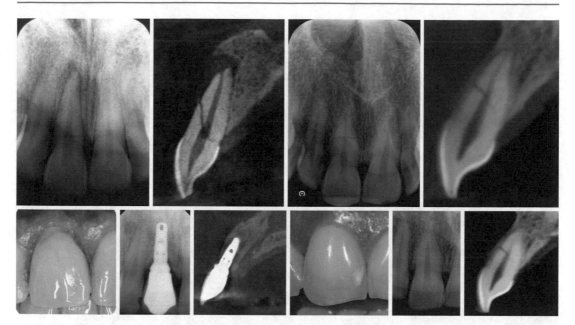

Fig. 1.6 CBCT analysis results quite useful to precisely evaluate cases where conventional X-rays failed to show relevant diagnostic information. These two horizontal fracture cases look quite similar on periapical X-rays: both shows evidence of the fracture and limited bone compromise. Maybe the experienced clinician could suspect these cases are completely different, but confirmation without further intervention is not guaranteed. As comparison CBCT sagittal slice show simply to anyone observing this a whole different situation for each case, regarding size, position and orientation of the dental fracture, and most important, the extension of the bone compromise, leading to two different and opposites approaches: extraction with later implant substitution on the first case, and simple observation with no intervention at all on the second one. Follow-up on each case is 6 years. Implant and regenerative procedures on left case is by Dr. Ernesto Muller & Dr. Luis Alberto García, Restoration by Dr. Tomás Seif (Caracas, Venezuela)

anatomy, as effective as histological sectioning of teeth [22] (Fig. 1.10).

1.2.1.3 Assessing Anatomical Details

Size and Position of the Pulp Chamber
Determination of the pulp chamber parameters is necessary for proper root canal access cavity, no matter which design is intended. Generally, clinicians rely on a tactile feel (the drop of a bur in the pulp chamber), but many teeth do not have enough chamber space for such sensation [23]. For these cases a different strategy is needed. Trying to measure the anatomic landmarks on an intraoral radiograph provides imprecise measurements. Data acquired from CBCT slices are confident to the level of resolution of the acquisition (up to 0.076 μm at this time) (Fig. 1.11). Preservation of the pulp chamber floor is crucial

considering that the dentin in this region is a part of the pericervical dentin.

Number of Roots and Root Canals
Preoperative assessment of the root canal anatomy is a key step in root canal treatment [24]. The 2D nature and the anatomical noise associated with intraoral radiographs result in limited information regarding the number and nature of root canals [25]. The etiology of endodontic failure is multifaceted, but a significant percent of failures is related to missed root canal system anatomy. Thus, in endodontic posttreatment failures, detecting missing roots and canals is the foremost issue. Investigations on the incidence of missed root canals in a population present missed canals in 23.04% of the endodontically treated teeth. Teeth with a missed canal were 4.38 times more likely to be associ-

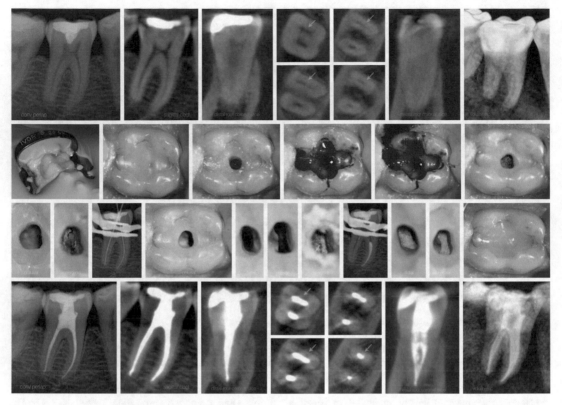

Fig. 1.7 CBCT use in primary root canal treatment provides significant information that leads to a novel procedure approach guiding diagnoses, access cavity design, anatomy recognition and analysis to decide conformation maneuvers, with later evaluation of performed procedures and reached goals. This type of procedure relies on detailed virtual analysis of the anatomical characteristics of the tooth candidate to endodontic therapy in order to know in advance relevant information that suppress clinical searching with structural loss, allowing concentrating on what is actually present

ated with a periapical lesion [26]. Intraoral radiographs have shown poor outcomes in identifying root canal configuration, whereas CBCT imaging showed no difference when compared with the gold standard, which is micro-computed tomographic imaging [27].

Currently, CBCT imaging is considered to provide an excellent, nondestructive, noninvasive imaging option with the potential to detect most anatomic variations, while creating an accurate representation of the external and internal dental anatomy. The quality of CBCT image resolution is sufficiently high to visualize root canal morphology for clinical endodontic treatment at low radiation and dosimetry [28]. It is as accurate as root canal staining and clearing techniques for identifying canal anatomy [29]. Studies have showed that CBCT imaging is more accurate than periapical radiographs in determining the number of root canals in mandibular molar teeth [30, 31]. This knowledge is necessary not to leave canals without approach as to preserve dental structure by not searching for possible anatomical configurations. A clear example of uncertainty is presented in the treatment of maxillary first molar. Reported incidence of two canals in the mesiobuccal root ranged from 18.6% to 96% [32], while weighted average of the incidence of two canals is 56.8% and for one canal 43.1% (Fig. 1.12).

Root Canal Configuration

The complexity of the root canal system and its internal morphology is directly related with root canal treatment planning strategy, therapy

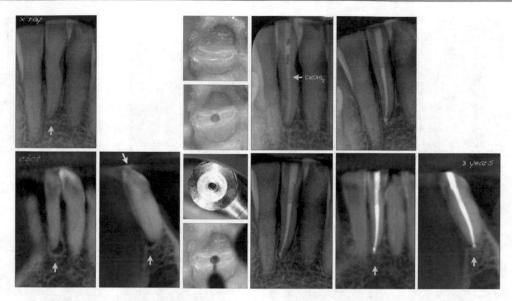

Fig. 1.8 Information provided by CBCT slices guides root canal planning in terms of access cavity design (from oval cingular to round incisal in this particular case) and by showing the indication for the use of medications in cases where the presence of periapical radiolucencies is not detectable on conventional X-rays. Other technological tools are used when structural preservation is a goal, like ultrasonic tips as example. High-speed burs are used without detailed visual control, where ultrasonic tips can be inserted, activated, and controlled through visual magnification aids, like loupes and microscopes, leading to a more selective dentin removal. Successful mandibular incisor case with apical periodontitis not detectable on intraoral X-ray, showing complete bone repair on a 3-year CBCT follow-up

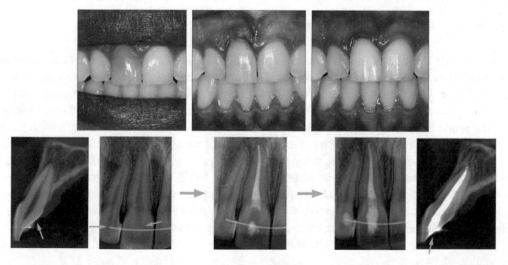

Fig. 1.9 Determination of the appropriate point of entry. In this particular case, conventional X-ray suggests that the traditional endodontic cingular cavity approach should be made under the orthodontic retainer due to the projected position of the wire related to the incisal pulp horns. However, CBCT results show a reality quite different: a cingular approach would not offer the correct approximation to the root canal axis, nor covering to the pulp horns. CBCT sagittal slice shows that a more incisal access over the orthodontic wire facilitates the biological, technical, and structural objectives

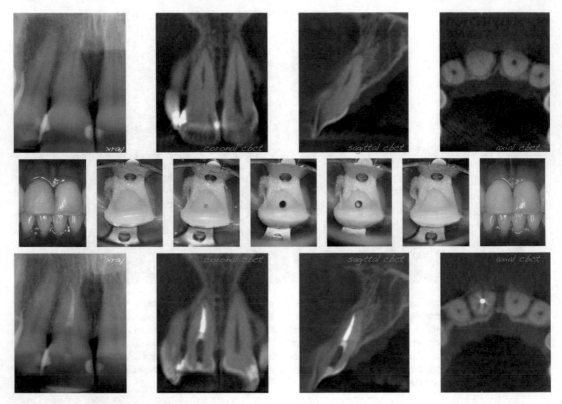

Fig. 1.10 In pretty calcified cases, CBCT helps by revealing the presence and position of the actual canal, providing hints in the design of the approach, like the access point. Instead of a conventional cingular triangular cavity, a more incisal and round approach centered in the root results far appropriate to catch the axis of the canal of this maxillary central incisor

execution, and outcome [34]. Comprehensive understanding of the root canal morphology in 3D is one of the key requirements for the treatment of infected root canal space. Deficiency in recognizing canal space morphology that leads to incomplete cleaning, shaping, and obturation maneuvers are all attributed as reasons for root canal treatment failures. Root canal morphology can include round, oval, ribbon, c-shaped canals, etc. Strategies conventionally used to identify it includes intraoral periapical radiographs and direct observation [35, 36]. Due to the 2D nature of the intraoral radiographs, it may show some clues to understand the root canal configuration. Canals not centered on the radiograph, distorted outline of the canal and/or the periodontal ligament and wider than usual canals may suggest the type of shape present. The use of radiopaque solutions inside the canals has also been proposed for such purposes

[37]. However, intraoral periapical radiographs have limitations, such as two dimensionality, anatomical noise, and geometric distortion that limit such purpose [38]. CBCT should overcome these limitations, eliminating superimposition of anatomical structures and by providing the appropriate slice to analyze root canal configuration at any given level. When compared, periapical radiographs presented low performance in the detection of root canal configurations, whereas CBCT imaging showed no difference compared with the gold standard of micro-computed tomographic (μCT) imaging [27] (Figs. 1.13 and 1.14).

Root Canal Curvatures

Understanding root curvatures is cumbersome while significant in order to safely maintain root canal anatomy during endodontic procedures. Root canal curvatures may affect access cavity

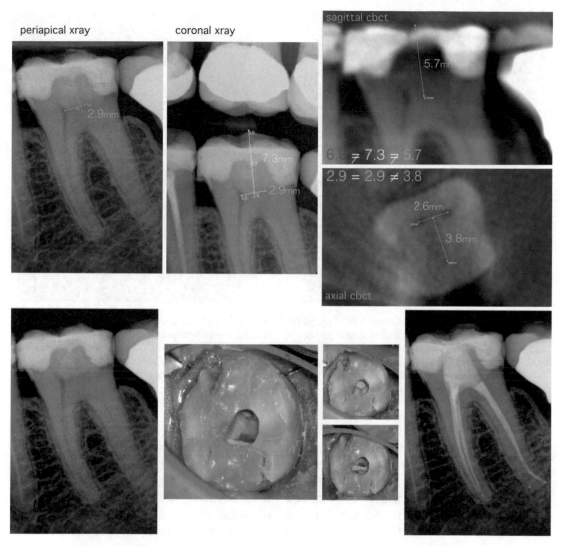

Fig. 1.11 Case presented shows vertical collapse of the pulp chamber space. Measurement of the distance from the central occlusal fossa to the pulp chamber floor differs from periapical X-ray (6.8 mm) to coronal X-ray (7.3 mm) to sagittal CBCT slice (5.7 mm). Intraoral X-rays show projection distortions. Being guided by intraoral X-ray measurements would end in a pericervical dentin reduction. Data acquired from CBCT slices are confident to the level of resolution of the acquisition, voxel size 0.076 mm for this study

design, instrument selection, instrumentation, and obturation techniques. Greater degree of root canal curvature predisposes to iatrogenic complications such as incomplete removal of pulp debris, instrument separation, post perforation, and canal transportation [39–41]. Traditional intraoral radiographs may not reflect all anatomical, morphological, and biological features. Ability of 2D images to appropriately reflect root canal curvatures depends on perpendicularity of the X-ray beam to the desired curvature. Considering that the root canal curvatures may be multiplanar, probabilities are that with 2D radiographic techniques curvature results are poorly represented. Since CBCT imaging has shown high correlation with histological determination of canal morphology [22], it has been successfully used for 3D analysis of the root canal curva-

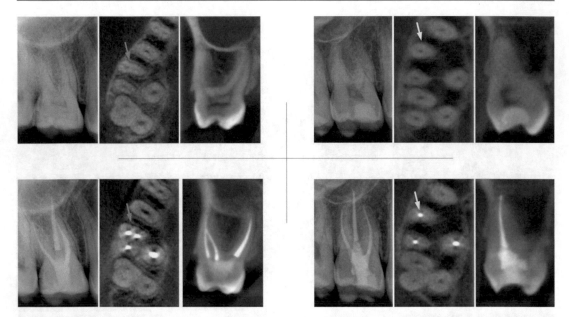

Fig. 1.12 Focalized high-resolution CBCT provides detailed information on the number of canals present in each particular endodontic case. This comparison of two maxillary first molars, where booth teeth, as part of Venezuelan population, has the same 47.1% probability of having an MB2 [33] reveals that a conventional X-ray is not determinant in revealing the actual number of canals present in each situation. The appropriate axial CBCT slice however shows quite easily the number and position of the canals. Certainty of information is useful not only for providing where and what to look. As important, by eliminating the need of search valuable pericervical structure is preserved

ture and the direction of roots [42] (Figs. 1.15 and 1.16). A specific software-based method to determine root curvature radius using CBCT images has also been described [43]. This method calculated the root curvature radius in both apical and coronal directions based on three mathematical points determined by the software. Similar software-based methods that extract more information from CBCT images can be valuable for endodontic treatment planning and for the preparation of curved root canals.

Working Length Determination

Precise determination of the working length is a principal step in performing accurate root canal treatment. Overestimation of the endodontic working length may cause over-instrumentation of the root canals, whereas underestimation of the working length may result in insufficient root canal preparation. Clinicians commonly rely on periapical radiographs and electronic apex locators to determine the working length distance.

Depending on intraoral radiographs for the working length measurement is insufficient, as this technique is sensitive and subjective, and the 2D representation of a 3D area increases the chances of miscalculation of the root canal length [44–46]. On the other hand, measurements reflected in electronic apex locators may provide inconsistencies in certain situations, such as partially or totally obliterated root canals [47]. Apical anatomical complexities may also affect the performance of electronic apex locators. It was also reported that the lateral positioning of the apical foramen or the presence of multiple apical foramen may negatively affect the measurement accuracy of electronic apex locators [48–50]. The combined use of these two resources allows for greater accuracy in working length determination than the use of intraoral periapical radiographs alone [51, 52].

Studies have compared the use of CBCT imaging with electronic apex locators for working length measurement in vivo [12, 53]. The

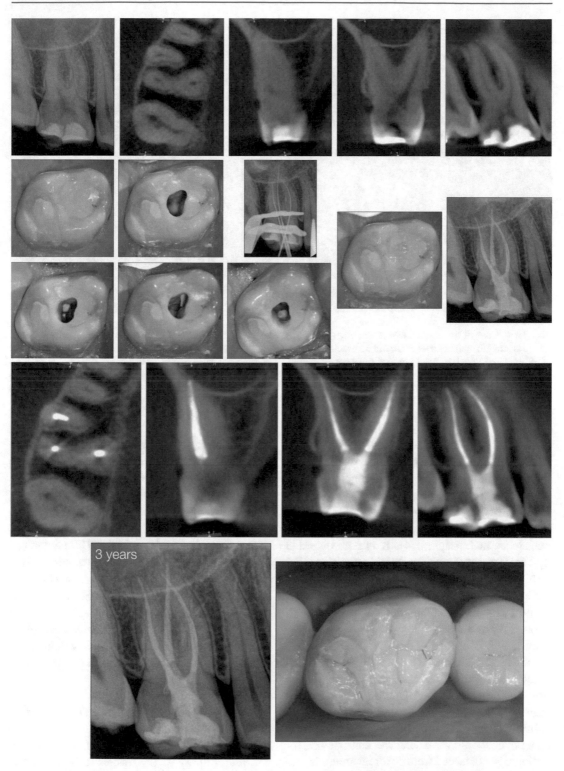

Fig. 1.13 Horizontal sizes and shape of the root canals are also relevant concepts in terms of adequately addressing the anatomical needs of the root canal procedure. The presence of isthmuses is important to consider and to treat when present. Appropriate CBCT slices are helpful to this objective. Note the isthmus present on the mesial root of this maxillary first molar. Follow-up 3 years. Restorative dentistry by Dr. Tomás Seif (Caracas, Venezuela)

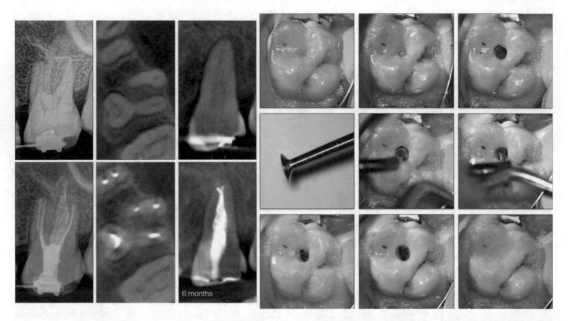

Fig. 1.14 Case of a maxillary first molar where the bone status around the palatal root could not be precisely evaluated on a periapical X-ray. Note that this root presents a c-shape configuration, easily detectable on the proper preoperative axial CBCT slice. Case solved with a less inva-sive procedure. One pointed concern about this approach is the possibility of tissue remains in the soffit around the contracted access cavity. In this case a special plate design ultrasonic tip was used for this purpose in order to assure proper cleaning of such space. Follow-up 6 months

findings from these studies support the use of CBCT images for endodontic working length determination. Another study concluded that when CBCT images were used for root canal length measurements of posterior maxillary teeth, they were significantly more accurate than periapical radiographs [54]. It is not suggested that intraoral radiographs should be replaced by CBCT scans for working length determinations exclusively, but if available, CBCT images can be helpful in establishing the working length (Figs. 1.17 and 1.18).

Root Canal Splitting

Anatomical variations, such as root canal splitting, can occur at a level where direct observation may not be possible. Interpretation of root canal splitting from intraoral periapical radiographs can be challenging. Therefore combination of radiographs obtained from different angles is recommended [55]. Two periapical radiographs with a 20° difference in angle combined with zooming have been suggested to assist in determining mul-

ticanal morphology of mandibular first premolars [56]. The disappearance of the root canal space and not having a continuous tapering canal have been traditionally pointed as characteristics to be observed to suspect and identify possible splitting of the root canal. However, reported success with such technique is limited [57]. In mandibular premolars, because their main variation is two canals in a bucco-lingual direction, a mesio-distal radiograph gives much more information for such purpose. However, a mesio-distal view is clinically impossible. CBCT provides visualization of fine dental anatomic details without overlapping of the tooth itself or adjacent structures [58] (Figs. 1.19 and 1.20).

Horizontal Root Bulk and Canal Dimension at Pericervical Region

Understanding the dimension of the anatomy and morphology of the tissues to be treated is paramount [59, 60]. Tooth anatomy and morphology have been investigated thoroughly. Many in vitro studies have recorded the anat-

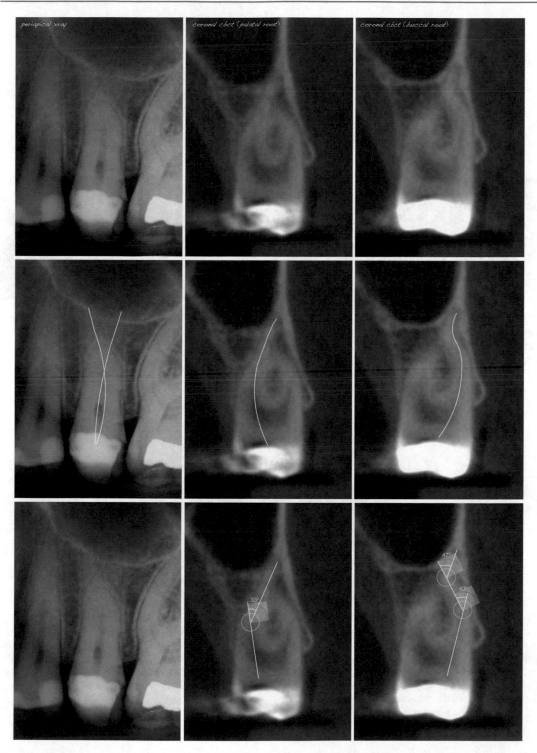

Fig. 1.15 Curvatures are most of the time poorly represented on conventional X-rays, considering that they occur
in multiple planes and positions, hardly interpretable on a
two plane view. CBCT slices can be analyzed from any
perspective, allowing the clinician to fully understand the
real orientation of roots and canals, making possible to
take the appropriate decisions to confront each situation.
This two rooted maxillary bicuspid is a clear example of
radicular curvatures not understandable in a periapical
X-ray. Even multiple X-rays would not be sufficient to
adequately evaluate it. Also, straight clinical view from
any kind of access cavity would not be helpful at all

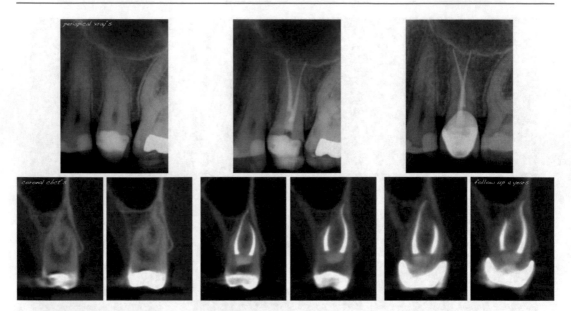

Fig. 1.16 Comparison of pre-op, post-op, and follow-up conventional X-rays and CBCT slices from the previous case. Note that the information obtained from the preoperative CBCT study results in the design and execution of a conservative procedure that correctly address the anatomical requirement of this multi-curved tooth. 4 years follow-up

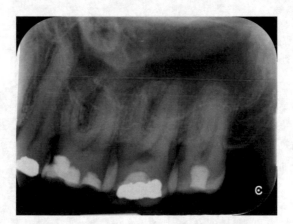

Fig. 1.17 Root length is also a characteristic hardly established with a periapical X-rays. Even with paralleling techniques, image distortion due to the nature of the projected image (elongation or shortening) makes inexact to translate conventional X-rays measurements to clinical procedures. Nowadays, clinicians have electronic apex locators that could work correctly in a vast number of clinical cases. However, there still are situations where such measurements are inaccurate or not relatable to what a conventional X-ray or the clinical approach suggests. This is the case with a third maxillary molar, where the palatal root is 6 mm shorter than their buccal ones. The conventional periapical image is unable to point this. Even a proper apex locator measurement would at least cause uncertainty to most clinicians

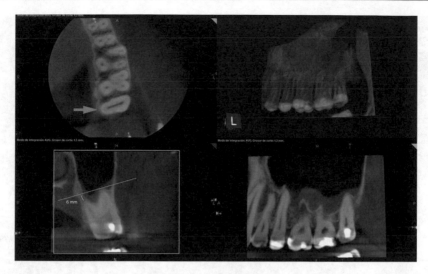

Fig. 1.17 (continued)

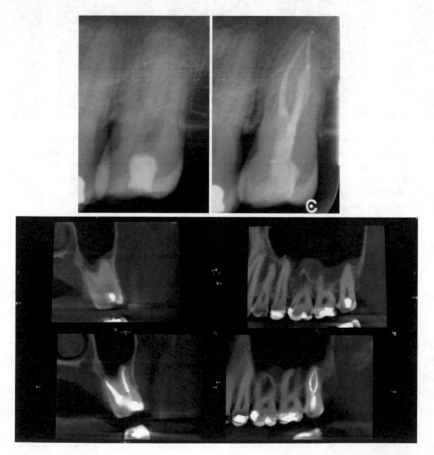

Fig. 1.18 Comparison of pre-op and post-op X-rays, with the post-op CBCT of the case shown in Fig. 1.17. Note that it is difficult to understand and accept the final X-ray as an appropriate procedure without further infor-mation of this particular situation, where the palatal root is considerably shorter than the buccals. CBCT slices explain correctly what this image is about

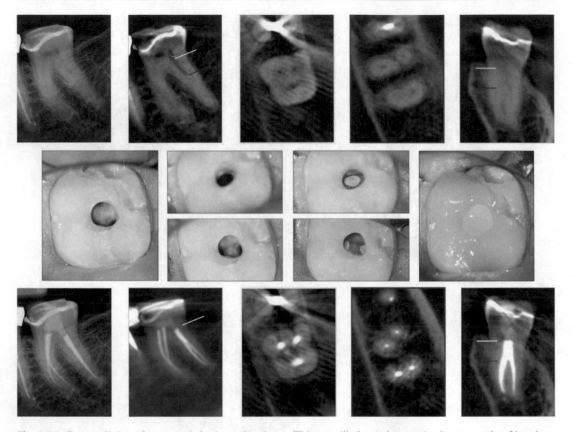

Fig. 1.19 Deep splitting of root canals is also a situation neither easily viewable on conventional X-rays nor findable through most clinical approaches. Despite the fact that studies show its occurrence, when present, major chances is not to found nor solve it. Preoperative CBCT studies should minimize not recognizing this situation. This mandibular molar case is clear example of it, where a split occurs deep in the distal root. By having this information preoperatively, appropriate measures could be regularly taken to address it without major structural compromise

omy, scales, and average sizes of root canals and roots at different levels. However, a valid method to determine the sizes or width of root canals and roots during clinical root canal treatment has not been established. Current literature failed to suggest an optimum canal preparation size, and it still remains a subject of uncertainty [61]. In the absence of the original canal width and optimal horizontal dimensions for the prepared canals, clinicians continue to make treatment decision without sound scientific basis [62].

Multiplanar radiographic imaging such as micro-CT (μ-CT) imaging has provided a comprehensive understanding of the root canal anatomy and the width of the root canals along its length, up to the apex [63–66]. However, due to the high dose of radiation, μ-CT is actually available only as an in vitro tool. CBCT appears to be the most promising preoperative investigation that delineates the canal width along the length of the tooth [67]. Pericervical dentin is the dentin located 4 mm above and 4 mm below the crestal bone [11], significant for the distribution of functional stresses in teeth. Preserving the pericervical dentin would aid in the biomechanical response of the tooth to chewing forces [68]. It has been suggested that no more than 10% of the pericervical dentin should be removed when working in this region of teeth [69] (Fig. 1.21). Root canal preparation at the pericervical level without precise guidelines

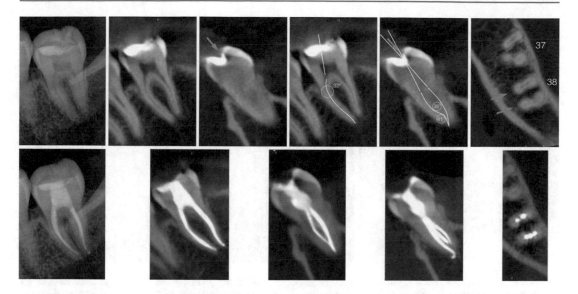

Fig. 1.20 Mandibular third molar with a variety of clinical anatomical variations not identifiable on a periapical X-ray. Lingual inclination, three canals, and a double curvature on the distal root make this one difficult to solve by conventional approach. With the proper preclinical information, a successful conservative approach could be executed

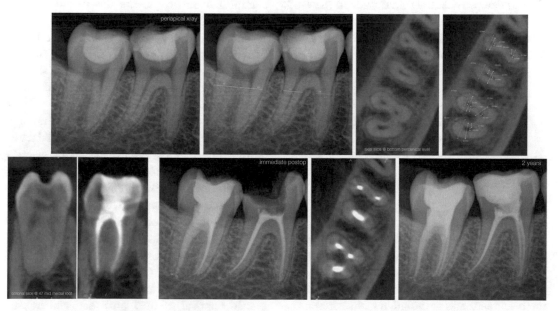

Fig. 1.21 With 3D CBCT imaging horizontal sizes become precisely measurable at any given level, providing valuable information that a 2D conventional X-ray image cannot offer. This becomes particularly valuable when directed size preparation is considered in the horizontal plane, mainly in the pericervical area. 2 years follow-up

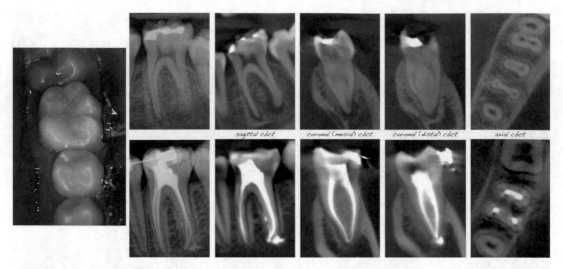

Fig. 1.22 Cases with thin roots, particularly in the peri-cervical area, undetected lesions, and apical curvatures could result in inadequate treatment by a conventional approach, mainly from a structural point of view. Such variables are precisely taken into consideration when a high-resolution focalized CBCT is analyzed previous to a primary endodontic procedure. 4 year follow-up

may render its preservation difficult. CBCT images can provide the actual sizes of the tooth at any given level. With this information, the pretreatment size and proposed controlled root canal preparation at the pericervical region may be performed (Fig. 1.22).

1.3 Technologies for Dentin Preservation: Phase 2—Treatment

1.3.1 Image-Guided Endodontic Access

Image-guided access employs image modalities such as 2D projection radiography as well as 3D CBCT images to precisely plan the access cavity and the root canal preparation. Instead of practicing a standard access design, a tooth specific and unique access design is proposed. The goal of the customize image-guided endodontic access design is to strategically remove and preserve dentin, and not to prepare the smallest access cavity possible.

There are two types of image-guided endodontic access preparations: (a) static and (b) dynamic. Static-guided access utilizes a stent or guide, which is fabricated using computer-aided design/computer-assisted manufacture (CAD/CAM) technology and/or 3D printing technology, based on the preoperative CBCT scans and a traditional or an optical impression giving an STL file that can be matched with the DICOM files originated by the CBCT. This system seems to be easy to use and very effective in predictable treatment of deeply calcified canals, guiding the operator who has to trust the precision of the system (Fig. 1.23) [70]. Other applications of such static guides have been described in identifying root canal orifices in teeth with crowns or bridge, guided removal of fiber post, and guided creation of the stage platform coronally to a fractured instrument fragment before attempting its removal. Advantages of this technique against classic throughing with ultrasonic tips are shorter operative time needed, less stress for the operator and the patient, it can be performed in absence of an operative microscope, and the absence of heat that a prolonged use of a ultrasonic vibration may cause. Some of the drawbacks of the static guides include: (1) the shape/dimensions of the guide cannot be changed easily after fabrication, (2) cost of production, (3) time required to plan and fabricate the guide, and (4) difficulty to use them in patients with limited mouth opening, or in the second molar regions where access is poor [71].

Dynamic guidance utilizes the computer-aided surgical navigation technology, which corresponds to the global positioning systems (GPS). Dynamic-guided access preparation uses CBCT image volume to plan an access cavity. The overhead tracking cameras in the system are used to relate the position of the jaw and the bur in a 3D space. During the therapeutic procedure, the clinician views the software interface and obtains immediate feedback on the bur position, which is related to the position of the planned access cavity in the tooth. Dynamic-guided access provides advantages such as: (1) the system integrates inter-occlusal distance in access plan, (2) it is compatible

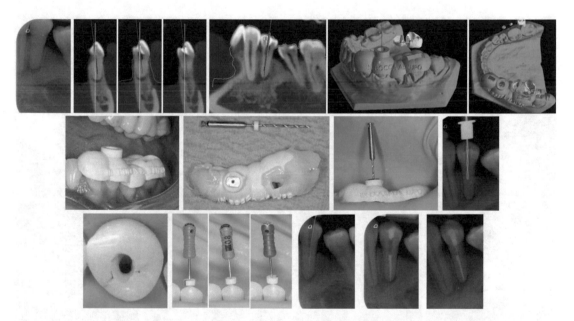

Fig. 1.23 Case of a severely calcified mandibular premolar. The canal was located using a static guide created via 3D project using a particular software starting from a CBCT volume. A specific bur was used oriented by the metal sleeve in the guide to the mid-apical portion of the root where the canal was located, negotiated, instrumented, and filled. The tooth was later reconstructed. Case courtesy of Dr. Gianluca Plotino (Rome, Italy)

with the high-speed handpiece burs, (3) it does not require wait time for the fabrication of static guides, and (4) allows treatment procedures to be changed if required [71, 72] (Fig. 1.24). Main disadvantages of this system are the high cost, the fact that the clinician should change its way to work by looking on a screen and being able to precisely follow the correct direction by free-hand; in fact this technique indicates the operator if he/she is making a directional error but does not guide operator's hand to the point to be reached. Furthermore, these systems are originally designed for guided implant placement giving a precision that is good enough for this purpose, but that should still be confirmed to be precise enough in smaller spaces as the endodontic anatomy.

1.3.2 Magnification Aids in Root Canal Treatment

Root canal procedures are performed in narrow spaces, where visual acuity is very demanding. Traditionally, locating all root canals during a treatment represent a principal step in endodontic therapy. Failing to locate all the root canals can compromise the outcome of the root canal therapy [73]. Therefore, visual aids represent a major help towards successful procedures, mainly if a conservative approach is intended. Clinicians with normal 20/20 visual resolution, those able to separate contours 1.75 mm apart at 20 ft. [74], find it challenging to identify relevant points inside a tooth since they are closer than what is normally discernible,

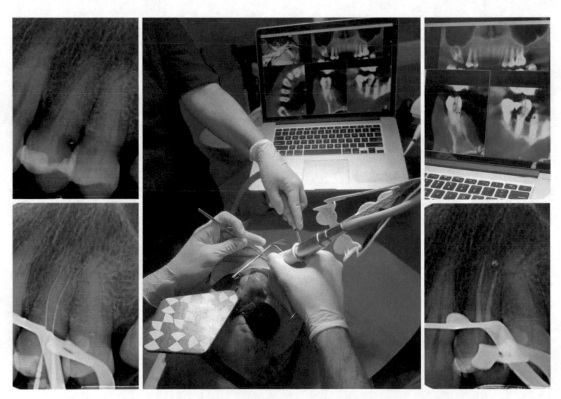

Fig. 1.24 Clinical case where the two calcified canals of a maxillary premolar with a distal caries penetrating the pulp chamber were located using a dynamic navigation system. The preoperative CBCT data is matched with the calibration system that guides the operator. The procedure is performed looking at the computer screen to monitor three-dimensionally the actual position of the bur. Case courtesy of Dr. Gianluca Plotino (Rome, Italy)

and/or the examining conditions with limited intra-canal illumination can be perplexing. The unaided eyes can only discern visually up to the level of canal orifice [75]. Introduction of varieties of magnification in endodontics, in the form of loupes and microscopes, in conjunction with increased illumination, has resulted in the improved clinical performances with enhanced technical accuracy [76].

All root canals are not visible at the base of the pulp chamber even after establishing a traditional access cavity. It was reported that additional root canals could be detected with the application of an operating microscope [77]. It has already been established that magnification can facilitate identification of difficult endodontic anatomy [78, 79]. The use of microscopes also has a positive impact towards improving access cavity preparations [80]. The application of microscope aided in avoiding unnecessary destruction of mineralized hard tissues. The use of magnification leads to a MB2

detection rate approximately three times more than that achieved without magnification [81]. The use of microscopes allows detection and negotiation of more accessory canals, both in mandibular [82] and in maxillary molars [83] (Fig. 1.25).

1.3.3   Ultrasonic Tips

Working under magnification requires direct visual control, not possible with the use of burs, despite the many variations available, just because is not possible to see when acting (Fig. 1.8). Refinement of access cavities, and, more important, searching for smaller canals require very selective actions quietly possible with appropriate energy activated inserts inside the root canal. Use of mechanical energy to produce microvibratory movements generated from electrical energy in ultrasonic tips, instead of tra-

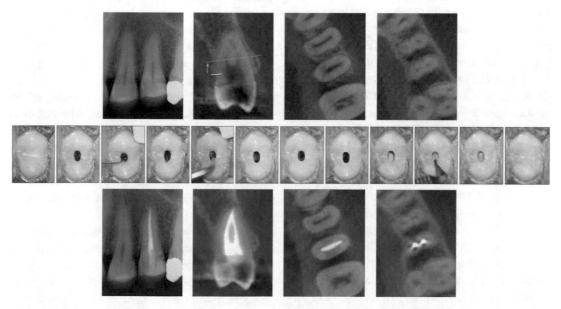

Fig. 1.25 Limited visibility and maneuverability through a contracted endodontic access cavity should not limit treatment goals when they are certainly determined via CBCT and taken into consideration prior to the procedure.

Magnification under a clinical microscope with 10× capability and proper light source provides enough visibility for most clinical situations

ditional burs, has improved clinical efficiency in endodontic therapy for a variety of purposes. The search for less invasive dentistry and evolving concepts to a smaller cavity preparation has included the use of sound energy with a frequency above the range of human earing (20 kHz) to make root canal insert to work in a linear back-and-forth motion within root canal lumen [84]. Ultrasonic tips have showed increased enhanced safety and control compared to burs as they do not rotate, making it easy to control while having a high cutting efficiency [84]. Use of ultrasonic tips in minimally invasive endodontics includes access refinement, search for smaller canals, removal of pulp stones and irrigant activation via acoustic streaming and cavitation [85].

Many advantages are found in the use of ultrasonic tips over burs. There is no obstruction of vision, since there is no headpiece head to block the view, better control, since its use under vibration represents a smaller risk of deviation compared to the rapid cutting effect of a bur, smaller area of action as many ultrasonic tips are smaller than the smallest bur [85], and ample area of action, because the neck of an ultrasonic tip is longer than most burs. When selecting ultrasonic tips, it is important to know that diamond-coated tips show significant better cutting efficiency, but are easier to break than either stainless steel or zirconium nitride [86]. The thinner the diamond coat, the more effective becomes the tip [87]. Cutting efficiency of ultrasonic tips is also dependent on the type of ultrasonic unit used [87] and the power setting [88]. Therefore, it is important to understand this synergy in order to produce only the desired effect. Furthermore, the use of ultrasonic tips is important to better clean the access cavity when a conservative approach is used and pulp horns and undercuts are left untouched.

However, it is significant to realize that ultrasonically activated inserts within the root canal can result in uncontrolled contact with root canal wall and subsequent dentin removal in the apical third, particularly in combination with root canal irrigant. This contact with root canal wall and dentin removal can occur even if the insert is applied within the manufacturer-recommended power settings and activation time [89].

1.3.4 Heat-Treated Ni-Ti Files

Root canal preparation techniques with modern nickel-titanium rotary and reciprocating instruments have shown the potential to avoid some of the major drawbacks of traditional instruments [90] that relied on conventional endodontic access cavity design and instrumentation techniques, particularly the strict requirement of straight-line access to enhance unimpeded entry of instruments into the canal curvatures. In a stainless steel world of instruments this was necessary to maximize the ability to reach and plane more canal walls, and to minimize procedural errors [91]. In order to obtain this objective, gates glidden and orifice openers drills were used as cervical actors, even to facilitate the appropriate selection of the first apical binding file. This raises the concern between the desired effect of orifice enlargement versus the undesired effect, orifice relocation created as a consequence of using such instruments. Orifice enlargement suggests uniform expansion in its original position, circumferentially on the entire canal wall. Use of gates glidden drills and orifices openers may result in non-uniform preparation circumferentially causing indiscriminate dentin removal and can result in thinning of the furcal side radicular dentin [92]. Any non-uniform removal of dentin around the centroid of the root canal lumen would reduce even more the resistance to root flexing. When exposed to chewing cycles, this repeated and increased root flexing (fatigue) may predispose root-filled teeth to vertical root fracture [8, 93].

More conservative access designs attempt to maintain original canal curvatures. If a decreased angle of curvature is intended, as with straight-line furcation and straight-line radicular access designs, greater amount of orifice relocation is needed, which can thin one side of the root more than the other sides [94]. Historically, straight-line endodontic access was proposed to reduce the difficulty in instrumenting curved root canals due to the limitations in the flexibility of endodontic instruments used. Teeth with inclinations of 30 or more degrees or S-shaped curves are considered as high difficulty by the

AAE endodontic case difficulty assessment form and guidelines. Modern alloys used for endodontic instruments have shown effective and safe for use in these conditions [95, 96]. Thermal treatment of NiTi alloys is used to increase their mechanical properties, resulting in increased flexibility [97, 98]. Maintaining canal curvature in order to eliminate transportation while avoiding instrument separation has always been one of the ideal requirements for endodontic files. Heat-treated NiTi instruments show adequate preparations of complex canals, even in cases with an S-shape canal morphology [90]. Modern NiTi heat-treated instruments come in a variety of designs, including multiples sizes and variable tapers. This facilitates instrument selection and instrumentation depending on the case-specific requirements

conceived by the clinician (Figs. 1.26, 1.27, 1.28, 1.29, 1.30, 1.31, and 1.32).

1.4 Conclusive Remarks

Preservation of residual tooth or dentin structure is of supreme importance in basic operative dentistry, endodontic therapy, or post-endodontic restorations. In conclusion, treatment modalities to maximize longevity of endodontically treated teeth include well-planned conservative access cavities that leverage caries and restorations, conservative root canal preparations and placement of immediate coronal restorations. Dentin preservation in root canal treatment can be implemented in two phases. Phase 1 is aimed towards patient-specific planning for access/canal preparation, while

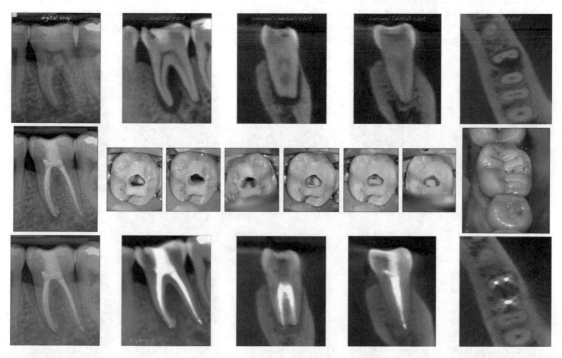

Fig. 1.26 Despite the fact that most teeth requiring endodontic treatment shows significant loss of enamel and coronal dentin, that is not always the case. When present, every dental structure should be preserved and only removed if strictly required to contribute to the procedure itself. Resources available heavily reduce the need of this removal, making possible successful endodontic treatments through contracted cavities and limited shaping even in the presence of bacterial proliferation in the root canal system. Infected mandibular molar case successfully treated through a less invasive approach. This also reduces the restorative need, making unnecessary the cusp protection to every posterior endodontically treated tooth, where the resulting cavity shows an ampleness smaller than one-third of the intercuspal distance, like the one presented. 3 years follow-up. Restorative dentistry by Dr. Tomás Seif (Caracas, Venezuela)

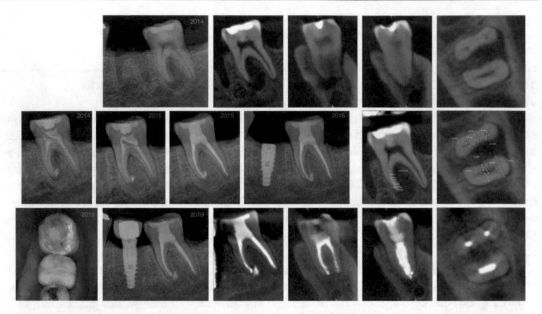

Fig. 1.27 Controlled shaping at the pericervical area. By measuring dental thickness and canal size at this level, preparation goals can be determined to ensure proper structural preservation and limiting chances of wall perforation, particularly in cases with increased risk due to their particular shape. By minimizing dentin removal, structural behavior is maintained. This tooth treated in a less invasive manner than with traditional maneuvers shows proper success in 5 years follow-up, even considering that is basically restored

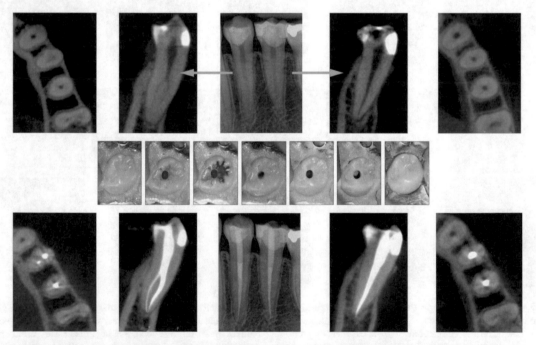

Fig. 1.28 Mandibular bicuspids in need of root canal treatment with different canal configurations. Without proper preoperative consideration, this case could easily end mistreated in one of the two canals present in the first mandibular bicuspid. Occasionally conventional X-rays suggest this canal configuration by mid root rapid disappearance of the radiolucency of the canal, as this one. Even though conventional X-rays may show this configuration, high-resolution CBCT slices give so much information quiet convenient for the proper resolution of the case: exact configuration, point of separation, sizes of each canal, length, curvatures, size, and convenient position of the access cavity. All this information taken into consideration should result in proper handling of the case with maximum dentin preservation

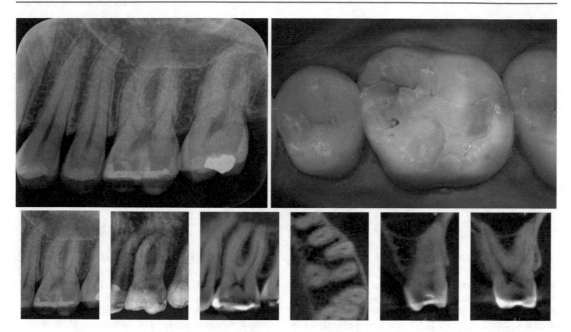

Fig. 1.29 Case of primary root canal treatment to resume concepts presented in this chapter. As a complement to conventional endodontic evaluation, a CBCT study provides relevant information not available by other noninvasive technique

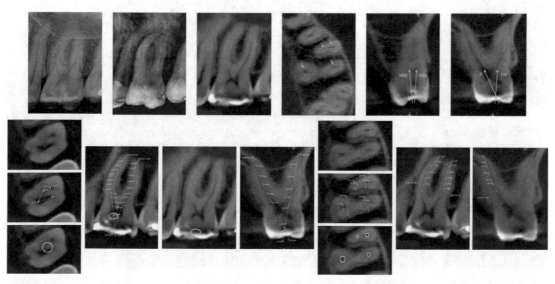

Fig. 1.30 Analysis of the information contained in the CBCT slices reveals for this maxillary first molar case the presence of three roots, two canals in the MB root, one in the DB and one in the palatal. Projection of the axis of the canals, as in majority of cases, points towards the center of the occlusal surface, allowing a contracted cavity to adequately provide enough access for all present canals. The pericervical bottom is located at 9 mm from the tip of the root for the DB and the P root, and at 10 mm to the MB root. At this point original canals measured 0.5 mm wide for the MB1 with a total thickness of the root of 2.8 mm, 0.2 mm for the MB2 (2.2 mm thickness of the root), 0.5 mm for the DB with 3.3 mm radicular thickness and 1.0 mm for the P canal in a 4.8 mm wide root. Distance between MB1 and DB is 2.4 mm, between MB1 and MB2 is 1.9 mm, between P and MB2 is 2.9 mm, and 3.9 mm from P to DB. Length of the canals measured in the CBCT slices are in the 22 mm in the buccal side and in the 23 mm for the palatal, to be precisely determined later in conjunction with an electronic apex locator

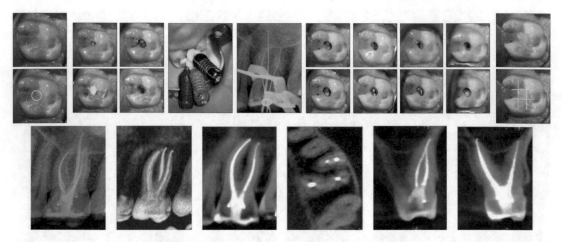

Fig. 1.31 Clinical sequence of the procedure performed. A contracted access cavity was created in the center of the occlusal surface, where all the four canals present joined and can be accessed following its particular axis. Note again that the projected canals converge freely to the access cavity. Length of the canals where electronically determined, cleaning and shaping procedures completed, preparation was set at 35/0.04 for the MB1 and DB, 35/0.03 for the MB2, and 40/0.05 for the P. The access cavity was sealed with fluid resin. No indication for cuspal protection post endodontic treatment since the access cavity is less than one-third of the intercuspal distance

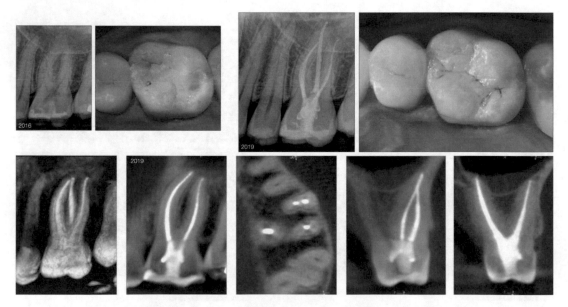

Fig. 1.32 Comparison of periapical X-ray and clinical view between the initial condition and 3 years later. Note the normal appearance of the supportive structures on the follow-up CBCT slices. Restorative procedure was limited to a new surface direct resin at the limit of the previous cavity prior to the endodontic procedure. Restorative dentistry by Dr. Tomás Seif (Caracas, Venezuela)

Phase 2 is aimed towards treatment steps that preserves root dentin. Preoperative limited FOV CBCT is recommended as a standard of practice. Information obtained from the preoperative CBCT volume can be used to plan minimally invasive endodontic procedures. The advent of new concepts and technologies that includes image-guided access and dynamically guided access appears to be promising technologies to preserve dentin tissue and improve patient-centered outcomes in root canal treatment.

References

1. Ng Y, Mann V, Rahbaran S, Lewsey J, Gulabivala K. Outcome of primary root canal treatment: systematic review of the literature—Part 1. Effects of study characteristics on probability of success. Int Endod J. 2007;40:921–39.
2. Kishen A. Mechanisms and risk factors for fracture predilection in endodontically treated teeth. Endod Top. 2006;13:57–83.
3. Wolcott J, Ishley D, Kennedy W, Johnson S, Minnich S, Meyers J. A 5 yr clinical investigation of second mesiobuccal canals in endodontically treated and retreated maxillary molars. J Endod. 2005;31:262–4.
4. Hoen MM, Pink FE. Contemporary endodontic retreatments: an analysis based on clinical treatment findings. J Endod. 2002;28:834–6.
5. Boutsioukis C, Kishen A. Fluid dynamics of syringe based irrigation to optimize antibiofilm efficacy in root canal disinfection. Roots. 2012;2012:22–6.
6. Abdo SB, Darrat AA, Masaudi SM, Luddin N, Husein A, Khamis MF. Comparison of over flared root canals of mandibular premolars filled with MTA and resin based material: an in vitro study. Smile Dent J. 2012;7:38–42.
7. Oliet S. Treating vertical root fractures. J Endod. 1984;10:391–6.
8. Ossareh A, Rosentritt M, Kishen A. Biomechanical studies on the effect of iatrogenic dentin removal on vertical root fractures. J Conserv Dent. 2018;21:290–6.
9. Paqué F, Balmer M, Attin T, Peters OA. Preparation of oval-shaped root canals in mandibular molars using nickel-titanium rotary instruments: a micro-computed tomography study. J Endod. 2010;36:703–7.
10. Goodacre CJ, Spolink KJ. Prosthodontic management of endodontically treated teeth: a literature review.

Part I. Success and failure data, treatment concepts. J Prosthodont. 1994;3:243–50.
11. Clark D, Khademi JA. Case studies in modern molar endodontic access and directed dentin conservation. Dent Clin N Am. 2010;54:275–89.
12. Patel S, Dawood A, Ford TP, Whaites E. The potential applications of cone beam computed tomography in the management of endodontic problems. Int Endod J. 2007;40:818–30.
13. Goldman M, Pearson AH, Darzenta N. Endodontic success—who's reading the radiograph. Oral Surg Oral Med Oral Pathol. 1972;33:432–7.
14. Boveda C. Clinical impact of cone beam computed tomography in root canal treatment. In: Basrani B, editor. Endodontic radiology. 2nd ed. Iowa: Wiley-Blackwell; 2012. p. 367–415.
15. AAE and AAOMR joint position statement in the Use of Cone Beam Computed Tomography in Endodontics - 2015/2016 Update.
16. Bender B, Seltzer S. Roentgenographic and direct observation of experimental lesions in bone I. J Am Dent Assoc. 1961;62:152–60.
17. Bender B, Seltzer S. Roentgenographic and direct observation of experimental lesions in bone II. J Am Dent Assoc. 1961;62:708–16.
18. Rai A, Burde K, Guttal K, Naikmasur VG. Comparison between cone-beam computed tomography and direct digital intraoral imaging for the diagnosis of periapical pathology. J Oral Maxillofac Radiol. 2016;4:50–6.
19. Lofthag-Hansen S, Huumonen S, Grondahl K, Grondahl H-G. Limited cone-beam CT and intraoral radiography for the diagnosis of periapical pathology. Oral Surg Oral Med Oral Pathol Oral Radiol Endod. 2007;103:114–9.
20. Friedman S. Prognosis of initial endodontic therapy. Endod Top. 2002;2:59–98.
21. Friedman S, Abitbol S, Lawrence HP. Treatment outcome in endodontics: the Toronto study. Phase 1: initial treatment. J Endod. 2003;29:787–93.
22. Michetti J, Maret D, Mallet JP, Diemer F. Validation of cone beam computed tomography as a tool to explore root canal anatomy. J Endod. 2010;36:1187–90.
23. Narayana P. Access cavity preparations. In: Schwartz R, Canakapalli V, editors. Best practices in endodontics. A Desk Reference. Batavia, IL: Quintessence; 2015. p. 89–103
24. European Society of Endodontology. Quality guidelines for endodontic treatment: consensus report of the European Society of Endodontology. Int Endod J. 2006;39:921–30.
25. Patel S, Durack C, Abella F, et al. Cone beam computed tomography in endodontics—a review. Int Endod J. 2015;48:3–15.

26. Karabucak B, Bunes A, Chehoud C, Kohli MR, Setzer F. Prevalence of apical periodontitis in endodontically treated premolars and molars with untreated canal: a cone-beam computed tomography study. J Endod. 2016;42:538–41.

27. Sousa T, Haiter-Neto F, Nascimento EH, Peroni L, Freitas D, Hassan B. Diagnostic accuracy of periapical radiography and cone-beam computed tomography in identifying root canal configuration of human premolars. J Endod. 2017;43:1176–9.

28. Silva EJ, Nejaim Y, Silva AV, Haiter-Neto F, Cohenca N. Evaluation of root canal configuration of mandibular molars in a Brazilian population by using cone-beam computed tomography: an in vivo study. J Endod. 2013;39:849–52.

29. Neelakantan P, Subbarao C, Subbarao CV. Comparative evaluation of modified canal staining and clearing technique, cone-beam computed tomography, peripheral quantitative computed tomography, spiral computed tomography, and plain and contrast medium-enhanced digital radiography in studying root canal morphology. J Endod. 2010;36:1547–51.

30. Blattner TC, George N, Lee CC, et al. Efficacy of cone-beam computed tomography as a modality to accurately identify the presence of second mesiobuccal canals in maxillary first and second molars: a pilot study. J Endod. 2010;36:867–70.

31. Ordinola-Zapata R, Bramante CM, Versiani MA, et al. Comparative accuracy of the clearing technique, CBCT and micro-CT methods in studying the mesial root canal configuration of mandibular first molars. Int Endod J. 2017;50:90–6.

32. Cleghorn BM, Christie WH, Dong CC. Root and root canal morphology of the human permanent maxillary first molar: a literature review. J Endod. 2006;32:813–21.

33. Martins JNR, Alkhawas MAM, Altaki Z, Bellardini G, Berti L, Boveda C, Chaniotis A, Flynn D, Gonzalez JA, Kottoor J, Marques MS, Monroe A, Ounsi HF, Parashos P, Plotino G, Ragnarsson MF, Aguilar RR, Santiago F, Seedat HC, Vargas W, von Zuben M, Zhang Y, Gu Y, Ginjeira A. Worldwide analyses of maxillary first molar second mesiobuccal prevalence: a multicenter cone-beam computed tomographic study. J Endod. 2018;44:1641–9.

34. Vertucci FJ. Root canal morphology and its relationship to endodontic procedures. Endod Top. 2005;10:3–29.

35. Trope M, Elfenbein L, Tronstad L. Mandibular premolars with more than one root canal in different race groups. J Endod. 1986;12:343–5.

36. Sert S, Bayirli GS. Evaluation of the root canal configurations of the mandibular and maxillary permanent teeth by gender in the Turkish population. J Endod. 2004;30:391–8.

37. Ruddle C (1998) Inventor applying an organic iodine solution in conjunction with a sodium hypochlorite solution USA. US Patent No. 5,797,745.

38. Abella F, Patel S, Durán-Sindreu F, Mercadé M, Bueno R, Roig M. An evaluation of the periapical status of teeth with necrotic pulps using periapical radiography and cone-beam computed tomography. Int Endod J. 2014;47:387–96.

39. Inan U, Aydin C, Demirkaya K. Cyclic fatigue resistance of new and used Mtwo rotary nickel-titanium instruments in two different radii of curvature. Aust Endod J. 2011;37:105–8.

40. Gao Y, Cheung GS, Shen Y, Zhou X. Mechanical behavior of ProTaper universal F2 finishing file under various curvature conditions: a finite element analysis study. J Endod. 2011;37:1446–50.

41. Vertucci FJ. Root canal anatomy of the human permanent teeth. Oral Surg Oral Med Oral Pathol. 1984;58:589–99.

42. Park PS, Kim KD, Perinpanayagam H, Lee JK, Chang SW, Chung SH, Kaufman B, Zhu Q, Safavi KE, Kum KY. Three-dimensional analysis of root canal curvature and direction of maxillary lateral incisors by using cone-beam computed tomography. J Endod. 2013;39:1124–9.

43. Estrela C, Bueno MR, Sousa-Neto MD, Pécora JD. Method for determination of root curvature radius using cone-beam computed tomography images. Braz Dent J. 2008;19:114–8.

44. Williams CB, Joyce AP, Roberts S. A comparison between in vivo radiographic working length determination and measurement after extraction. J Endod. 2006;32:624–7.

45. ElAyouti A, Weiger R, Löst C. The ability of root ZX apex locator to reduce the frequency of overestimated radiographic working length. J Endod. 2002;28:116–9.

46. ElAyouti A, Weiger R, Löst C. Frequency of over instrumentation with an acceptable radiographic working length. J Endod. 2001;27:49–52.

47. ElAyouti A, Dima E, Ohmer J, et al. Consistency of apex locator function: a clinical study. J Endod. 2009;35:179–81.

48. Pagavino G, Pace R, Baccetti T. A SEM study of in vivo accuracy of the root ZX electronic apex locator. J Endod. 1998;24:438–41.

49. Piasecki L, Carneiro E, da Silva Neto UX, et al. The use of micro-computed tomography to determine the accuracy of electronic apex locators and anatomic variations affecting their precision. J Endod. 2016;42:1263–7.

50. Meder-Cowherd L, Williamson AE, Johnson WT, et al. Apical morphology of the palatal roots of maxillary molars by using micro-computed tomography. J Endod. 2011;37:1162–5.

51. Haffner C, Folwaczny M, Galler K, et al. Accuracy of electronic apex locators in comparison to actual length—an in vivo study. J Dent. 2005;33: 619–25.

52. Gordon MP, Chandler NP. Electronic apex locators. Int Endod J. 2004;37:425–37.

53. Shemesh H, Cristescu R, Wesselink PR, et al. The use of cone-beam computed tomography and digital periapical radiographs to diagnose root perforations. J Endod. 2011;37:513–6.

54. Metska ME, Liem VM, Parsa A, Koolstra JH, Wesselink PR, Ozok AR. Cone-beam computed tomographic scans in comparison with periapical radiographs for root canal length measurement: an in situ study. J Endod. 2014;40:1206–9.

55. Zaatar EI, al-Kandari AM, Alhomaidah S, al-Yasin IM. Frequency of endodontic treatment in Kuwait: radiographic evaluation of 846 endodontically treated teeth. J Endod. 1997;23:453–6.

56. England MC Jr, Hartwell GR, Lance JR. Detection and treatment of multiple canals in mandibular premolars. J Endod. 1991;17:174–8.

57. Sun Y, Lu TY, Chen YC, Yang SF. The best radiographic method for determining root canal morphology in mandibular first premolars: a study of Chinese descendants in Taiwan. J Dent Sci. 2016;11:175–81.

58. Cotton TP, Geisler TM, Holden DT, Schwartz SA, Schindler WG. Endodontic applications of cone-beam volumetric tomography. J Endod. 2007;33:1121–32.

59. Bjorndal AM, Skidmore AE. Anatomy and morphology of human teeth. 2nd ed. Iowa City: University of Iowa Press; 1987.

60. Weine FS, Healey HJ, Gerstein H, et al. Canal configuration in the mesiobuccal root of the maxillary first molar and its endodontic significance. Oral Surg Oral Med Oral Pathol. 1969;28:419–25.

61. Albuquerque D, Kottoor J. Working width, a deserted aspect of Endodontics. Restor Dent Endod. 2015;40:334–5.

62. Jou YT, Karabucak B, Levin J, Liu D. Endodontic working width: current concepts and techniques. Dent Clin N Am. 2004;48:323–35.

63. Paqué F, Zehnder M, Marending M. Apical fit of initial K-files in maxillary molars assessed by micro-computed tomography. Int Endod J. 2010;43:328–35.

64. Markvart M, Darvann TA, Larsen P, Dalstra M, Kreiborg S, Bjørndal L. Micro-CT analyses of apical enlargement and molar root canal complexity. Int Endod J. 2012;45:273–81.

65. Peters OA, Arias A, Paqué F. A micro-computed tomographic assessment of root canal preparation with a novel instrument, TRUShape, in mesial roots of mandibular molars. J Endod. 2015;41:1545–50.

66. Paqué F, Ganahl D, Peters OA. Effects of root canal preparation on apical geometry assessed by micro-computed tomography. J Endod. 2009;35:1056–9.

67. Scarfe WC, Farman AG. What is cone-beam CT and how does it work? Dent Clin N Am. 2008;52:707–30.

68. Gluskin AH, Peters CI, Peters OA. Minimally invasive endodontics: challenging prevailing paradigms. Br Dent J. 2014;216:347–53.

69. Boveda C, Kishen A. Contracted endodontic cavities: the foundation for less invasive alternatives in the management of apical periodontitis. Endod Top. 2015;33:169–86.

70. Connert T, Krug R, Eggmann F, Emsermann I, ElAyouti A, Weiger R, Kühl S, Krastl G. Guided endodontics versus conventional access cavity preparation: a comparative study on substance loss using 3-dimensional-printed teeth. J Endod. 2019;45:327–31.

71. Ahn SY, Kim NH, Kim S, et al. Computer-aided design/computer-aided manufacturing-guided endodontic surgery: guided osteotomy and apex localization in a mandibular molar with a thick buccal bone plate. J Endod. 2018;44:665–70.

72. Nadeau B, Jung D, Vora V. Trends towards conservative endodontic treatment. Oral Health. 2019;109:30–45.

73. Tabassum S, Raza KF. Failure of endodontic treatment. The usual suspects. Eur J Dent. 2016;10:144–7.

74. https://www.aao.org/eye-health/tips-prevention/what-does-20-20-vision-mean.

75. Perrin P, Neuhaus KW, Lussi A. The impact of loupes and microscopes on vision in endodontics. Int Endod J. 2014;47:425–9.

76. Carr G. Microscopes in endodontics. J Calif Dent Assoc. 1992;20:55–61.

77. Kulild JC, Peters DD. Incidence and configuration of canal systems in the mesiobuccal root of maxillary first and second molars. J Endod. 1990;16:311–7.

78. de Carvalho MC, Zuolo ML. Orifice locating with a microscope. J Endod. 2000;26:532–4.

79. Schwarze T, Baethge C, Stecher T, Geurtsen W. Identification of second canals in the mesiobuccal root of maxillary first and second molars using magnifying loupes or an operating microscope. Aust Endod J. 2002;28:57–60.

80. Rampado ME, Tjaderhane L, Friedman S, Hamstra SJ. The benefit of the operating microscope for access cavity preparation by undergraduate students. J Endod. 2004;30:863–7.

81. Buhrley LJ, Barrows MJ, BeGole EA, Wenckus CS. Effect of magnification on locating the MB2 canal in maxillary molars. J Endod. 2002;28:324–7.

82. Karapinar-Kazandag M, Basrani B, Friedman S. The operating microscope enhances detection and negotiation of accessory medial canals in mandibular molars. J Endod. 2010;36:1289–94.

83. Görduysus MÖ, Görduysus M, Friedman S. Operating microscope improves negotiation of second mesiobuccal canals in maxillary molars. J Endod. 2001;27:683–6.

84. Plotino G, Pameijer CH, Grande NM, Somma F. Ultrasonics in endodontics: a review of the literature. J Endod. 2007;33:81–95.

85. Ansar A, Shetty KH. Uses of ultrasonics in endodontics, a review. Int J Adv Res. 2017;6:1448–59.

86. Lin YH, Mickel AK, Jones JJ, Montagnese TA, Gonzalez AF. Evaluation of cutting efficiency of ultrasonic tips used in orthograde endodontic treatment. J Endod. 2006;32:359–61.

87. Paz E, Satovsky J, Moldauer I. Comparison of the cutting efficiency of two ultrasonic units utilizing two different tips at two different power settings. J Endod. 2005;31:824–6.

88. Waplington M, Lumley PJ, Bunt L. An in vitro investigation into the cutting action of ultrasonic radicular access preparation instruments. Endod Dent Traumatol. 2000;16:158–61.

89. Boutsioukis C, Tzimpoulas NJ. Uncontrolled removal of dentin during in vitro ultrasonic irrigant activation. J Endod. 2016;42:289–93.

90. Gu Y, Kum KY, Perinpanayagam H, Kim C, Kum DJ, Lim SM, Chang SW, Baek SH, Zhu Q, Yoo YJ. Various heat-treated nickel–titanium rotary instruments evaluated in S-shaped simulated resin canals. J Dent Sci. 2017;12:14–20.

91. Walton RE. Current concepts of canal preparation. Dent Clin N Am. 1992;36:309–26.

92. Wu MK, Vander Sluis LW, Wesselink PR. The risk of furcal perforation in mandibular molars using Gates-Glidden drips with anticurvature pressure. Oral Surg Oral Med Oral Pathol Oral Radiol Endod. 2005;99:378–82.

93. Ossareh A, Kishen A. Effect of endodontic chemicals on the ultrastructure, chemical and mechanical characteristics of dentin hard tissue. J Endod. 2014;40:6.

94. Eaton JA, Clement DJ, Lloyd A, Marchesan MA. Micro-computed tomographic evaluation of the influence of root canal system landmarks on access outline forms and canal curvatures in mandibular molars. J Endod. 2015;41:1888–91.

95. Plotino G, Grande NM, Cordaro M, Testarelli L, Gambarini G. A review of cyclic fatigue testing of nickel-titanium rotary instruments. J Endod. 2009;35:1469–76.

96. Bhagabati N, Yadav S, Talwar S. An in vitro cyclic fatigue analysis of different endodontic nickel-titanium rotary instruments. J Endod. 2012;38:515–8.

97. Hayashi Y, Yoneyama T, Yahata Y, et al. Phase transformation behaviour and bending properties of hybrid nickel-titanium rotary endodontic instruments. Int Endod J. 2007;40:247–53.

98. Yahata Y, Yoneyama T, Hayashi Y, et al. Effect of heat treatment on transformation temperatures and bending properties of nickel-titanium endodontic instruments. Int Endod J. 2009;42:621–6.

Vital Pulp Therapy

2

Stéphane Simon

Contents

2.1   Introduction

Recent research advances demonstrating that the dentin-pulp complex is capable of repairing itself and regenerating mineralized tissue offer hope of new endodontic treatment modalities that can protect the vital pulp, provoke reactionary dentinogenesis, and stimulate revascularization of a damaged root canal [1]. The dental pulp is a complex and highly specialized connective tissue that is enclosed in a mineralized shell and has a limited blood supply; these are only a few of the many obstacles faced by the clinicians and researchers attempting to design new therapeutic strategies for its regeneration.

The primary aim of pulp capping is to protect the underlying tissue from any external stress, especially bacteria, meaning that the quality of the filling and its seal are of the utmost importance. For many years, only this seal was thought to determine the success of the procedure. In the 1990s, direct pulp caps with adhesive seemed to deliver good medium-term results [2]. However, the deterioration of the material, especially the sealing junctions, had not been taken into account. Although the results proved acceptable over a

S. Simon (✉)
INSERM, UMR 1138, Team Berdal, Paris, France

Endodontics and Oral Biology, Paris Diderot
University, Paris, France

period of months, the destruction of the seal and subsequent infiltration of bacteria prompted either acute inflammatory responses several months after treatment or 'low-level' pulpal necrosis [3].

These shortcomings caused a paradigm shift in the underlying biological concepts. A complete, biological closure of the wound comprising a long-term seal came to be seen as essential. To do this, materials with bioactive properties were used and eventually others were developed with the explicit goal of inducing dentin-bridge formation. For years, calcium hydroxide was used as a capping material, either undiluted or in combination with resins for easier manipulation [4]. The best-known product of this kind is Dycal® (Dentsply, De Trey). Though applying this material directly to the pulp causes a mineral barrier to form, this barrier is neither uniform nor bonded to the dentin wall; thus, a long-lasting seal cannot be formed [5]. Since this material tends to dissolve over time, after a matter of months the clinical situation would be the same as that of a treatment involving no capping material. While calcium hydroxide was the pulp-capping material of choice for many years, this is no longer the case today.

Of the many traits a given capping material should have, the following three are essential [6]:

- Creates an immediate seal of the dental cavity in order to protect the pulp in the first few weeks before the dentin bridge is formed.
- Meets all non-toxicity and biocompatibility criteria.
- Has bioactive properties that trigger the biological principles involved in forming a mineralized barrier between the pulp being treated and the material itself.

After pulp exposure, the odontoblasts layer is damaged. But these cells are the only dentin-producing cells. Then, to form the mineralized barrier, it is necessary to induce the growth of neo-odontoblasts, the only cells that can secrete dentin. Since these highly differentiated cells are post-mitotic (so no renewal by simple mitosis as for the other tissues), the healing process requires regenerative processes [7].

In a reparative process, progenitor cells are recruited on the wound site by chemotaxis or plithotaxis [8]. As soon they are in contact with the capping material, these cells differentiate into dentin-secreting cells and biological activity is stimulated and activated (Fig. 2.1).

Ideally, the biomaterial used should have these three abilities: chemiotaxis, stimulation of

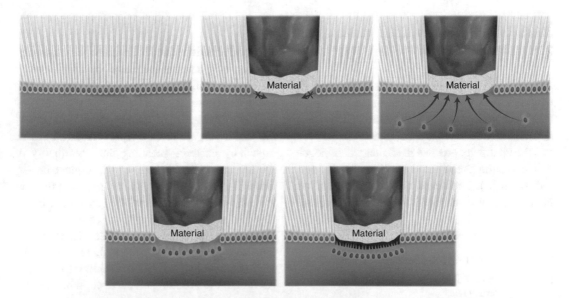

Fig. 2.1 The pulp healing process occurs in a three-step process after pulp capping with a dedicated material: progenitors recruitment, cell-differentiation and dentinogenesis stimulation

differentiation and activation of dentin synthesis. The results obtained from biomaterials until now have often been discovered by chance, once the dental device is on the market.

Dentin is a partially mineralized tissue whose organic phase consists of a matrix of collagen I enriched with a number of non-collagen matrix proteins. These proteins are initially secreted by the odontoblasts and then fossilized during the mineralization process [9]. The many matrix proteins include a large number of growth factors, including TGF Beta, VEGF and ADM.

Any biological (carious) or therapeutic process (etching) that demineralize dentin will release these growth factors from the matrix [10]. Even if most of the growth factors disappear into the saliva, some will diffuse through the dentinal tubules and reach the dental pulp [11].

Another way for stimulating growth factors release from dentin is to use a biomaterial that triggers partial but fairly controlled demineralization when the biomaterial comes into contact with dentin. The Dentine Matrix Proteins can be released from dentin by using calcium hydroxide [12], mineral trioxide aggregate [13] or any etching substance used during bonding [14]. The dentin matrix proteins boost chemotaxis, angiogenesis (18) and the differentiation of progenitor cells into dentinogenic cells [15]. Nevertheless, there are currently no viable therapeutic solutions available that can make use of these proteins' properties.

Odontoblasts are best known for their role in producing dentin, for both secreting it and mineralizing it during primary and secondary dentinogenesis [16]. When a carious lesion occurs, odontoblasts asleep and the 'quiescent' phase of synthesis can be reactivated to synthesize tertiary dentin, known as reactionary dentin [17].

If the secretion activity of odontoblasts is the most described, these cells have two other special roles: one in immunocompetence in relation with the Toll-like receptors (TLRs) on their membranes which transform the bond of bacteria toxins into a cellular signal that is communicated to the underlying connective tissue [18]; the second one is mechanosensation due to the presence of cils on the surface of the membrane [19]. Thanks to these two abilities, odontoblasts act as a protective barrier for the pulp by fending off aggressors and producing a suitable, intelligible signal for immune cells residing therein. Odontoblasts can transform information they receive into transmissible information that the underlying tissue can interpret. Odontoblasts are also especially sensitive to growth factors and biostimulators. When dental tissue is demineralized due to caries, dentin matrix proteins are released and can circulate freely in the dentinal tubules [15].

2.2 Pulp Inflammation and Healing

In dentistry, inflammation has a strong negative connotation. Pulpitis is immediately associated with pain and adverse effects leading to destroyed and necrotic pulp tissue. Treating this pain requires removing the inflamed tissue with a surgical procedure which is often quite invasive, and difficult to find the limit in accordance with minimally invasive treatments. Because of the difficulties to find the limits of the disease, the majority of cases end in a complete pulpectomy and root canal treatment.

However, the adverse effects of inflammation should be contrasted with its benefits. Inflammation marks the first step of tissue healing. Inflammation helps by cleaning and disinfecting the wound to be healed on one hand, and on the other hand by secreting a variety of substances (cytokines) that help in the healing and regeneration process [20].

In a clinical setting, pulpal inflammation is commonly referred to as 'reversible' or 'irreversible'. The process of inflammation exists or not and then, cannot be reversible. This idea of reversibility means that the process is controlled well enough that it can be stopped, and then guided to aid in healing. When the inflammation is too advanced to be controlled, the inflammation process is called 'irreversible'. This term refers to a certain clinical situation associated with relatively basic diagnostic elements (type of pain, persistence, etc.) which are poorly related to the right histo-physio-pathological status of the tissue. This lack of correlation has been demonstrated for years [21] and has been confirmed with some additional nuances multiple times [22]. Some studies have looked into markers of pulp inflammation and their potential use in diagnosis or treatment [23]. Although these markers are known to exist, more specific information remains elusive and more robust studies are still required to eventually imagine reliable diagnostic tools and reproducible use-cases.

So far, without more biological help, practitioners must do with what is available now: tooth anamnesis to define the patient's pain as well as heat and electrical tests whose reliability is still suboptimal. More options based on observation, including controlling haemostasis at the time of pulp exposure and/or partial pulpectomy, can be used as clinical marker. Inflammation is associated with hypervascularization, which could be identified by the bleeding. Nevertheless, the same bleeding may arise when vascular connective tissue is cut. To understand the difference, the lesion can be packed with a damp cotton pellet placed

directly on the tissue with pressure applied for 1–2 min. This is enough time to achieve haemostasis under physiological conditions. If bleeding persists, it may be assumed that some of the pulp tissue is still inflamed and partial removal is necessary until healthy tissue is exposed.

Given the huge difference from one situation to another one, and because of the variability from one practitioner to another one, these markers are not reliable enough to state on the inflamed pulp tissue status. Thus, it becomes clear that the means for identifying and testing the presence of inflamed tissue in exposed pulp are both arbitrary and inadequate. Despite the binary description (reversible versus irreversible), histological section observations confirm that it is not so easy to differentiate the first one from the second one. Indeed, a precise observation of an inflamed pulp confirms that all the pathological status (necrosis, irreversible inflammation and reversible inflammation) of the tissue are present on the same disease on different layers (Fig. 2.2).

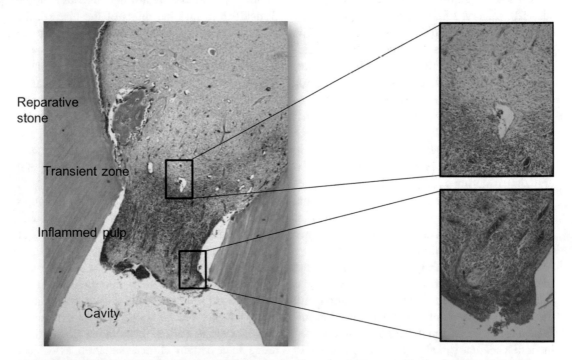

Fig. 2.2 Pig dental pulp exposed to the oral cavity for 7 days. This was done for miming the pulp inflammation. This histological slice (7 microns cut, haematoxylin-eosin staining) clearly shows that on the same tissue, all the disease levels are present (necrosis, irreversible inflammation, reversible inflammation, pulp stone given by a low level of inflammation)

Additional research is therefore necessary to identify more specific markers (biological or clinical) to develop suitable, accurate diagnostic tools and improve long-term results. This is an important point to consider because controlling inflammation remains the key for the success of pulp capping therapies.

2.3 Pulp Capping and Biomaterials

Mineral trioxide aggregate (MTA), marketed under the name ProRoot MTA® (Dentsply Sirona), gradually became the material of choice over the years, as scientific evidence mounts [3]. Sold as a powder to be mixed with water, the substance is placed onto a glass tray and applied directly to the pulp using a dedicated instrument, such as the MAP System® (PDSA, Vevey, Switzerland). The material is not packed in but placed into direct contact with the pulp, lightly tapped into the dentin wall using a bit of thick paper or a cotton pellet. It is now recommended to amend the usage protocol for this specific circumstance and restore the tooth immediately with bonded composite resin. Since the material takes over 4 h to set, it requires taking all necessary precautions because spraying water to rinse the cavity, for example, would wash away the material that has just been applied. If the restoration protocol includes spraying dental tissue with water, we recommend completing this step first before applying the capping material (Fig. 2.3).

The advantage of biological properties of this material has been shown with in vitro and in vivo studies, as well as in clinical trials comparing it to other materials [24]. The higher histological quality of the dentin bridges formed using this material compared with calcium hydroxide has been demonstrated.

One of the most common disadvantages of this material is the difficulty to manipulate it and the risk to induce dyschromia of the tooth, given to the presence of bismuth oxide added in the material to improve its radio-opacity. Multiple manufacturers have developed during the years some similar materials (hydraulic cements) trying to limit its inconvenience by replacing bismuth oxide by zirconium oxide.

Some years ago, a tricalcium silicate-based material (Biodentine®, Septodont, France) has been launched on the market. Initially developed as a dentin substitute for coronal fillings, it demonstrated effects on biological tissues that led to an extension of its indications to include pulp capping [25]. One of its notable qualities is its effect to start mineralization [26] and cellular differentiation [25]. These results provide excellent proof for optimism about its long-term clinical potential.

In addition to their sealing ability (to protect the pulp) and their biological activity (inflammation control), these capping materials also have the ability to release the dentin matrix proteins from the dentin upon contact with such a material. In particular, this has been demonstrated for calcium hydroxide [12] and MTA [13]. Therefore, these substances combine a direct biological effect on the pulp with an indirect effect by causing a gradual, delayed release of growth factors, including some anti-inflammatories. It may therefore be worthwhile in the future to extend the application area of these materials to include the adjacent dentin walls where preparation of the cavity has made the dentin thinner. The material in contact with the dentin can extract the matrix proteins, which could travel through the dentinal tubules (which are quite large at this depth) and help to heal the pulp [27] (Fig. 2.4). This is an application in which the use of Biodentine may have a real potential, as it may be used to fill an entire coronal cavity, which is not the case for MTA. However, the mechanical behaviour of the material still necessitates an additional procedure in which it is coated with a bonded composite which both makes the restauration more aesthetically pleasing and keeps the substitution material from dissolving.

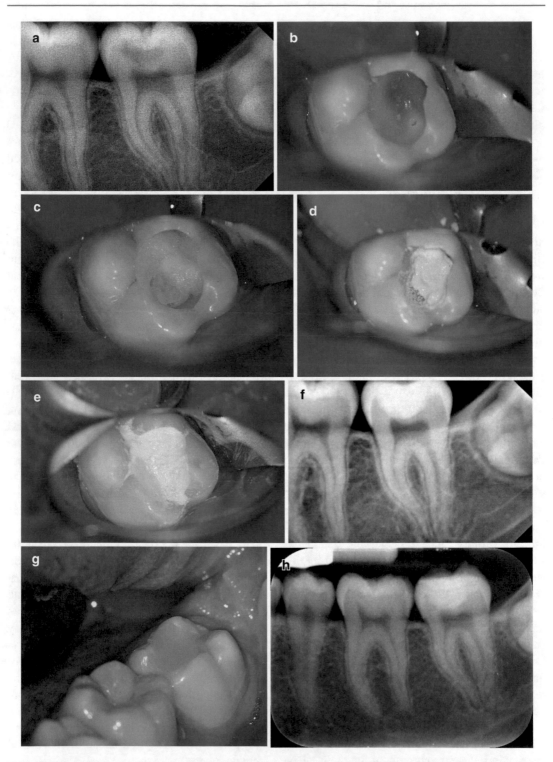

Fig. 2.3 Pulp capping on a permanent tooth suffering of deep carious lesion. (**a**) pre-operative X-ray; (**b**) cavity after removal of the carious tissue; (**c**) cavity disinfection with a 2% chlorhexidine solution; (**d**) placement of the pulp capping material in direct contact with the pulp and also used for a bulk coronal restoration; (**e**) final view before bonded composite resin restoration will be placed. (**f**) Post-operative X-ray; (**g**) clinical image at 10 months recall, the tooth responds normally to pulp sensitivity tests; (**h**) 10 months recall radiograph

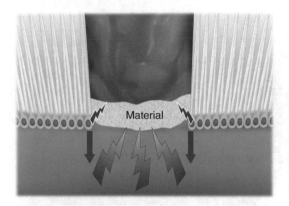

Fig. 2.4 The bioactive material can act in two ways for pulp healing: with a direct effect onto the pulp tissue and with an indirect pathway by controlled dissolution of the dentin leading to growth factors release

2.4 Step-by-Step Procedure

2.4.1 Pulp Capping (Fig. 2.3)

The objective is to cap the pulp when it is exposed, with a dedicated material. The following step by step can be used in most of the clinical situations.

1. Anaesthesia of the tooth is completed first as for a restorative procedure. The use of a vasoconstrictor is possible, but must be considered for the rest of the treatment (bleeding control step).
2. Placement of the rubber dam and disinfection.
3. Remove the carious tissues and clean the cavity with sterile excavators and burs under cooling water. It is recommended to remove first most of the carious tissue before exposing the dental pulp.
4. When the cavity is very deep, the pulp is exposed.
5. Control the bleeding with a moist sterile cotton pellet (with sterile water) placed into the cavity with a gentle compression.
6. Remove the cotton pellet and control the stop of the bleeding. Do not use other product to stop the bleeding (ferric sulphate, laser, etc.). Indeed, the control of the haemorrhage is the only reliable technique to evaluate the inflam-

mation status of the pulp. If the pulp is not inflamed, the bleeding due to the wound only can be stopped with a gentle compression.

7. If the bleeding cannot be controlled, the exposed pulp must be removed with a sterile bur under copious water to process a partial pulpotomy. Then try again to control the bleeding with the same technique than before. At this stage it is important to keep in mind that the bleeding control is necessary, being a poor clinical diagnostic tool, but the only one we have until new diagnostic tools will be developed. One more limiting factor is the use of a vasoconstrictor for anaesthesia; then the blood stream into the pulp is modified. Furthermore, bleeding can also be restricted leading to a good control even if the pulp is inflamed.
8. The exposed pulp can be inflamed, but is not infected. The dentine can be disinfected with a 2% chlorhexidine solution left into the cavity for 2–3 min. Laser (Er-Yag) can also be considered. Sodium hypochlorite is not recommended, as it modifies the dentinal structure and interferes with the bonding process to follow.
9. Place the capping material directly in contact with the pulp with a dedicated device, but do not plug it.
10. The cavity is filled out with the same material, if it is dedicated or the bonded restoration covering the capping material can be done in the same session.
11. The post-operative X-ray is then taken and the occlusion is checked.
12. Follow the patient at short (1–3 months) and long term (every 6 months). The pulp sensibility is checked with a cold test and a recall X-ray is also recommended.

2.4.2 Pulp Chamber Pulpotomy (Fig. 2.5)

The clinical procedure is similar. The pulp chamber pulpotomy is indicated when the bleeding control of the pulp exposure site is not possible or in case of any doubt of the inflammation status

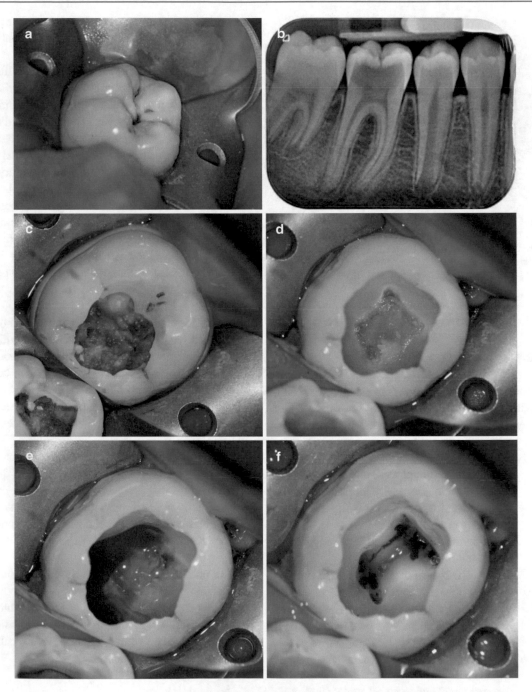

Fig. 2.5 Full pulp chamber pulpotomy. (**a**) pre-operative image; (**b**) pre-operative X-ray; (**c**) view after enamel removal; (**d**) coronal view after full carious tissue removal, some carious tissue remains in direct contact with the pulp; (**e**) after complete affected dental tissue removal the pulp is exposed and bleeding is difficult to control; (**f**) it was decided to remove the full pulp of the pulp chamber instead of doing a conventional pulp capping; (**g**) after control of the bleeding, capping material is placed into the cavity with an amalgam carrier; (**h**) the material is gently packed on the floor of the cavity with an amalgam plugger; (**i**) the full cavity is filled with the material; (**j**) the 10 months recall associated to normal clinical tests confirm the short-term success of the treatment

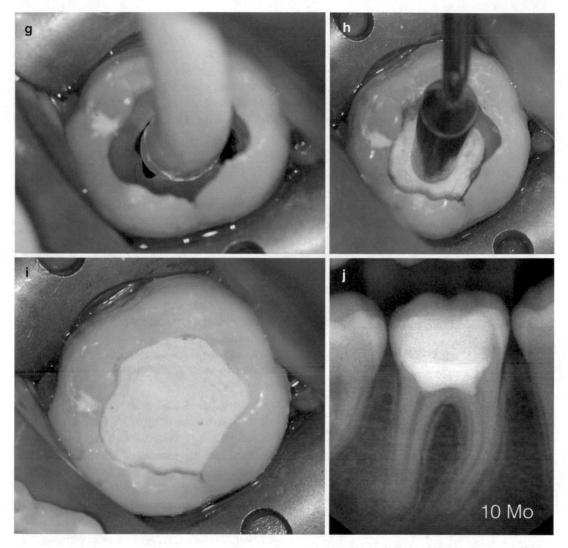

Fig. 2.5 (continued)

of the pulp. In that case, it is probably safer to process a deep pulpotomy. The six first steps of the pulp capping remain the same. Then the following steps are performed:

1. The pulp chamber is emptied of the whole coronal pulp with a sterile carbamide bur used with a low-speed handpiece under copious water cooling.
2. The pulp is cut with a sharp and sterile excavator at the entrance of the root canal.

3. The bleeding is controlled by a gentle pressure with a moist sterile cotton pellet.
4. Radicular pulp stamps are capped with the capping material as described before.
5. Fill the rest of the coronal cavity with the same material or with a bonded composite resin.
6. Control the quality of treatment with a postoperative X-ray and check the occlusion.
7. Recall the patient for short- and long-term checks. Note that in the case of a pulp chamber pulpotomy, the sensibility tests are not reliable.

2.5 Application of Pulp Capping and 'Bio-Products' to Stimulate Regeneration

The extracellular matrix (ECM) of dentin contains a variety of molecules involved in regulating dentinogenesis. Attempts have been made to use ECM proteins (expressed in recombinant bacteria) to stimulate pulp regeneration [28]. The biological effects of several other ECM molecules have also been examined, including dentonin, an acid synthetic peptide derived from matrix extracellular phosphoglycoprotein (MEPE), and A + 4 and A−4, two splice products of the amelogenin gene. Each molecule induced regeneration of a superficial pulp [29].

Such biological approaches helped to elucidate what is occurring during pulp capping and regeneration; however, before their clinical application, more studies are necessary to confirm the advantages and safety of such bio-products versus mineral hydraulic cements.

2.6 Short- and Long-Term Future Developments

Progress in developments of capping biomaterials in the past 10 years helped to reawaken interest in techniques to preserve pulp vitality. Our understanding of pulp biology continues to progress, which makes it possible to explain the reason for certain failures because the Achilles heel of these procedures remains the assessment of the state of inflammation of the pulp in need of treatment. Clinically, it remains difficult to know exactly how deep down the pulp tissue needs to be removed, in order to eliminate the risk of leaving any inflamed tissue.

A suggestion deriving from this idea was recently made in which a larger portion of the pulp may be removed, thus ensuring that all of the inflamed tissue has been eliminated, but without resulting in a complete pulpectomy of the tooth.

Until now, this treatment was restricted to primary teeth or certain immature teeth. However, in the coming years, pulp chamber pulpotomies might come to be seen as an endodontic therapeutic alternative to pulpectomies and root canal treatment. In this procedure, the whole tissue of the pulp chamber is removed and the radicular stumps are capped with a capping material (Fig. 2.5). Preliminary studies have shown promising results [30], but these must be supplemented with more formal studies before it can be proposed as a generally viable procedure.

2.7 Conclusions

The aim of any endodontic treatment is to prevent the bacterial leakage from the mouth (which is infected with commensal flora), up to the maxillary bone underneath, which is free of any infection and must be prevented to any bacterial contamination.

Based on this postulate, every clinical process permitting to block the bacteria progression must be considered.

Pulp capping and pulp chamber pulpotomy allow to close the door of bacterial penetration, by just placing a material in direct contact with the pulp connective tissue. This material ensures the sealing of the wound in few minutes/hours and will create a double protection by inducing the setting of a mineralized barrier between material and pulp tissue. Thus, partial and full chamber pulpotomies followed by pulp capping must be considered as minimally invasive endodontic treatments. Furthermore, the new strategies of coronal restoration with bonded composite resins or bonded prosthetic restoration allow now to minimize the root canal treatment indication, at least for restorative reasons.

References

1. Simon S, Smith AJ. Regenerative endodontics. Br Dent J. 2014;216:E13.
2. Cox CF, Hafez AA, Akimoto N, Otsuki M, Suzuki S, Tarim B. Biocompatibility of primer, adhesive and resin composite systems on non-exposed and exposed pulps of non-human primate teeth. Am J Dent. 1998;11. Spec No::S55–63.

3. Nair PN, Duncan HF, Pitt Ford TR, Luder HU. Histological, ultrastructural and quantitative investigations on the response of healthy human pulps to experimental capping with mineral trioxide aggregate: a randomized controlled trial. Int Endod J. 2008;41:128–50.
4. Heys DR, Cox CF, Heys RJ, Avery JK. Histological considerations of direct pulp capping agents. J Dent Res. 1981;60:1371–9.
5. Goldberg F, Massone EJ, Spielberg C. Evaluation of the dentinal bridge after pulpotomy and calcium hydroxide dressing. J Endod. 1984;10:318–20.
6. Witherspoon DE. Vital pulp therapy with new materials: new directions and treatment perspectives—permanent teeth. J Endod. 2008;34(7 Suppl):S25–8.
7. Simon S, Cooper P, Isaac J, Berdal A. Tissue engineering and endodontics. In preprosthetic and maxillofacial surgery biomaterials, bone grafting and tissue engineering woodhead publishing series in biomaterials. 2011;336–62. ISBN 9781845695897.
8. Hirata A, Dimitrova-Nakov S, Djole S-X, et al. Plithotaxis, a collective cell migration, regulates the sliding of proliferating pulp cells located in the apical niche. Connect Tissue Res. 2014;55(Suppl 1):68–72.
9. Smith AJ, Duncan HF, Diogenes A, Simon S, Cooper PR. Exploiting the bioactive properties of the dentin-pulp complex in regenerative endodontics. J Endod. 2016;42:47–56.
10. Simon SRJ, Berdal A, Cooper PR, Lumley PJ, Tomson PL, Smith AJ. Dentin-pulp complex regeneration: from lab to clinic. Adv Dent Res. 2011;23:340–5.
11. Sloan AJ, Shelton RM, Hann AC, Moxham BJ, Smith AJ. An in vitro approach for the study of dentinogenesis by organ culture of the dentine-pulp complex from rat incisor teeth. Arch Oral Biol. 1998;43:421–30.
12. Graham L, Cooper PR, Cassidy N, Nor JE, Sloan AJ, Smith AJ. The effect of calcium hydroxide on solubilisation of bio-active dentine matrix components. Biomaterials. 2006;27:2865–73.
13. Tomson PL, Grover LM, Lumley PJ, Sloan AJ, Smith AJ, Cooper PR. Dissolution of bio-active dentine matrix components by mineral trioxide aggregate. J Dent. 2007;35:636–42.
14. Ferracane JL, Cooper PR, Smith AJ. Can interaction of materials with the dentin-pulp complex contribute to dentin regeneration? Odontology. 2010;98:2–14.
15. Liu J, Jin T, Ritchie HH, Smith AJ, Clarkson BH. In vitro differentiation and mineralization of human dental pulp cells induced by dentin extract. Vitr Cell Dev Biol Anim. 2005;41:232.
16. Simon SR, Smith AJ, Lumley PJ, et al. Molecular characterisation of young and mature odontoblasts. Bone. 2009;45:693–703.
17. Stéphane S, Cooper Paul R, Lumley Philip J, Berdal A, Tomson PL, Smith Anthony J. Understanding pulp biology for routine clinical practice. Endod Pract Today. 2009;3:171–84.
18. Farges JC, Keller JF, Carrouel F, et al. Odontoblasts in the dental pulp immune response. J Exp Zool B Mol Dev Evol. 2009;312B:425–36.
19. Magloire H, Couble ML, Thivichon-Prince B, Maurin JC, Bleicher F. Odontoblast: a mechano-sensory cell. J Exp Zool B Mol Dev Evol. 2009;312B:416–24.
20. Cooper PR, Takahashi Y, Graham LW, Simon S, Imazato S, Smith AJ. Inflammation-regeneration interplay in the dentine-pulp complex. J Dent. 2010;38:687–97.
21. Dummer PM, Hicks R, Huws D. Clinical signs and symptoms in pulp disease. Int Endod J. 1980;13:27–35.
22. Ricucci D, Loghin S, Siqueira JF. Correlation between clinical and histologic pulp diagnoses. J Endod. 2014;40:1932–9.
23. Zanini M, Meyer E, Simon S. Pulp inflammation diagnosis from clinical to inflammatory mediators: a systematic review. J Endod. 2017;43:1033–51.
24. Hilton TJ, Ferracane JL, Mancl L. Comparison of CaOH with MTA for direct pulp capping: a PBRN randomized clinical trial. J Dent Res. 2013;92(7 Suppl):16S–22S.
25. Zanini M, Sautier JM, Berdal A, Simon S. Biodentine induces immortalized murine pulp cell differentiation into odontoblast-like cells and stimulates biomineralization. J Endod. 2012;38:1220–6.
26. Laurent P, Camps J, About I. Biodentine induces TGF-β1 release from human pulp cells and early dental pulp mineralization. Int Endod J. 2012;45:439–48.
27. Simon Stéphane R, Smith Anthony J, Lumley Philip J, Cooper Paul R, Berdal A. The pulp healing process: from generation to regeneration. Endod Top. 2012;26:41–56.
28. Rutherford RB, Spångberg L, Tucker M, Rueger D, Charette M. The time-course of the induction of reparative dentine formation in monkeys by recombinant human osteogenic protein-1. Arch Oral Biol. 1994;39:833–8.
29. Goldberg M, Six N, Chaussain C, DenBesten P, Veis A, Poliard A. Dentin extracellular matrix molecules implanted into exposed pulps generate reparative dentin: a novel strategy in regenerative dentistry. J Dent Res. 2009;88:396–9.
30. Simon S, Perard M, Zanini M, et al. Should pulp chamber pulpotomy be seen as a permanent treatment? Some preliminary thoughts. Int Endod J. 2013;46:79–87.

Minimally Invasive Access to the Root Canal System

Antonis Chaniotis and Gianluca Plotino

3

Contents

A. Chaniotis
Private Practice, University of Athens, Attica, Greece

G. Plotino (✉)
Private Practice, Grande, Plotino & Torsello – Studio di Odontoiatria, Rome, Italy
e-mail: endo@gianlucaplotino.com

3.1 Introduction

Traditionally endodontic access cavity designs were dictated by the underlying anatomy and the need to facilitate all the subsequent stages of

© Springer Nature Switzerland AG 2021
G. Plotino (ed.), *Minimally Invasive Approaches in Endodontic Practice*,
https://doi.org/10.1007/978-3-030-45866-9_3

root canal treatment. In this regard, the outline form of the access cavities was guided by the operator convenience through the extension for prevention form. Although such access designs offered many advantages to the operator needs, they disregarded the need to preserve sound tooth structure to allow the long-term function of the tooth. Recently, minimal invasive dentistry concepts highlighted the importance of dentin preservation for the longevity of endodontically treated teeth. Traditional access cavity designs were questioned, regarded as legacy concepts, and modified to fit the current trends of tissue preservation in endodontics. Current technological advancements enabled this process. This chapter will describe the advantages and disadvantages of traditional and conservative access cavity designs and will suggest modifications that will lead to the concept of dynamic access cavity design dictated by the anatomy, the pathology, and the available equipment.

3.2 Access Cavity Designs in Endodontics

The first step of the endodontic treatment procedures is always the creation of an access cavity to the internal anatomy of the tooth to be treated. Access cavity designs in endodontics are geometrically predesigned shapes dictated by the underlying chamber anatomy of the tooth to be treated [1]. Therefore the alliance between access cavity design and anatomy is inflexible and inseparable [2]. This means that in order to master the anatomic concept of cavity preparation the operator should develop a clear mental three-dimensional image of the inside of the tooth from pulp horns to the apical foramen. Unfortunately, for many years periapical radiographs only provided a two-dimensional blue print of pulp chamber and canal anatomy. It was the third dimension that we should visualize as a supplement to the two dimensional thinking in order to locate and negotiate the aberrant canal system (Fig. 3.1).

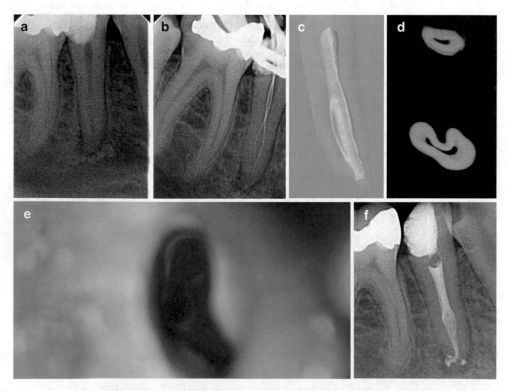

Fig. 3.1 (a) C-shape canal anatomy in a mandibular premolar as seen in the two-dimensional preoperative periapical radiograph; (b) working length radiograph revealing the anatomy in two dimensions; (c, d) micro-CT images of a similar anatomy on scanned extracted teeth (courtesy of dr. Ronald Ordinola Zapata); (e) access cavity extended accordingly in order to negotiate the middle third c-shape; (f) postoperative radiograph

Knowledge of the most common anatomical patterns of pulp chamber spaces and projecting these anatomical patterns through a traditional access cavity was the main focus for many years to facilitate clinical exploration and negotiation of the deeper parts of root canal anatomy.

3.3 Anatomy of the Pulp Chamber

The pulp chamber is located in the center of the tooth crown and its anatomy under no pathological conditions resembles the shape of the crown surface.

Based on the anatomical study of 500 teeth, Krasner and Rankow [3] proposed some laws for aiding the determination of the pulp chamber position as well as the location and number of root canal entrances in each group of teeth (Fig. 3.2):

- **Law of centrality**: The floor of the pulp chamber is always located in the center of the tooth at the level of the cemento-enamel junction (CEJ).
- **Law of concentricity**: The walls of the pulp chamber are always concentric to the external surface of the tooth at the level of the CEJ, i.e., the external root surface anatomy reflects the internal pulp chamber anatomy.
- **Law of the CEJ**: The distance from the external surface of the clinical crown to the wall of the pulp chamber is the same throughout the circumference of the tooth at the level of the CEJ.
- **Law of symmetry 1**: Except for maxillary molars, the orifices of the canals are equidis-

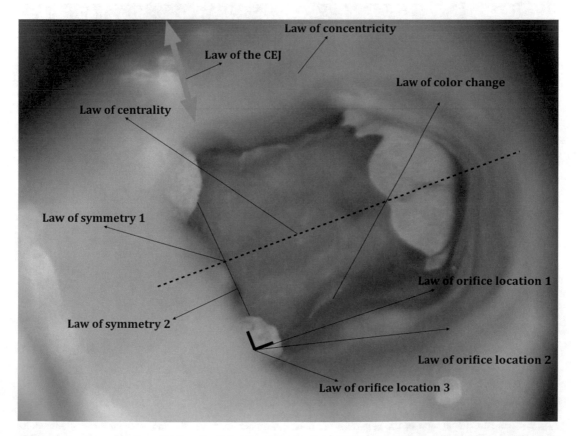

Fig. 3.2 Krasner and Rankow [3] laws for aiding the determination of the chamber position as well as the location of canal entrance

tant from a line drawn in a mesial-distal direction, through the pulp chamber floor.

- **Law of symmetry 2:** Except for the maxillary molars, the orifices of the canals lie on a line perpendicular to a line drawn in a mesial-distal direction across the center of the floor of the pulp chamber.
- **Law of color change**: The color of the pulp-chamber floor is always darker than the walls.
- **Law of orifice location 1**: The orifices of the root canals are always located at the junction of the walls and the floor.
- **Law of orifice location 2**: The orifices of the root canals are located at the angles in the floor-wall junction.
- **Law of orifice location 3**: The orifices of the root canals are located at the terminus of the root developmental fusion lines.

In addition of knowing these laws, the use of illumination and magnification through an access cavity would provide the best approach to explore all anatomic variations of the pulp chamber in order to locate all canal orifices and avoid missed canals, which has been considered one of the main causes of endodontic failure.

3.4 Traditional Access Cavity
(Fig. 3.3)

For more than 50 years, the "traditional" access cavity designs were subjected to some principles that were left unchanged over the time. The traditional endodontic access cavities principles include [2, 4]:

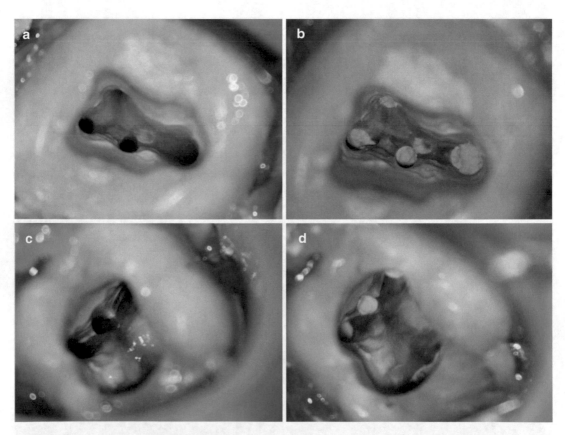

Fig. 3.3 (**a, b**) Clinical view of the pulp chamber floor after shaping procedures and after completion of obturation in a maxillary molar with fused roots as seen through a traditional access cavity; (**c, d**) clinical view of the chamber floor after shaping procedures and after completion of obturation in a mandibular molar with middle mesial canal as seen through a traditional access cavity

- The removal of all carious dentin and defective restorations.
- The outline form that is dictated by the occlusal extent of the prepared cavity with divergent axial walls.
- The convenience form that is dictated by the degree of dentin to be removed at specific locations so as to achieve a straight-line access to root canal orifices.
- The "toilet" cleaning of the cavity.
- The extension for prevention that is dictated by the removal of dentin obstructions to extend the straight line access to the apical foramen or the primary curvature of the root canal.

These traditional access cavities offered some inherent advantages, such as the enhanced visibility, the improved clinical exploration of the floor anatomy and canal openings, the facilitation of cleaning, shaping, and obturation procedures, and the alteration of root canal curvature parameters in a way that would minimize complications [4].

Traditionally the instrumentation difficulty of a given canal was assessed by the arbitrary Schneider angle of curvature [5]. The angle of curvature as described by Schneider is the angle forming by the interception of a line passing through the long axis of the root and a line passing through the apical foramen to the point that the canal starts to deviate. Increase in angle of curvature results in increased instrumentation difficulty. Some years later, Pruett et al. [6] noticed that two roots can have the same angle of curvature, but totally different abruptness of curvature. In order to describe the abruptness of curvature they introduced the radius of curvature. Radius of curvature is the radius of a circle passing through the curved part of the root. A decrease in radius of curvature results in increased abruptness of curvature and increased instrumentation difficulty. Additionally to these parameters, Schafer et al. [7] stated that, in order to define mathematically and unambiguously the canal curvature, the length of curve should be reported as well. An increase in length results in increased instrumentation difficulties. Finally, Gunday

et al. [8] introduced the concept of the location of the curve by describing the canal access angle (CAA) parameter. Canal access angle is the angle forming from the intersection of a line passing through the long axis of the root with a line drawn from the apical foramen to the canal entrance. Curvature height and distance together with the CAA define the instrumentation difficulty. The more the curvatures are located coronally, the more stressful they are for the endodontic instruments [9]. A traditional access cavity with convenience form and extension for prevention can shift the aforementioned parameters in a way that facilitates instrumentation as shown in Fig. 3.4. Especially for the curvature parameters, convenience form and extension for prevention will decrease the angle of curvature, increase the radius of curvature, shorten the curved part of the canal, and relocate the curvature apically facilitating root canal instrumentation to a great extent (Fig. 3.4). Although access cavities with convenience form and extension for prevention improve the parameters of curvature, unfortunately they selectively remove dentin from the cervical tooth area. However the benefits of fewer complications in endodontic instrumentation outweighed the drawbacks of tissue removal for many years, until minimal invasive treatment concepts affected dentistry.

3.5 Minimal Invasive Dentistry

Recently medicine and dentistry in general moved towards minimal invasive concepts that might benefit most the patients. This patient-centered approach affected also endodontic concepts. Minimal invasive dentistry concepts seek to bridge the gap between prevention and dental intervention. They highlight the application of a systematic respect for the original tissue. This implies that the dental profession recognizes that an artifact is of less biological value than the original tissue. The common delineator is tissue preservation preferably by preventing disease from occurring and intercepting its progress, but also by removing and replacing as little tissue as possible [10].

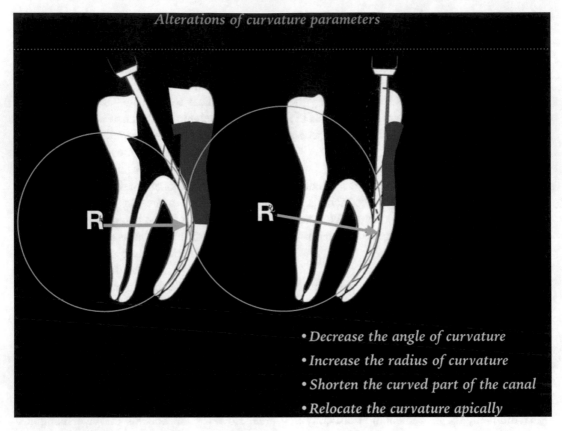

Alterations of curvature parameters

- *Decrease the angle of curvature*
- *Increase the radius of curvature*
- *Shorten the curved part of the canal*
- *Relocate the curvature apically*

Fig. 3.4 Alteration of curvature parameters after creating convenience form and extension for prevention form in a traditional access cavity

In endodontology, minimal invasiveness is defined as the process of achieving the objectives of endodontology by removing and replacing as little tissue as possible. These objectives include not only the prevention and treatment of apical periodontitis but also the lifetime retention of the natural teeth. Especially with regard to the last objective, the traditional endodontic access cavity concepts were questioned and modified.

The most frequent reason for the failure of endodontically treated teeth was reported to be the pronounced loss of dental tissues due to non-restorable caries and fractures [11]. The fracture of endodontically treated teeth is suggested to be directly related to the quantity of tissue lost and to the specific cavity configuration [12]. The more the tissue removed, the more the weakening of the tooth structure and the reduction of tooth stiffness and resistance to fracture [13]. In fact, it was showed since late 80s that access cavity and endodontic procedures per se had only a small effect on the tooth, reducing the relative stiffness by 5%, compared with 20% reduction in tooth stiffness because of restorative procedures for an occlusal restoration or 63% if both marginal ridges were lost in an MOD cavity [14], suggesting that the marginal ridges are very important elements for the fracture resistance of the tooth. In agreement with the above findings, Lang et al. [15] reported that access preparation (removal of the pulp chamber roof), as well as post preparation, resulted in a significant increase in deformability of the tooth, while the removal of dentin at the wall of the canal without extensive alteration of the root canals' outline (by manual widening) resulted in no significant increase of deformability.

However, in molars cuspal deflection always increased with increasing cavity size and was greatest following endodontic access cavity preparation [16], suggesting that a cuspal coverage protective restoration was always needed in molars after endodontic access cavity preparation. Over the years different types of restoration were developed and recommended for the endodontically treated teeth [17]. According to the clinical situation the objective was always to compensate for tissue loss and design a restoration that might protect the remaining tooth from fracturing. The reason that endodontically treated teeth can fracture is because of trauma or fatigue failure from repeated stress overloading. With normal functional stresses a tooth can fracture because of the reduced mechanical properties of teeth with incomplete root formation, caries, wear, and highly invasive operative dentistry procedures and because of the changes in tooth structure that happen due to aging, vitality loss, and endodontic treatment [18].

Considering all the aforementioned growing evidence, an attempt to minimize tissue loss in all aspects of dentistry was initiated and rapidly became very popular and evolved in a trend. This attempt was triggered with the introduction of new cutting edge technological advancements.

The current technological advancements that enabled the process of tissue preservation in endodontics can be summarized as follows:

- *Dental operating microscopes (DOM)*
  The DOM, although not new, provide visual feedback, depth perception, magnification, coaxial illumination, and improved ergonomics for use in all stages of dental treatment [19].
- *Small field of view cone-beam computed tomography (CBCT) imaging*
  Current advancement in CBCT imaging resulted in visualization of the three-dimensional root canal anatomy for most configurations [20].
- *Ultrasonic (US) tips and devices*
  US may guarantee clinicians with an increased visibility and precision during the operating procedures, thus promoting more conservative treatments.
- *Martensitic flexible and resistant files*
  Current advancements in thermo-mechanical processing of NiTi alloys resulted in the manufacturing of extremely resistant and flexible instruments. These instruments can be pre-curved and they can be used safely through confined spaces without the need for convenience form and extension for prevention [21].
- *Evolution of irrigation techniques*
  Recent advancements in irrigant activation techniques (ultrasonic, high-power-sonic, multisonic or laser-assisted activation) suggest that disinfection of the root canal system may be possible with minimal or even no instrumentation [22].
- *Evolution of biocompatible root canal filling materials*
  Recent evolutions in bioactive obturation materials resulted in the development of simplified techniques to fill the root canal system [23].
- *3D fixed (static) and/or dynamic guidance* [24]
  These new technologies may help the clinician to perform conservative treatments even in the most difficult cases, such as completely calcified canals or access through crown and bridges.
- *Adhesive dentistry procedures*
  Increase in the quality of the restorative procedures may help to achieve a better prognosis even with partial adhesive restorations of endodontically treated teeth.

Under this framework, removing tissue to facilitate the stages of root canal treatment seems obsolete in endodontics. Tissue preservation emerges as the new paradigm shift that might result in the lifetime retention of natural teeth. Tissue preservation in endodontics can take various forms including prevention, early diagnosis, vital pulp therapy concepts, access cavity designs, canal preparation sizes, irrigation techniques, and microsurgical endodontics. This chapter will deal only with access cavity designs and tissue preservation.

3.6 Conservative Access Cavity

According to Boveda and Kishen [4], conservative endodontic access shapes are geometrical shapes that prioritize the removal of (i) restorative material ahead of tooth structure, (ii) enamel ahead of dentin, and (iii) occlusal tooth structure ahead of cervical dentin. The objective is to increase the mechanical stability of the tooth and its fracture resistance resulting in long-term survival and function. The common delineator of all conservative access cavities is the creation of a shape that:

- Overlooks the traditional requirements of extension for prevention and convenience form.
- Overlooks straight-line access and complete unroofing of the pulp chamber.
- Emphasizes the importance of preserving the pericervical dentin in posterior teeth (pericervical dentin is the dentin located 4 mm above and 4 mm below the CEJ).
- Emphasizes the importance of preserving the pericingulum dentin in anterior teeth.

A dynamic approach is needed to perform a conservative access cavity, opening it in a conservative way without performing a predefined shape from the beginning, until an enlargement of the cavity becomes necessary to ensure a greater visibility.

3.7   Access Cavity Terminology

When discussing new concepts of access cavity design, it is important to define the common new terminology that will help the clinician communicate in a common ground.

The Traditional Endodontic Cavity (TEC) has been defined as a cavity that "aims to perform a complete unroofing of the pulp chamber, exposure of all the pulp horns and a straight-line access to the root canals with coronally divergent walls without undercuts, to visualize the pulp chamber floor and all the root canal orifices from the same visual angulation" [25] (Fig. 3.5).

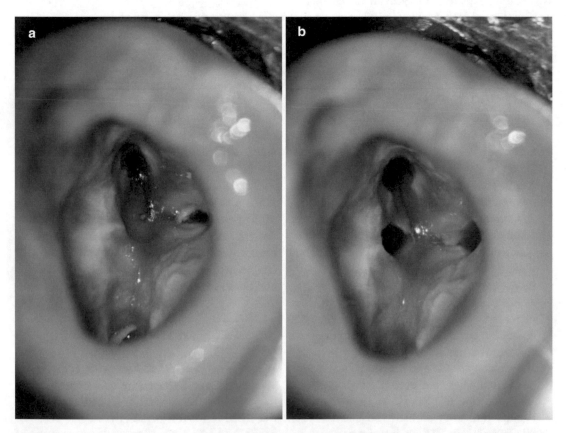

Fig. 3.5 (**a**) Typical traditional extended access cavity design in a maxillary first molar before the negotiation of the MB2 canal and (**b**) after finding and shaping the MB2 canal

The **Conservative Endodontic Cavity (CEC)** "aims to perform a partial unroofing of the pulp chamber with preservation of the pulp horns, with slightly convergent walls occlusally beveled, to visualize the pulp chamber floor and all the root canal orifices from different visual angulations" [25], following the principles given by Clark and Khademi [26]. It means that clinicians can visualize the chamber space and the floor even if not by the same angulation, but also tilting the mirror (Fig. 3.6).

The **Ultra-Conservative Endodontic Cavity or Ninja Endodontic Cavity (NEC)** "aims to perform an ultra-conservative cavity just locating the orifices, with an extreme unroofing of the pulp chamber and preservation of all the pulp horns, extremely convergent walls and preservation of the occlusal enamel" [25] (Fig. 3.7).

The **Orifice-Directed Endodontic Cavity or TRuss Endodontic Cavity (TREC)** is "an orifice-directed access, in which separate cavities are prepared to negotiate the different roots of molars avoiding removal of the central part of the pulp chamber's roof" [27] (Fig. 3.8).

The **Opportunistic Endodontic Cavity or Caries-Driven Endodontic Cavity (CDEC)** is "a strategic interproximal (Fig. 3.9) or buccal (Fig. 3.10) access aiming to remove all the carious tissue and the entire old fillings, taking advantage of the loss of tooth structure to enter the root canal system from the pre-existing cavity without enlarging it with a predefined shape."

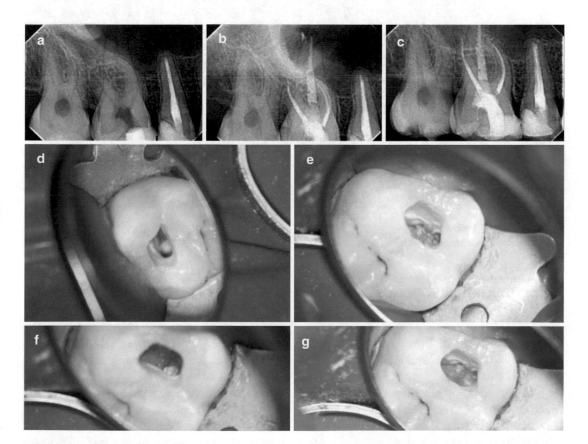

Fig. 3.6 (**a**) Preoperative periapical radiograph of a maxillary molar with previously initiated root canal treatment; (**b**, **c**) postoperative radiographs with different angulations after completed the root canal treatment through a conservative access cavity; clinical view of palatal canal (**d**), mesio-buccal canals (**e**), and disto-buccal canal (**f**) through the conservative access cavity; (**g**) lower magnification of the conservative access cavity for the estimation of the coronal tooth structure removal

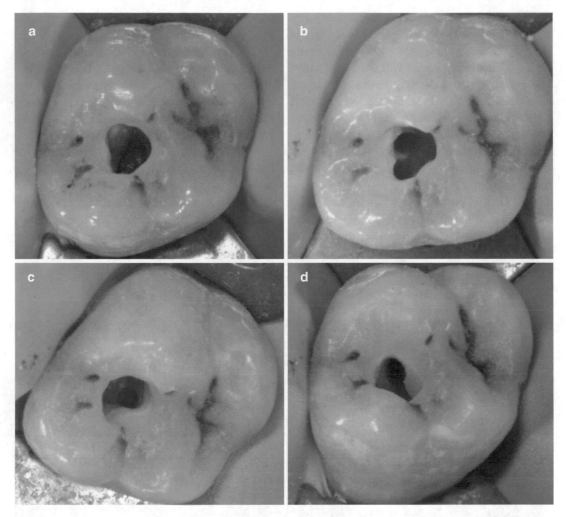

Fig. 3.7 (**a**) Preoperative occlusal image of an ultra-conservative "ninja" access cavity; clinical view of the MB1 and MB2 (**b**), DB (**c**) and P (**d**) canals after instrumentation through the ultra-conservative access cavity

3.8 Conservative Access Cavity Equipment

The review article of Bóveda and Kishen [4] describes the contracted endodontic cavities and the foundation for less invasive alternatives in the management of apical periodontitis. The specific equipment needed to apply the conservative access cavity concepts in the clinical practice include specially designed and miniaturized burs, thin and double curved endodontic explorers, reflective miniaturized mirrors, endodontic file holders, magnification and coaxial illumination equipment, ultrasonic tips, and diagnostic tools.

3.8.1 Burs

The main instrument available to penetrate the pulp chamber of all the teeth is a diamond, slightly tapered, round ended, gross grain (blue, green or black) bur.

This bur can be conical or even cylindrical.

There are different sizes available depending on the size of the tooth. Usually, a size #10–12 bur can be used to access smaller teeth, like lower incisors, upper lateral incisor, lower canine, or calcified pulp chambers, and the size #12 and #14 ones to access bigger teeth, like molars, bicuspids, upper central incisors, or "young teeth" with large pulp chambers.

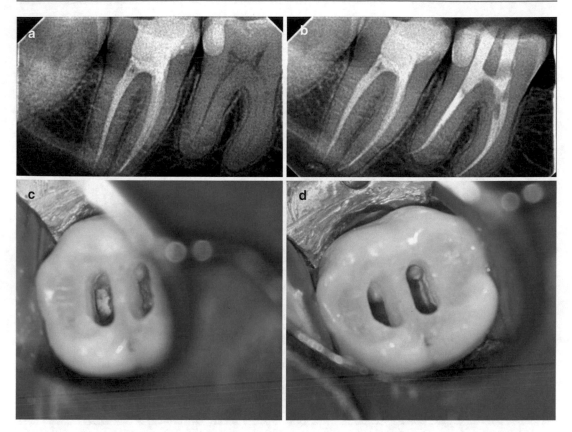

Fig. 3.8 (**a**) Preoperative periapical radiograph of the first mandibular molar diagnosed with acute pulpitis; (**b**) postoperative periapical radiograph after the completion of root canal treatment through an orifice directed or truss access cavity; (**c**) clinical view of distal (**c**) and mesio-buccal (**d**) canal through the orifice-directed-truss access cavity

The round characteristic end of this bur creates smoother cavities and it lasts more in time, because of less consumption. Flat-end bur may create more steps. High-speed ball bur is effective, but it does not have a great directional control and cuts indiscriminately even laterally. It can also create undercuts and a ball-shaped access cavity with unnecessary removal of pericervical dentin; in non-expert hands it can lead to iatrogenic damages. The only recommended ball bur is a multiblade carbide stainless-steel bur for low-speed handpiece, in #12 or #14 size, ideally with long neck for a better visibility: it can be used after the diamond-coded bur as above, only for caries and pulp removal and to access the orifices. The low-speed ball multiblade bur must not be used touching the axial walls nor to remove undercuts, in order to avoid a round-shaped access cavity and the removal of pericervical dentin. As already mentioned, a conservative access does not require the removal of every undercut, because the canal should be just entered following its projection on the occlusal surface and not straight on the occlusal surface. A possible solution is to bevel occlusal enamel and this is a paradigm shift in changing the access cavity.

There are some carbide multiblade burs with non-cutting tips, like Batt's bur type, that can be useful in refining access cavities. These burs were designed to remove all the pulp horns and interferences, so they tend to create traditional, excessively tapered cavities and increase the

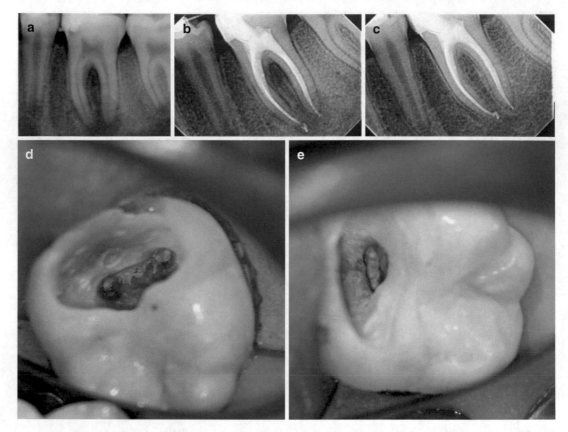

Fig. 3.9 (**a**) Preoperative radiograph of a first mandibular molar diagnosed with acute pulpitis; (**b**) postoperative periapical radiograph after the completion of root canal treatment through an opportunistic or caries-driven mesial access cavity; (**c**) 1-year follow-up periapical radiograph after the completion of root canal treatment; clinical view of mesial canals (**d**) and distal canal (**e**) through the opportunistic access cavity

possibility of over-enlarging cavities. Furthermore, they can create extra-smooth surfaces on the axial walls, but the roughness of axial walls is not as important as the preservation on sound structure.

For a deeper search of root canals through the pulp chamber floor, smaller and longer burs may be suggested, such as the conical diamond-coded Clark's EG3 micro-access bur and the round-end low-speed Munce discovery burs. These burs may be helpful to clean pulp horns, open the orifices area, and in all the situations in which dentin should be saved, because they increase visibility, permit a directional control, and reduce the risk to indiscriminately remove the axial dentin. The small Munce discovery burs are used to reach deep areas under the orifices and isthmuses and

they are useful in difficult cases when it is needed to discover canals deep inside the root.

Gates-Glidden (GG) burs have been introduced to be used inside the root canals, but they are too demolitive for the pericervical dentin down the orifice. In a minimal invasive approach, GG burs should be only used inside the pulp chamber but outside the root canal, with lateral brushing movements to selectively remove some coronal interference and refine the dentin up to the orifice, on the axial walls or in the pulp horns. Usually, a GG n°3 (0.90 mm) or n°4 (1.10 mm) may be used for this purpose.

Football-end small grain (yellow or red) burs may be used to create the enamel/dentinal occlusal bevel to avoid interferences in the coronal part of the instruments.

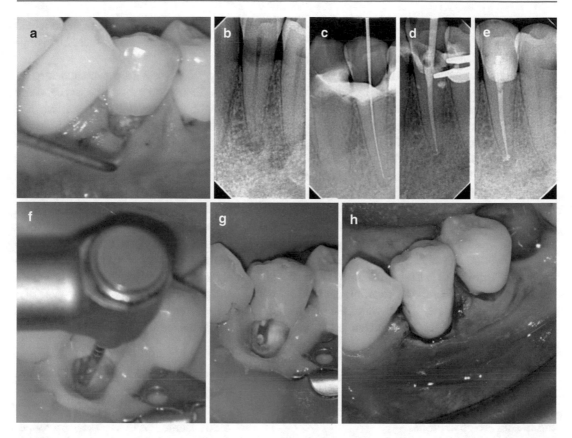

Fig. 3.10 Preoperative clinical view (**a**) and periapical radiograph (**b**) of a buccal carious lesion in the first mandibular premolar; working length determination (**c**), cone-fit (**d**), and postoperative (**e**) radiograph of the root canal treatment through the buccal opportunistic access; (**f**) clinical view of rotary file negotiation through the buccal opportunistic caries-driven access cavity; (**g**) clinical view after the completion of root canal treatment (**g**) and post-endodontic restoration (**h**) through the opportunistic buccal access cavity

About the handpieces, the low-speed 1:1 contra-angle is necessary for round multiblade burs or Gate Glidden burs, while the high-speed 1:5 contra-angle can be helpful for high-speed burs, but at a lower speed than turbine. High-speed contra-angle is not mandatory rather than turbine, but it is suggested to reduce the risk to remove too much dentine.

image and refraction. A black contour usually indicates rhodium surface.

Magnifying mirrors are not suggested, because they increase distortion. If magnification is needed, it is better to use loupes or microscopes. The key is magnification, illumination, and reflection through a high-quality clean mirror.

3.8.3 Endodontic Explorers

Endodontic explorers are useful in the location and determination of direction of the root canals. In everyday clinical practice standard straight explorers are enough effective, but there are also specialized endodontic explorers (DG-16 and JW-17) that can be useful.

3.8.2 Mirrors

The best mirror possible is needed to increase visibility. Rhodium surface mirrors give the best visibility and light transmission, especially through small access cavities and avoid double

3.8.4 Handle Files

These files are attached to a handle. Clinicians can easily use them like probes to go inside the orifices. There are different types, sizes, and tapers. Some examples of these instruments are the MC K-files and H-files (VDW, Munich, Germany), in the sizes 0.08, 0.10, and 0.15, taper 0.04, the Micro-Openers K-files, in the sizes 0.10 and 0.15/taper 0.04 and 0.10/taper 0.06 (Maillefer, Baillagues, Switzerland) and the Micro-Debriders H-files (Maillefer, Baillagues, Switzerland), in the sizes 20 and 30, taper 0.02. They may act like probes, because they are tapered and so resistant to axial pressure and can be used to clean the root canal walls going in lateral brushing motion if there are some pulp or filling material remnants.

They are particularly useful under the microscope, because they let the clinician not to use fingers to handle the files, thus increasing visibility during the procedures.

Existing alternative solutions are also to have a handle where to mount the hand files and that support any kind and size of endodontic files, acting like an effective probe.

3.8.5 Microscopes and Loupes

Magnifications are helpful to be more conservative. In authors' opinion, at least loupes are mandatory, in particular 4.5× to 5× magnification loupes may help to solve nearly 80% of all endodontic case, but there are some specific cases that can be solved only with microscope.

Prismatic magnification loupes, with different kind of support on glasses or head-set, are the ideal initial solution for regular cases. Galilean loupes have usually a lower magnification and a different transmission of the light.

It is important to select the appropriate loupes for personal working distance. If young practitioners want to start from lower magnifications to have a contact with the magnification field, 3.5× magnification Galilean loupes can act as a starting point, to pass then to 4.5–6× magnification prismatic loupes that are more indicated for endodontic cases.

LED lights are also available to be mounted on loupes. They are important to increase visibility of loupes.

Normally, access cavity preparation step of the endodontic treatment may be successfully performed with loups and lights even when a conservative approach is attempted. In these cases, the microscope may be mainly useful in the control phase of what clinicians are doing or in particularly difficult cases. When, instead, clinicians have to perform procedures deep inside the root, such as to search for calcified root canals, attempt the removal of fractured fragments or remove fiber posts or even just try to locate difficult root canal orifices, it is difficult to do it safely and effectively with the use of loupes with LED lights only. In these cases the use of a microscope with coaxial light is mandatory to see so deep inside the tooth.

3.8.6 Ultrasonic Devices and Ultrasonic Tips

The use of ultrasonic tips in access cavity refinement and orifice location permit to be less aggressive and more conservative than when using high- or low-speed handpieces, because of better control and greater visibility. Ultrasonic tips help to remove calcifications of the pulp chamber without touching the walls or the pulp chamber floor. Furthermore, when ultrasonic tips are associated to microscope to locate root canal orifices, the accessory anatomy may be discovered more easily [28].

Diamond-coated or the less aggressive non-diamond-coated tips should be mainly used on the pulp chamber floor to search root canals or to refine the orifices. Their use should be limited to dentin when refining the access cavity walls, to avoid contact with the enamel that may crack under the vibration produced [29].

The endo-chuck is a device with different angulation (90° and 120°) in which some tips or files can be mounted to search for root canals or to go through isthmuses. There are some chucks, in which burs may be also mounted on to clean pulp horns and remove pulp remnants from the access cavity. For this purpose, there are also microsurgical bendable tips that may be adapted to clean pulp horns and undercuts.

3.8.7 CBCT

Despite this 3D diagnostic tool is regularly used in retreatment cases and endodontic surgery, because it is helpful to study if there are missed anatomy, problems inside the root canals, like ledges, perforations and fractured files or the relationship between teeth and the surrounding anatomical structures, standard primary treatments may be usually completed without CBCT, unless the clinician finds difficulties to understand root canal anatomy in three dimensions and the relationship between teeth and lesions or to study the anatomy of completely calcified root canals. These are the cases in which a 3D planning of the access cavity based on the CBCT scan may be more useful. In fact, in case of completely calcified canals, it is possible to design silicon-metal guides for special burs, like those used in implantology, following the indications of the CBCT. Microguided endodontics provides an accurate technique for the preparation of access cavities and is therefore of high clinical relevance [24, 30–32].

Intraoperatory 3D navigation is also an innovative experimental method to perform endodontic access. This idea is borrowed from the implant-guided surgery, so that in endodontics the operator can see the progression of the bur inside the tooth crown and roots directly in a screen in real time on the CBCT images. So, the "CBCT-based cavity access" may represent the future.

In any case, treatment planning of the access cavity and of all the treatment may be also done in standard cases by dedicated 3D software with the rendering of the 3D CBCT exam, to perform a tridimensional examination of the tooth anatomy.

3.8.8 Time

The most important "special equipment" the clinicians need to perform a conservative access cavity and endodontic treatment in general, aim-

ing to preserve as much sound tooth structure as possible is the time. In fact, the canal preparation time was significantly increased when working through a conservative access design rather than traditional cavities [33].

3.9 Conservative Access Cavity Drawbacks

Although conservative access cavities have the potential of preserving tooth structure that might result in better long-term prognosis, some concerns may be raised.

Conservative access cavities might:

- Jeopardize disinfection of the pulp chamber [34].
- Increase the risk of missed canals [28].
- Increase the untouched canal walls [35].
- Increase the stress on the mechanical files [36].
- Compromise irrigant penetration, needle wedging, vapor lock, dampening of ultrasonic energy [4].
- Complicate root canal obturation and coronal restoration (existence of under cuts that make the utilization of some techniques and materials difficult).
- Increase the time span of the treatment to unacceptable level [33].

The benefits and the possible drawbacks of conservative access cavities have become the topic of extensive research effort in order to formulate the best available evidence for the clinical endodontic practice.

3.10 Research Evaluation of Conservative Access Cavities

New research focuses on the comparison between different access modalities as they were defined earlier. In the first study recently published on this topic [35], the fracture resistance of unrestored molars and premolars with CEC was about 2.5-fold and 1.8-fold more, respectively, than in matched teeth with TEC but comparable for incisors with both cavity designs. The fact that in this study teeth were unrestored reduced its clinical relevance, so Moore et al. [37] repeated the study on restored maxillary molars and reported that the fracture strength with CECs and TECs was comparable and consistently lower than that of intact molars. Thus, CECs in restored maxillary molars did not positively impact fracture strength, suggesting no apparent benefit in this regard. Considering that maxillary molars present with particularly challenging root canal systems in mesio-buccal roots, where secondary canals are difficult to locate and negotiate, the application of CECs in these teeth merits careful consideration. Similar to the previous findings, Corsentino et al. [27] reported that the endodontic access cavity design and the loss of one or two walls reduce the fracture strength of intact teeth. The access cavity designs tested (CEC, TREC) did not influence the fracture strength of treated teeth that was reduced by the loss of two marginal walls. Similarly, CEC preparation did not increase the fracture strength of teeth with class II cavities compared with TEC preparation in a study by Ozyurek et al. [38]. In the same line with the above findings the results of Rover et al. [28] did not show any benefits associated with CECs. They noted that this access modality in maxillary molars resulted in less root canal detection when no ultrasonic troughing associated to an OM was used and did not increase fracture resistance.

Sabeti et al. [39] reported that increasing the taper of the root canal preparation to 0.08 can reduce the fracture resistance of teeth. Although they reported that access cavity preparation can reduce the resistance, CEC in comparison with TEC had no significant impact. In addition, instrumentation time in teeth with CECs was found to be 2.5-fold longer than in teeth with non-extended TECs, reflecting the typical challenges associated with constricted access [33].

Although most of the initial in vitro studies suggested minimal effect of access cavity dimensions in the fracture strength of human teeth, other studies reported conflicting results. The most important variation in the published studies is that there is no consensus how to define the different type of access cavities and in some studies what is defined TEC instead correspond more to

a CEC and what is defined CEC correspond more to a NEC. For this reason several studies that found no differences have instead compared CEC to NEC instead of the declared TEC and CEC. The article which more clarify this aspect and better classify the different access cavity is the study by Plotino et al. [25], in which teeth with TEC access showed lower fracture strength than the ones prepared with CEC or NEC. Ultraconservative "ninja" endodontic cavity access did not increase the fracture strength of teeth compared with the ones prepared with CEC. Following this study, the same authors are trying to standardize the dimensions of the different type of access cavities for a research point of view [40]. The authors showed a significantly different percentage of volume of dentin and enamel removed in molars and premolars measured by CBCT among the groups analyzed, being teeth with NEC < CEC < TEC and a new classification of access cavity preparation has been proposed according to percentage of volume of dentin and enamel removed: NEC less than 6%, CEC up to 15%, and TEC more than 15%.

In Fig. 3.11 the superimposition of these three different types of access cavity is visualized in a simulation that clearly underlines the differences from an occlusal and a lateral point of view.

Unfortunately no randomized controlled trials exist at the moment to support or reject the effect that minimal invasive access cavity concept exert on the longevity of the teeth. Up to now the best available evidence indicates that the difference is very small to be relevant.

3.11 The "Less Is More" Concept in Endodontics

Although clear benefits of conservative access cavities are yet to be supported by randomized clinical trials, clinicians tend to embrace the concept of *less is more* when it comes to tissue removal during access cavity preparation. Through the long history of endodontology the vision was always the lifetime retention of the natural dentition. However, lifetime is not always the same because the life expectancy of humans at birth is not a stable parameter. The estimate of the average number

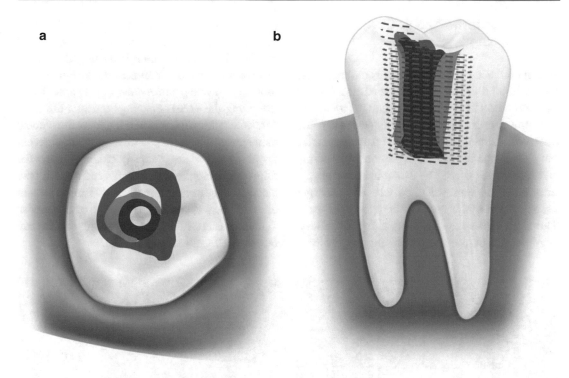

Fig. 3.11 Superimposition of TEC (purple), CEC (green), and NEC (red) access cavity in a three-dimensional simulation that clearly underline the differences from an occlusal (**a**) and a lateral (**b**) visualization

of years a newborn infant would live if prevailing patterns of mortality at the time of birth were to stay the same throughout its life increased dramatically through the years, from 20 years of age in 1548 to nearly 85 years in some countries in 2015 (https://ourworldindata.org) [41]. Aging population results in huge challenges for the lifetime retention of the natural dentition. Dentin is subjected to physiological and pathological changes that can affect the lifetime teeth retention. Physiological changes of dentin are age related and result in increased mineralization, increased dentinal hardness, peritubular occlusion, 40% lower fatigue crack growth, 48% lower endurance strength, over 100 times faster fatigue crack propagation, reduction of flexure strength by 20 Mpa/decade, increased collagen cross-link, and loss of matrix-degrading enzymes [42]. The caries associated pathological changes of dentin include the lowering of its mineral content, the increase in dentin porosity, the altering of collagen structure and distribution, the altering of non-collagenous proteins, the increase in wetness, the reduction of dentin hardness, stiffness and tensile strength, the

reduction in the modulus of elasticity, the reduction in fatigue strength, the drying shrinkage, and the increase in fatigue crack growth [42].

Taken all these changes together it becomes evident that the less tissue is removed during operative dental procedures and endodontics, the more the chances of avoiding catastrophic tooth fractures might be. Especially in endodontics, tissue removal in combination with the age- and caries-related changes in dentin composition and structure that cannot be avoided may have deleterious consequences. It is suggested that such catastrophic tooth fractures might be avoided if the endodontic and restorative procedures are performed not only to repair and limit the damage from caries but also to protect and preserve the tooth structure. Under this context minimizing tissue removal during access cavity preparation seems logical as far as the objectives of root canal treatment are not jeopardized. This means that clinicians need to adapt their skills and equipment to work more effectively through confined spaces. Under this framework the introduction of the concept of a customized dynamic access cavity design seems extremely relevant.

3.12 Dynamic Access Cavity Design

A dynamic access cavity design is different from the traditional predesigned shapes dictated by the most common anatomical variations of root canal anatomy. A dynamic access cavity design can take different forms according to the pathology, anatomy assessment and the evolution in materials and techniques used. The dynamic access always prioritizes the removal of carious and damaged tissues ahead of the negotiation to the pulp space. The pulp space negotiation that follows always starts from a pinpoint exposure and progressively

is enlarged to facilitate the removal of all irreversibly inflamed pulp tissue or the removal of all necrotic tissues. Difficulties in the negotiation and disinfection of the anatomical extensions of the root canal system are managed by strategically extending the access openings towards the most convenient direction that will facilitate the clinical management. The shapes of the dynamic access openings will be continuously modified under the future technological developments that will take place in diagnosis, prevention, and management of apical periodontitis. An example of a stepwise dynamic access cavity in a mandibular molar can be seen in Figs. 3.12 and Fig. 3.13.

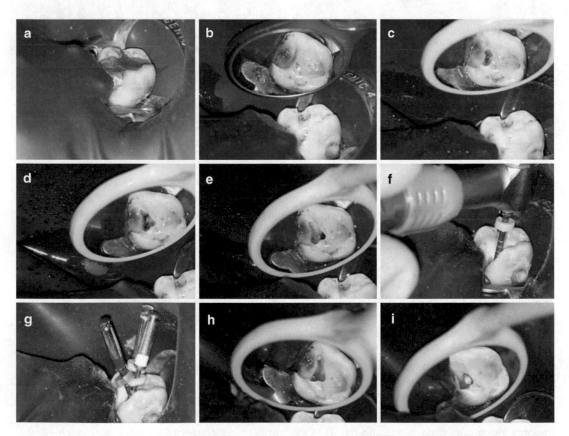

Fig. 3.12 (a) Preoperative clinical view of a second mandibular molar diagnosed with acute pulpitis; (b) stepwise removal of amalgam filling prior to dentine removal; (c) caries removal and initial access to the pulp chamber; (d) dynamic stepwise enlargement of the access to negotiate the mesial root canal system; (e) dynamic strategically extended access cavity to negotiate the distal root canal (to note the distal groove); (f) unobstructed negotiation of the engine-driven file in the mesio-buccal canal; (g) unobstructed negotiation in all three canals; postoperative clinical view of the mesial root canals (h) and the distal canal (i)

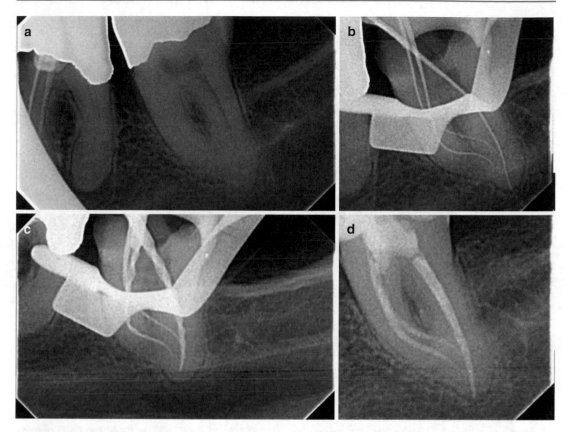

Fig. 3.13 (a) Preoperative periapical radiograph of a second mandibular molar suffering acute pulpitis; (b) working length determination radiograph after performing a dynamic access to the root canal system; (c) unobstructed negotiation of the rotary files after strategically extension of the access cavity; (d) postoperative radiograph

3.13 The Future Concept of Biological Repair of Access Cavities

Recently, the concept of the biological repair of the access openings after regenerative endodontic procedures was introduced [43]. The removal of tooth tissue, despite its subsequent restoration with dental materials, weakens the tooth by changing the stress intensity and distribution through tooth structures [44]. Moreover, the replacement of missing tissue with artificial means cannot possibly compete with the biological replacement of the missing tissue with natural dental structures. Regenerative endodontics has the potential to induce not only continuous root development and dentin wall thickening but also the biological repair of access openings in close continuity with the axial walls and resistant to displacement forces [43]. This biological repair might account for true fortification of endodontically treated teeth (Fig. 3.14). This area of research should continue to have a high priority for support because of this potential. The modulation of this potential and the development of clinical protocols that can result in this biological repair might eliminate the need to create durable interfaces between the artificial materials and natural dentin, which remains a challenge. However, until such a time comes when these techniques will become predictable and mainstream, there will be interest in alternative methods of root fortification [45].

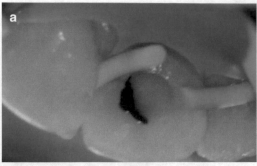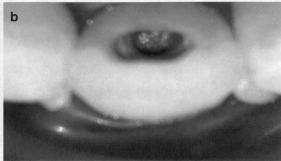

Fig. 3.14 (a) Palatal access in a necrotic draining maxillary central incisor; (b) hard tissue biological repair of the access cavity in a cervical level 10 years after the application of regenerative endodontic procedures (published with permission from [43])

References

1. Ordinola-Zapata R, Versiani MA, Bramante CM. Root canal components. In: Versiani MA, Basrani B, Sousa-Neto MD, editors. The root canal anatomy of permanent dentition. 1st ed. Cham: Springer; 2019.
2. Ingle J. Endodontic cavity preparation. In: Ingle J, Bakland LK, editors. Endodontics. 5th ed. Philadelphia: BC Decker; 2002.
3. Krasner P, Rankow HJ. Anatomy of the pulp chamber floor. J Endod. 2004;30:5–16.
4. Boveda C, Kishen A. Contracted endodontic cavities: the foundation for less invasive alternatives in the management of apical periodontitis. Endod Topics. 2015;33:169–86.
5. Pruett JP, Clement DJ, Carnes DL Jr. Cyclic fatigue testing of nickel-titanium endodontic instruments. J Endod. 1997;23:77–85.
6. Schneider SW. A comparison of canal preparations in straight and curved root canals. Oral Surg Oral Med Oral Pathol. 1971;32:271–5.
7. Günday M, Sazak H, Garip Y. A comparative study of three different root canal curvature measurement techniques and measuring the canal access angle in curved canals. J Endod. 2005;31:796–8.
8. Schäfer E, Diez C, Hoppe W, Tepel J. Roentgenographic investigation of frequency and degree of canal curvatures in human permanent teeth. J Endod. 2002;28:211–6.
9. Lopes H, Vieira MVB, Elias C, Goncales L, Siqueira JF, Moreira EJL, Vieira VTL, Souza LC. Influence of the geometry of curved artificial canals on the fracture of rotary nickel-titanium instruments subjected to cyclic fatigue tests. J Endod. 2013;5:704–7.
10. Ericson D. What is minimally invasive dentistry? Oral Health Prev Dent. 2004;2(Suppl 1):287–92.
11. Tsimpoulas NE, Alisafis MG, Tzanetakis GN, Kontakiotis EG. A prospective study of the extraction and retention incidence of endodontically treated teeth with uncertain prognosis after endodontic referral. J Endod. 2012;38:1326–9.
12. Rocca T, Krejci I. Crown and post-free adhesive restorations for endodontically treated posterior teeth: from direct composite to endocrowns. Eur J Esthet Dent. 2013;8:156–79.
13. Dietschi D, Duc O, Krejci I, Sadan A. Biomechanical considerations for the restoration of endodontically treated teeth: a systematic review of the literature, part I. Composition and micro- and macrostructure alterations. Quint Int. 2007;38:733–43.
14. Reeh E, Messer H, Douglas W. Reduction in tooth stiffness as a result of endodontic and restorative procedures. J Endod. 1989;15:512–5.
15. Lang H, Korkmaz Y, Schneider K, Raab WH. Impact of endodontic treatments on the rigidity of the root. J Dent Res. 2016;85:364–8.
16. Panitvisai P, Messer H. Cuspal deflection in molars in relation to endodontic and restorative procedures. J Endod. 1995;21:57–61.
17. Dietschi D, Duc O, Krejci SA. Biomechanical considerations for the restoration of endodontically treated teeth: a systematic review of the literature, Part II (Evaluation of fatigue behavior, interfaces, and in vivo studies). Quint Int. 2008;39:117–29.
18. Tang W, Wu Y, Smales RJ. Identifying and reducing the risks for potential fractures in endodontically treated teeth. J Endod. 2010;36:609–17.
19. Rampado ME, Tjäderhane L, Friedman S, Hamstra SJ. The benefit of the operating microscope for access cavity preparation by undergraduate students. J Endod. 2004;30:863–7.
20. Sousa TO, Haiter-Neto F, Nascimento EHL, Peroni LV, Freitas DQ, Hassan B. Diagnostic accuracy of periapical radiography and cone-beam computed tomography in identifying root canal configuration of human premolars. J Endod. 2017;43:1176–9.
21. Shen Y, Zhou HM, Zheng YF, Peng B, Haapasalo M. Current challenges and concepts of the thermomechanical treatment of nickel-titanium instruments. J Endod. 2013;39:163–72.

22. Chan R, Versiani MA, Friedman S, Malkhassian G, Sousa-Neto MD, Leoni GB, Silva-Sousa YTC, Basrani B. Efficacy of 3 supplementary irrigation protocols in the removal of hard tissue debris from the mesial root canal system of mandibular molars. J Endod. 2019;45:923–9.

23. Chaniotis A, Zervaki A. Minimally invasive microsurgical management of the necrotic immature apex tooth: case report and treatment recommendations. Quint Int. 2013;44:429–36.

24. Connert T, Zehnder MS, Amato M, Weiger R, Kuhl S, Krastl G. Microguided endodontics: a method to achieve minimally invasive access cavity preparation and root canal location in mandibular incisors using a novel computer-guided technique. Int Endod J. 2018;51:247–55.

25. Plotino G, Grande NM, Isufi A, Ioppolo P, Pedullà E, Bedini R, Gambarini G, Testarelli L. Fracture strength of endodontically treated teeth with different access cavity designs. J Endod. 2017;43:995–1000.

26. Clark D, Khademi J. Modern molar endodontic access and directed dentin conservation. Dent Clin N Am. 2010;54:249–73.

27. Corsentino G, Pedulla E, Casteli L, Liguori M, Spicciarelli V, Martignoni M, Ferrari M, Grandini S. Influence of access cavity preparation and remaining tooth substance on fracture strength of endodontically treated teeth. J Endod. 2018;44:1416–21.

28. Rover G, Belladonna FG, Bortoluzzi EA, De-Deus G, Silva EJNL, Teixeira CS. Influence of access cavity design on root canal detection, instrumentation efficacy and fracture resistance assessed in maxillary molars. J Endod. 2017;43:1657–62.

29. Zoghein C, Roumi R, Bourbouze G, Plotino G. The formation of coronal enamel and dentinal defects after access cavity preparation and refinement. Submitted for publication 2020.

30. Krastl G, Zehnder MS, Connert T, Weiger R, Kuhl S. Guided endodontics: a novel treatment approach for teeth with pulp canal calcification and apical pathology. Dent Traumatol. 2016;32:240–6.

31. Zehnder MS, Connert T, Weiger R, Krastl G, Kuhl S. Guided endodontics: accuracy of a novel method for guided access cavity preparation and root canal location. Int Endod J. 2016;49:966–72.

32. Buchgreitz J, Buchgreitz M, Mortensen D, Bjorrndal L. Guided access cavity preparation using cone-beam computed tomography and optical surface scans—an ex vivo study. Int Endod J. 2016;49:790–5.

33. Marchesan MA, Lloyd A, Clement DJ, McFarland JD, Friedman S. Impacts of contracted endodontic cavities on primary root canal curvature parameters in mandibular molars. J Endod. 2018;44:1558–62.

34. Neelakantan P, Khan K, Hei Ng GP, Yip CY, Zhang C, Pan Cheung GS. Does the orifice-directed dentin conservation access design debride pulp chamber and mesial root canal systems of mandibular molars similar to a traditional access design? J Endod. 2018;44:274–9.

35. Krishan R, Paque F, Ossareh A, Kishen A, Dao T, Friedman S. Impacts of conservative endodontic cavity on root canal instrumentation efficacy and resistance to fracture assessed in incisors, premolars, and molars. J Endod. 2014;40:1160–6.

36. Alovisi M, Pasqualini D, Musso E, Bobbio E, Giuliano C, Mancino D, Scotti N, Berutti E. Influence of contracted endodontic access on root canal geometry: an in vitro study. J Endod. 2018;44:614–20.

37. Moore B, Verdelis K, Kishen A, Dao T, Friedman S. Impacts of contracted endodontic cavities on instrumentation efficacy and biomechanical responses in maxillary molars. J Endod. 2016;42:1779–83.

38. Ozyurek T, Ulker O, Demiryerek EQ, Yilmaz F. Preparation design on the fracture strength of endodontically treated teeth: traditional versus conservative preparation. J Endod. 2018;44:800–5.

39. Sabetti M, Kazem M, Dianat O, Bahrololumi N, Beglou A, Rahimipour K, Dehnavi F. Impact of access cavity design and root canal taper on fracture resistance of endodontically treated teeth: an ex vivo investigation. J Endod. 2018;44:1402–6.

40. Isufi A, Plotino G, Grande NM, Testarelli L, Gambarini G. A new classification of endodontic access cavities based on 3D quantitative analysis of dentine and enamel removed. Submitted for publication 2020.

41. https://ourworldindata.org.

42. Tjaderhane L. Dentine basic structure composition and function. In: Root canal anatomy of permanent dentition. 1st ed. Cham: Springer; 2019.

43. Chaniotis A, Petridis X. Cervical level biological repair of the access opening after regenerative endodontic procedures: three cases with the same repair pattern. J Endod. 2019;45:1219–27.

44. Zelic K, Vukicevic A, Jovicic G, Aleksandrovic S, Filipovic N, Djuric M. Mechanical weakening of devitalized teeth: three-dimensional Finite Element Analysis and prediction of tooth fracture. Int Endod J. 2015;48:850–63.

45. Seghi RR, Nasrin S, Draney J, Katsube N. Root fortification. Pediatr Dent. 2013;35:153–9.

Minimally Invasive Root Canal Instrumentation

4

Gustavo De-Deus, Emmanuel J. N. L. Silva,
Jorge N. R. Martins, Daniele Cavalcante,
Felipe G. Belladonna, and Gianluca Plotino

Contents

G. De-Deus (✉) · D. Cavalcante · F. G. Belladonna
Endodontics, Fluminense Federal University,
Niterói, RJ, Brazil

E. J. N. L. Silva
Endodontics, Fluminense Federal University,
Niterói, RJ, Brazil

Endodontics, Rio de Janeiro State University,
Rio de Janeiro, RJ, Brazil

Endodontics, Grande Rio University,
Rio de Janeiro, RJ, Brazil

J. N. R. Martins
Endodontics, Faculdade de Medicina Dentária da
Universidade de Lisboa, Lisbon, Portugal

G. Plotino
Private Practice, Grande, Plotino & Torsello – Studio
di Odontoiatria,
Rome, Italy

4.1 Minimally Invasive Shaping: A Matter of Size

Vertical root fractures (VRFs) are defined as longitudinal fractures that follow the vertical axis of the root [1]. VRFs can occur in both endodontically and non-endodontically treated teeth; however, the root canal treatment has been associated with the incidence of this phenomenon since 1931 [2]. Even after almost a century, it is still a clinical complication of utmost importance, as it often leads to tooth extraction [3]. The current understanding points out a multifactorial basis for the causes of fractures in endodontically treated teeth [1]. Unfavourable occlusal load,

© Springer Nature Switzerland AG 2021
G. Plotino (ed.), *Minimally Invasive Approaches in Endodontic Practice*,
https://doi.org/10.1007/978-3-030-45866-9_4

steep cuspal incline, deep fissures on the crown, overflared canals and supraosseous post and dowel placement have been traditionally related to VRFs [1]. In a broader sense, these factors can be considered as iatrogenic and non-iatrogenic causes, but the weakening of the teeth by dentin mass loss is supported by logical reasoning and by the weak scientific evidence that is currently available. The logical reasoning on this topic is plain and says that overall dentin mass loss, mitigates the ability of the tooth to resist intermittent masticatory forces in the long term. There is laboratory evidence showing a direct correlation between the amount of dentin removed and root strength [4–6]. Disease processes or clinical procedures that lead to dentinal loss or eccentric canal shaping result in more stress in the apical direction and in the bucco-lingual plane of the root, which may impact the overall resistance to root flexure. Rundquist and Versluis [7] called attention to the influence of the taper on the root stress during masticatory loading. They concluded that, in a tooth under compressive force, the maximum stress resulting from bending is predominantly observed at the cervical aspect of the root (cervical dentin), which may be related to coronal pre-flaring procedures. While it is undeniable that unnecessary loss of dentin tissue should be avoided, other factors such as root canal geometry and volume also impact on the resistance to fracture [8]. Therefore, it is understandable why the resistance of the root to flexion depends upon the distribution of dentin tissue around the canal wall.

Despite the passionate way that some defend that conventional canal mechanical instrumentation decreases the resistance of teeth to fracture, the current literature is composed by a limited amount of laboratory studies [9, 10], which means low-quality evidence to shape and guide the clinical decision-making process. Therefore, the idea of providing optimum dimensions for root canal mechanical preparation is one current ongoing concern in endodontic practice and science.

The degree of mechanical shaping is determined by the pre-operative dimensions of the root canal, the obturation technique, and the restorative treatment plan. However, the greatest focus today is being able to clean the root canal space while preserving maximum strength of the tooth. Within this framework, one may argue that current mechanical preparations should keep the canal dimensions as small as possible, since instrumentation per se is ineffective in cleaning and disinfecting the inner dentinal walls in irregular and hard-to-reach areas, such as fins and isthmuses of oval-shaped canals [11–16]. On the other hand, mechanical preparation needs to suffice for creating an operational pathway to irrigate the root canal space. For that, a minimal but optimal size/taper is necessary to be set, which was not currently supported by reliable documented formal evidence.

Considering the as yet unclear situation of the minimal invasive approaches and rationales proposed to render an endodontically treated tooth predictably functional, the present text focuses on the optimal size/taper relationship necessary to avoid unnecessary overflared canals and, at the same time, to allow the turbulence and solution exchange indispensable for the minimal cleaning and disinfection conditions to assure healing. The big picture is to address and discuss the close-to-optimum operative conditions to maximize tooth strength and longevity. Moreover, advances and developments in nickel-titanium (NiTi) technology have allowed endodontics to move towards the minimally invasive dentistry paradigm.

4.2 Limitations of the Current Technology for Mechanical Shaping

The ongoing debate around the so-called minimally invasive canal shaping is indeed a matter of physical size, and it can be summarized into a single question: What's the optimal minimal canal size preparation?

The problem emerges with the limitations of current technology for canal shaping. Ideally, adequate mechanical instrumentation should uniformly plane the entire perimeter of the root canal—a kind of scrubbing action on the canal walls—thus completely removing the inner layers of heavily contaminated dentinal tissue. This, in turn, will ensure an effective removal of as much of the remaining soft tissue and bacterial biofilm as possible, which may predispose to cause or perpetuate disease, influencing the outcome of treatment [17–19]. However, current rotary and reciprocating NiTi systems are only able to prepare the main root canal space into a circular final shape, because the instrument cannot adapt to the irregular cross-section area of the canal; thus, they leave most buccal and lingual extensions unprepared [11–16, 20]. It is of note that this phenomenon cannot be observed in two-dimensional clinical periapical radiographs, which represent only the bucco-lingual projection. On the other hand, it can be easily observed in histological cross-sections and in the results from high-definition microtomography (micro-CT) studies [11–16, 20], which have underlined the suboptimal standard of mechanical preparation by the current NiTi systems. Using non-destructive micro-CT technology, it has been systematically shown that the amount of mechanically prepared root canal surface is frequently below 60% [11–16, 20–22].

In short, available NiTi systems leave a substantial amount of untreated dentin areas; therefore, it is possible to say that the current technology for canal shaping is satisfactory from a mechanical point of view, but way limited from a biological standpoint. This situation is illustrated in the sequence of Fig. 4.1. The first image (a) shows a histological cross-section of a given oval-shaped canal and the black line in the second image (b) roughly shows what the original anatomy of this canal should be—the canal before mechanical preparation. The green circle shows what is possible to obtain with the available NiTi preparation systems. The debrided area always follows this very same pattern, because, as far as the NiTi instrument penetrates towards the apex, the resulting force pushes the instrument towards a single direction, where circular cutting occurs. This means that a lot of sound dentinal tissue is cut (as shown in blue in [c]) and, at the same time, a lot of contaminated

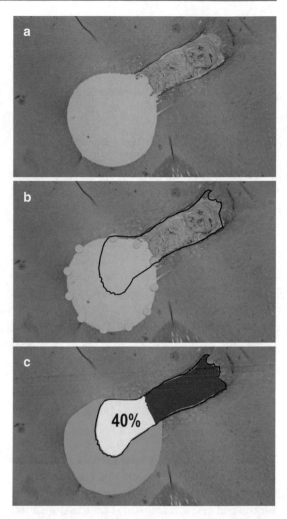

Fig. 4.1 Graphic illustration that exemplifies the dynamics that affect all mechanized systems currently available in the preparation of oval-shaped canal. In (**a**), we have a histological section of the canal with oval section. In (**b**), the black line illustrates what the original canal anatomy looked like. The green area shows the region of dentin that the mechanized system has cut. Any commercially available rotary or reciprocating system penetrates into the root space, following the same pattern as the resulting forces of this process require the instrument to settle and press on one side of the canal and only touching a fraction of the original root space (**c**). This process reveals that much healthy dentin tissue is eliminated (**c**, blue area), while a considerable area that should be mechanically debrided is not removed due to the limitation of NiTi instrument technology (**c**, red area). Thus, the so-called real efficiency area of the mechanical debridement process is only 40%, in a hypothetical situation of an oval canal like this example (**c**, yellow area)

dentin is left behind, as shown in the red area in (c). Only the yellow area is the effective cutting promoted by the NiTi preparation, which typically means that only around 40% of the effectiveness of mechanical debridement is possible in a typical oval-shaped canal like the current example.

Accordingly, the messages are crystal clear:

1. NiTi instruments only act on the central body of the canal, leaving almost all irregular areas untouched and undebrided. As such, the bacteria biofilm cannot be scrubbed out from most dentinal walls in a normal oval-shaped canal.
2. This background puts too much responsibility on the shoulders of irrigation, which has its own limitations.
3. Sound dentinal tissue is unnecessarily lost during shaping procedures. Future developments on mechanical shaping should be strictly focused on improving the scrubbing action and being able to uniformly plane the entire perimeter of the canal as much as possible.

Mechanical canal preparation is invasive in nature and different degrees of dentin removal may occur as different instrumentation techniques and systems are used, which may alter the biomechanical response of teeth [23]. So, future work should focus on the quest for a balance in the ratio of canal enlargement to close-to-optimal irrigation.

4.3   Preservation of Pericervical Dentin—Is Coronal Pre-flaring Still Necessary?

Coronal pre-flaring, canal scouting and glide path are early steps in mechanical canal preparation. Coronal pre-flaring can be defined as an extension of the access cavity into the cervical-most third of the canal space. Flaring the coronal portion of a narrow, calcified or difficult-to-access root canal affords several benefits by the relocation of the canal pathway, such as:

1. Improving tactile sensation and control by removing cervical calcifications and dentin overhangs, which allows unimpeded access for the apical third stream, canal scouting and apical patency procedures.
2. Facilitating larger instruments to reach the apical critical zone more loosely.
3. Reducing procedural errors such as loss of working length and canal transportation.
4. Optimization of infection control for twofold reasons: (a) most of bacteria is located in cervical and middle thirds of the root canal. Thus, coronal pre-flaring removes most of bacteria present in the root canal space early in treatment, contributing to the optimization of infection control and (b) coronal pre-flaring also allows deeper insertion of the irrigation needle in the earlier stages of cleaning and shaping procedures, which optimizes the irrigation. The enlarged area created by coronal pre-flaring acts as an escape space for the irrigating solution, enabling a better flow and reflux of the irrigating solution [24–26].
5. Better control of the incidence of postoperative pain due to less bacterial extrusion through the apical foramen.
6. Better control of instrument fracture. Ehrhardt et al. [27] performed 556 treatments and demonstrated that the use of MTwo system (VDW, Munich, Germany) after coronal pre-flaring revealed a low fracture rate, even reusing the instrument five times.
7. Coronal pre-flaring leads to more accurate apical sizing [28], and this information can be useful to define an appropriate final diameter for apical shaping.

Independently of all aforesaid advantages of the pre-flaring procedure, overflaring of canals by unbalanced enlargement of its coronal region through overusing large instruments can weaken the root. Ultimately, it can compromise the outcome of the root canal treatment due to the amount of dentinal tissue removed in this key and strategic structural region, the so-called pericervical dentin (PCD). The preservation of this region can be even more important to maintain strength of endodontically treated teeth as compared to very reduced occlusal access preparations [29]. Overall, logical reasoning claims that the loss of PCD implies in the weakening of root structure and decreased resistance to VRF. Actually, the more a canal is tapered and flared in the coronal region, the weaker the root tends to be. PCD was defined by Clark and Khademi [30] as "the dentin near the alveolar crest. This critical zone, roughly 4 mm coronal to the crestal bone and extending 4 mm apical to it, is crucial to transferring load from the occlusal table to the root, and much of the PCD is irreplaceable". The authors move ahead saying that no man-made material can compensate the tooth structure lost in key areas of the PCD.

With all exposed plus the popularization of NiTi rotary files, it is easy to understand the rapid influx of new instruments specifically designed to perform a better-balanced coronal pre-flaring procedure. The introduction of superelastic alloys associated with variable taper instruments (not following the international ISO standardization system) and an improved cutting ability by an S-shape design has opened up a new technical possibility for the coronal pre-flaring procedure. Besides being specially designed to perform coronal pre-flaring procedures, some NiTi rotary instruments—defined as orifice shapers such as ProFile (Dentsply Tulsa Dental; Tulsa, OK, United States) or Vortex orifice openers (Dentsply Tulsa Dental)—have never really become popular, and none of them has become the archetypal instrument for the coronal pre-flaring procedure.

The introduction of reciprocating systems in late 2010 brought the possibility of a new approach for the coronal pre-flaring procedure, as a single variable regressive taper reciprocating NiTi instrument is able to enlarge the main root canal space into a minimum acceptable taper size. This approach is able to perform a significantly more conservative coronal pre-flaring procedure.

Coronal pre-flaring performed with a single reciprocating instrument is done synchronously with the canal glide path. This way, it is possible to didactically list four advantages of coronal pre-flaring directly performed with a single reciprocating instrument:

1. More conservative coronal preparation due to the regressive taper of the single reciprocating instrument.
2. Better technical workflow as a function of less transoperative stages and few instruments used.
3. Shorter learning curve.
4. Improved safety by the use of the reciprocating movement per se.

Thus, it is not erroneous to consider the coronal pre-flaring done with a single regressive taper reciprocating instrument as an efficient technical approach, aligning the most up-to-date concepts of mechanical shaping and also valuing preservation of unreplaceable dental tissues.

4.3.1   The Role of the Danger Zone

One of the critical points of the mechanical damage normally caused by over-instrumentation on an already thin dentinal wall is that it may seriously compromise the outcome of root canal treatment [31]. This kind of damage is essentially mid-root perforations or excessive loss of dentin, which have been historically related to the distal area of mesial roots of mandibular molars and, based on that, Abou-Rass et al. [32] introduced the concept of the "danger zone" (DZ) in the early 1980s. In fact, these authors formally reported what experienced clinicians already knew-often: mesial canals of mandibular molars do not assume a central position in the root with the distal area between the canal and root bifurcation being relatively thin, the so-called DZ, which is more vulnerable to strip perforations. On the other hand, the safety zone was described as the mesial area of the mesial root with a thicker dentine layer, which is often minimally instrumented by endodontic instruments.

In short, Abou-Rass et al. [32] pointed out the importance of this anatomical area during canal shaping. Nowadays, the concerns around the DZ have moved towards dentinal preservation of the critical cervical region since this over-weakening of the root seems to mitigate the overall fracture resistance standard of teeth. This topic is addressed further where the taper of the mechanical preparation is discussed.

4.4 Evolution of NiTi-Based Preparations

4.4.1 NiTi Alloys

The use of NiTi alloy to produce instruments for root canal mechanical preparation has raised endodontic practice to a new level, revolutionizing it conceptually, practically and also economically. The NiTi technology made it possible to relate the geometric configuration of the instrument with the main anatomical features of the root canals, such as the angle and radius of curvature. Moreover, canal shaping became more centralized, giving a more precise adjustment to the canal anatomy and adequate modelling [33, 34] (Fig. 4.2). In addition, the mechanical properties and intrinsic characteristics presented by the NiTi alloy made it possible to use safety-mechanized canal shaping in a reduced treatment time with shorter learning curve [35, 36].

The NiTi alloy was developed by William Buehler in the United States in 1960, and it was firstly named NiTiNOL, an acronym for nickel (Ni), titanium (Ti) and Naval Ordinance Laboratory (NOL) [37]. In dentistry, Andreasen and Morrow [38] performed its initial application in orthodontics due to its low modulus of elasticity, shape memory effect and super flexibility. In 1975, Civjan and colleagues [39] published a manuscript containing suggestions for applying this new alloy in different dentistry specialties, including endodontics. The authors concluded that, due to the low modulus of elasticity, the construction of instruments with this alloy would allow the mechanical preparation of curved canals more efficiency and with less iatrogenic risks than using conventional manual stainless-steel instruments. The first experimental endodontic instruments made from NiTi orthodontic wires were found to have two to three times more elastic flexibility in bending, as well as superior resistance to torsional fracture, when compared to similar instruments manufactured using stainless-steel [40].

The NiTi alloys used in the manufacturing of endodontic instruments have near-equiatomic nickel and titanium proportions [40]. NiTi alloys contain three microstructural phases named austenite, martensite and R-phase, and the amounts of these phases determine the overall mechanical properties of the alloy [41]. The transformation of austenite into martensite (classic martensitic transformation) is caused by the alloy's ability to modify its atomic arrangement. The alteration of its crystalline microstructure and transformation characteristics directly influence the mechanical properties. Martensite, the low-temperature phase, is relatively soft and ductile, can be easily deformed and possesses the shape memory effect (SME) [41, 42]. In contrast, austenite, the high-temperature phase, is relatively stiff and hard, and possesses superior superelasticity (SE) [41–43]. The phase composition of the NiTi alloy is dependent on the ambient temperature and whether the alloy is cooled or heated to this temperature (Fig. 4.3). If the temperature is above the austenite finish temperature (A_f), the NiTi alloy is in the austenitic state. If the temperature is below the martensite finish temperature (M_f), the NiTi is in the martensitic state [41–43].

Among the main characteristic properties of the NiTi alloy used to manufacture endodontic instruments are the SME and SE [43–45]. SME is characterized as a property that, after relatively high deformations at temperatures below the full formation of martensite, instruments use to regain their original shape and size through subsequent heating at temperatures where austenite formation occurs (Figs. 4.4 and 4.5). In other words, SME is the ability of the NiTi alloy to recover its original shape when heated above the martensite-to-austenite transformation temperature. While the SE is characterized by the ability of the alloy to recover its original shape, even after large strains, it only occurs with the removal of tension without the need for heating (Fig. 4.6). Bending instrument and after applying forces, the instrument regains its original shape [44, 46].

In the last years, manufacturers have been performing additional metallurgical treatments on the NiTi alloys of instruments in order to improve their clinical performance. Among the most used

Fig. 4.2 Representative 3D reconstructions of the external and internal anatomy of curved mesial roots of mandibular molars, before and after root canal preparation. Changes in overall canal shape are visible in the superimposed root canals before (green) and after (red) mechanical preparation

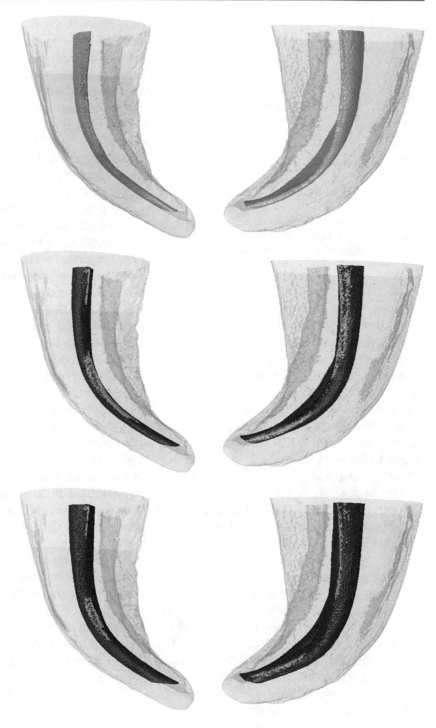

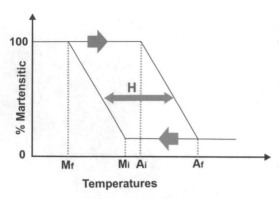

Fig. 4.3 Temperature hysteresis diagram of NiTi alloy. *Mi* martensite start temperature, *Mf* martensite finish temperature, *Ai* austenite start temperature, *Af* austenite finish temperature

treatment procedures are electropolishing and heat treatment. Electropolishing is the process of electrolytically removing components from metal parts in a highly ionic solution using an external source of electrical current. In this process, a very thin layer of material on the surface is removed, resulting in the reduction of microasperities that characterizes metal surfaces. The electropolishing of NiTi mechanized instruments, besides improving the finish of its metallic surface, also makes it more rigid [47–49].

Moreover, technological advances in the thermal management of NiTi alloy have allowed the development of instruments with altered crystalline compositions, which means alloys in intermediate stages between the austenitic and martensitic phases, containing substantial stable martensite phase under clinical conditions [50]. Some examples of thermal treatments are the M-wire (Dentsply Tulsa Dental), R-phase (SybronEndo, Orange, USA), CM-wire (DS Dental, Johnson City, USA), EDM (Coltene/ Whaledent AG, Altstätten, Switzerland), Gold and Blue treatments (Dentsply Tulsa Dental), T-wire (MicroMega, Besancon, France), and MaxWire (FKG Dentaire, La Chaux-de-Fonds Switzerland). While M-wire and R-phase instruments maintain an austenitic state, CM-Wire, Gold and Blue heat-treated instruments are composed of substantial amounts of martensite.

MaxWire is in the martensitic state at room temperature and changes to the austenitic state at intracanal temperature.

From a practical point of view, all new thermo-mechanically treated NiTi alloys available on the market demonstrated increased fatigue resistance and flexibility when compared to conventional NiTi alloys [51–57]. It is well known that martensitic alloys also possess higher flexibility than austenitic ones [42, 56]. Due to its improved flexibility, these martensitic instruments are indicated in the presence of extreme curvatures (Fig. 4.7). Another advantage of heat treatment is that these instruments can better maintain the root canal anatomy, so they are supposed to have an equal or better quality of root canal preparation [15, 58–60]. A recent study from Bürklein et al. [61] has demonstrated that both M-wire instruments and their Gold and Blue corresponding files have maintained the original canal curvature well with no significant differences and without fracturing. This means that M-wire files are already flexible enough to maintain root canal curvature, but presumably in most difficult root canals, the more flexible Gold and Blue alloys would better maintain the anatomy. Gold and Blue thermo-mechanically treated files also have better centring ability in both coronal and apical portions with minimal transportation [61], which is a clear advantage from a minimally invasive perspective (Fig. 4.8). The pre-bendability of a martensitic file is helpful to have better access in difficult cases. In a small mouth opening, a martensitic instrument can be pre-bent to have an easier direction, being more conservative in the coronal portion without performing early coronal enlargement and straight-line access. In addition, pre-bending these files for difficult cases permits to overcome ledges or complicated apical anatomy, such as abrupt curvatures.

However, there are also some limitations of heat-treated alloys. The major limitation of a martensitic state instrument is that the martensitic phase has a low transitional temperature, so it requires less energy for deformation. This means that plastic deformation and unwinding of these instruments can be more often experienced

Fig. 4.4 (**a**) NiTi alloy
wire in the original
shape; (**b**) deformed
NiTi alloy; (**c**) NiTi
alloy recovering the
original shape after
being heated above the
martensite-to-austenite
transformation
temperature

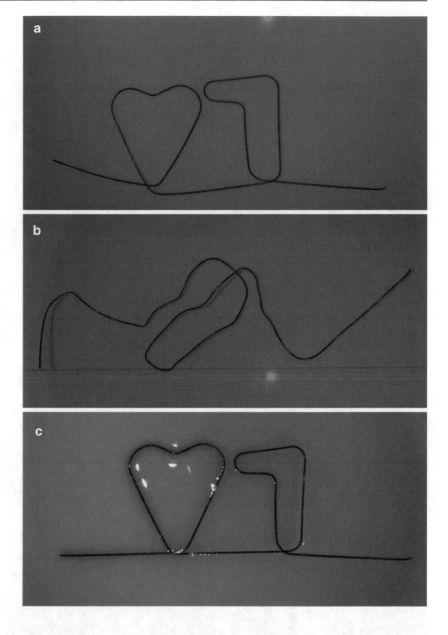

(Fig. 4.9). Martensitic thermally treated instruments have a higher angle of rotation to fracture, so they can be rotated more before fracture; the force needed to deform and fracture them is lower [57, 62, 63]. Less stress is needed to deform these files inside the root canals; however, even deformed, they will fracture later. Martensitic files are very flexible and therefore perfect for highly curved root canals; however, extremely flexible instruments may have less cutting ability. For this reason, these types of instruments may be difficult to advance in very strict root canals, enhancing the risk of distortion. In contrast, austenitic instruments reveal high torque values at fracture; thus, these files might be useful to shape straight or slightly curved constricted root canals. Therefore, it is important to find a balance between mechanical properties and flexibility and the resistance to torsion.

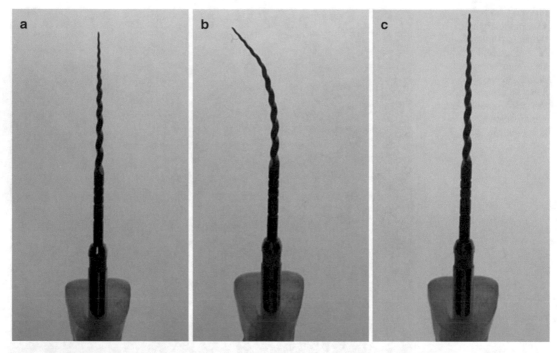

Fig. 4.5 (a) NiTi martensitic instrument in the original shape; (b) deformed NiTi instrument; (c) NiTi instrument recovering the original shape after being heated above the martensite-to-austenite transformation temperature

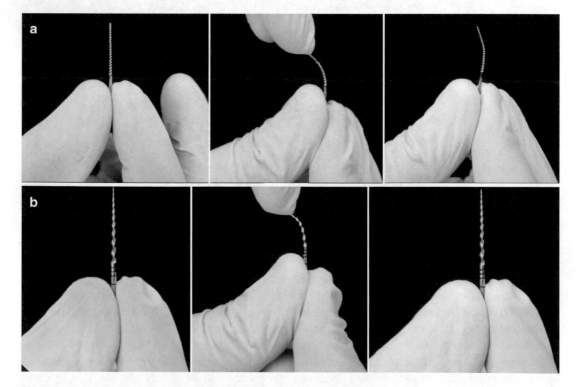

Fig. 4.6 (a) Stainless-steel instrument after the application of tension being plastically deformed; (b) NiTi instrument recovering its original shape after applying forces

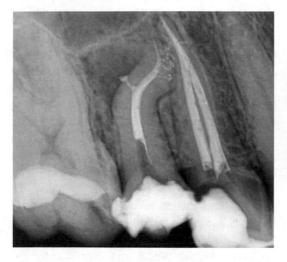

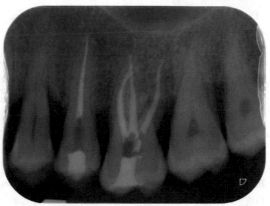

Fig. 4.8 A first upper molar treated with martensitic Blue files demonstrating respect of the original anatomy and a conservative approach

Fig. 4.7 An upper premolar with an extreme double curvature

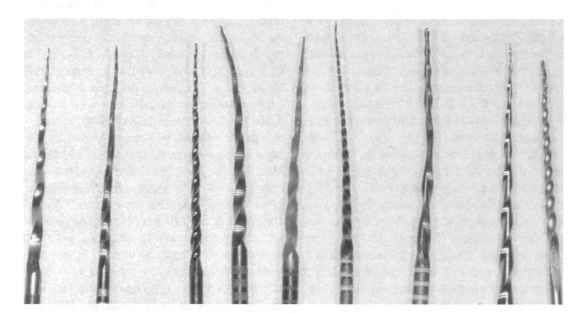

Fig. 4.9 Deformed files from several different brands

4.4.2 Shaping Kinematics

In addition to the advancements related to NiTi alloys, innovative kinematics were developed with the purpose of overperforming the conventional continuous rotation. Nowadays, reciprocating movement stands as a reliable and feasible alternative to the conventional continuous rotation [64]. In fact, reciprocating kinematics have been extensively described and tested in mechanical endodontic procedures for stainless-steel files since the 1960s [65–74]. This "first mode" of reciprocating movement is based on symmetrical oscillation, in which the forward cutting angle is the same as the backward release angle (i.e. 30° clockwise followed by 30° counterclockwise or 45° clockwise followed by 45° counterclockwise). This kinematic was basically used for stainless-steel instruments and now it is mainly used for mechanical scouting with stainless-steel instruments. In 2008, Yared proposed an approach to the use of the ProTaper F2 instrument (Dentsply Maillefer, Baillagueis, Switzerland) in a reciprocating movement [75] as an alternative to the conventional continuous rotation. This "second mode" of reciprocating kinematics is a partial or asymmetrical reciprocation, in which the forward angle is bigger than the backward angle. Doing this movement continuously generates a positive angle, so that a "rotary effect" can be maintained. This means that the reciprocating movement maintains the tendency to naturally advance towards the apex because of the "rotary effect".

Asymmetrical reciprocation kinematics can be performed using different types of angle combinations (e.g. 60–40°, 108–72° or 150–30°), which overall relieves stress on the instrument by a forward (cutting action, the instrument advances in the canal and engages dentin to cut it) and a backward (release of the instrument, which is immediately disengaged releasing the stress) movement [64]. This new kinematics extended the lifespan of NiTi instruments when compared to continuous rotation [36, 76, 77]. When actioned in reciprocating kinematics, the instruments travel a shorter angular distance than continuous rotation instruments, being subject to lower stress values, which extends its fatigue life [36, 76, 77]. Reciproc (VDW), Reciproc Blue (VDW), WaveOne (Dentsply Maillefer) and WaveOne Gold (Dentsply Maillefer) are the main examples of modern commercially available NiTi systems for root canal preparation using asymmetric reciprocating motion.

There are several advantages of using reciprocating kinematics instead of continuous rotary kinematics. The opening is the possibility of a single variable tapered reciprocating NiTi instrument able to enlarge the root canal into a minimally acceptable taper size, which is indeed appealing by the oversimplification of technical workflow procedure and reducing the overall learning curve. Under a cost-effective perspective, the use of a single disposable NiTi instrument is also advantageous over conventional multi-file rotary systems.

In addition, there is a strong body of evidence showing that reciprocating-based mechanical preparations are safer than conventional continuous rotation [36, 76–79]. Studies reported a lower incidence of fracture for reciprocating instruments (0.13–0.26%) rather than rotary files; thus, reciprocation is considered a safer movement [80–82]. It is of note that this safer shaping in clinical usage is directly related to an improved fatigue resistance shown by reciprocation over conventional continuous rotation. Actually, this was an unexpected but welcome "side-effect" once reciprocation was introduced to reduce torsional failures, but it also increased the resistance to cyclic fatigue failure and consequently the lifespan of instruments [36, 76–78]. Torsional failure occurs when the tip of the instrument is locked in the canal, while the shaft continues to rotate. If the elastic limit of the metal is exceeded, the instrument undergoes plastic deformation, which can be followed by fracture if the load is high enough. When submitted to reciprocation kinematics, an instrument has reduced torsional stress, since during the reciprocating movement the instrument engages dentin during the cutting movement, whereas the opposite movement disengages the instrument immediately afterwards. Moreover, an instrument used in reciprocation lasts longer used in a curvature rather than the same instrument used in rotation [77]. A rearrangement of the NiTi molecular structure of the instrument during the forward and backward movements may happen. Moreover, the backward movement tends to reduce the propagation of initial cracks in metal, thus reducing the possibility of fracture by cyclic fatigue [77]. The more bent the curvature is, the higher the risk of fracture for cyclic fatigue. But reciprocating files are safe to be used in most curved root canals. Since the instrument's lifespan is increased by the reciprocating movement [36, 76–78], a higher number of root canals can be prepared in a safer way than under continuous rotary movement.

The reciprocating movement has the same or even more cutting efficiency than full rotation. Since the first moment, doubts were raised if the reciprocating movement would reduce cutting efficiency as, until that moment, continuous rotation was considered the optimal movement from a cutting efficiency point of view. However, evidence demonstrated that the same file used both in rotation and in reciprocation has the same cutting ability [83, 84].

Moreover, reciprocating kinematics allows an equal or better quality of preparation. An instrument used in reciprocation has an improved shaping ability as compared to the same instrument used in continuous rotation. A recent study demonstrated that a reciprocating file remains better centred inside the root canals when compared to a rotary file [85]. The superior shaping ability promoted by the reciprocating movement is especially true for instruments with bigger sizes, which yields less canal transportation [86]. Smaller files are not the problem, as they are flexible enough to be used in both rotation and reciprocation without any clue of canal transportation. For single-file techniques, the main reason for these results is that a single-file is usually bigger than the root canal, so it can touch at least two of the opposite sides of the canal walls, the inner and the outer portion, cutting them equally. It resembles the classical "balanced force" technique by Roane et al. [87] for stainless-steel manual files, which was proposed to allow bigger instrument sizes going beyond the canal curvature with controlled canal transportation.

There are two main criticisms of reciprocation preparations: (i) instruments would be more prone to promote the development or propagation of dentinal microcracks and dentinal damage than conventional full-sequence rotary systems and (ii) the accumulation and apical extrusion of debris.

The idea that the reciprocating preparation is more related to root dentinal defects is based on the rationale that using only a single, large-tapered reciprocating instrument, which cuts substantial amounts of dentin in a short period of time, is more aggressive than conventional rotary preparation, which comprises a more progressive and slower cutting of the root dentinal tissue. However, the scenario was created by studies based only on root sectioning methods and direct observation by optical microscopy [88–94] (Fig. 4.10). These methods undoubtedly have a noteworthy drawback related to the destructive

nature of the experiment. Despite the fact that the control groups, which used unprepared teeth, seemed to validate these results because no dentinal defects could be detected, this sort of control does not take into account the potential damage produced by the interplay among three sources of stresses on the root dentin [95]:

1. The mechanical preparation.
2. The chemical attack with sodium hypochlorite-based irrigation.
3. The sectioning procedures per se.

As time went by, it was demonstrated that the correct technology to study microcracks is the 3D micro-CT non-destructive analysis. By using this method, De Deus et al. [95] showed a clear lack of causal relationship between dentinal microcracks development and canal preparation with both rotary and reciprocating systems (Fig. 4.11). This conclusion was later confirmed by other studies from different groups worldwide using the same methodology [96–100]. In addition, more recently, it was demonstrated by the association between the micro-CT analytical platform and a cadaveric experimental model that the so-called root dentinal microcracks, observable in the cross-sectional images, are indeed a phenomenon that belongs to the framework of extracted storage teeth [101] (Fig. 4.12). In other words, root dentinal microcracks are not a true clinical phenomenon, and as such, there is no more room for concerns.

The worldwide rise of reciprocating systems led to another potential drawback: single-file mechanical preparations cutting significant amounts of dentin in short periods of time are prone to force more debris, dentin chips, irrigants, remaining pulp tissue, bacteria, and their by-products through the apex. The basis for this assumption is the clinical impression that reciprocation is an overall forceful movement, which may act as a mechanical piston, pumping debris and irrigants through the apex. However, at least to some measure, this assumption may not have a well-built background, since reciprocation tries to mimic balanced force technique kinematics, which is well known as being a pressureless movement pushing less material periapically [102].

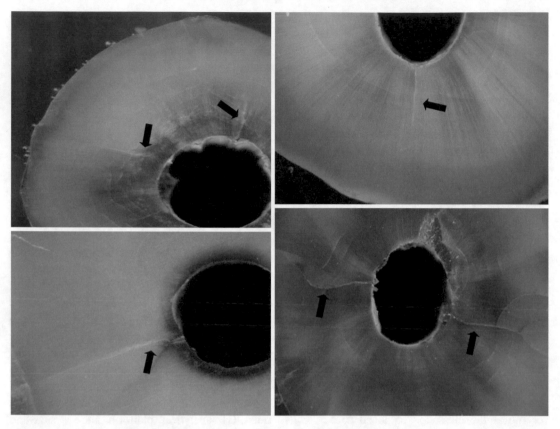

Fig. 4.10 Representative images of root canal slices showing the presence of cracks (arrows) after root canal preparation

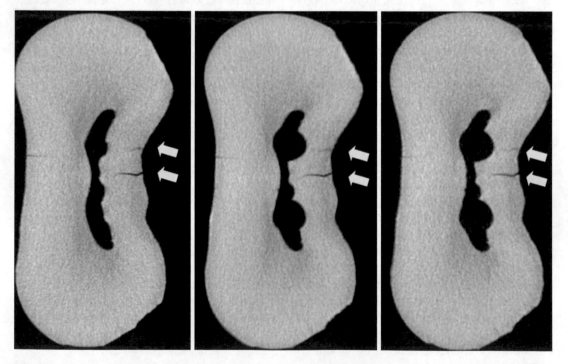

Fig. 4.11 Representative cross-section images of mesial roots of mandibular molars showing the presence of cracks (arrows) before and after preparation of the mesiobuccal and mesiolingual canals

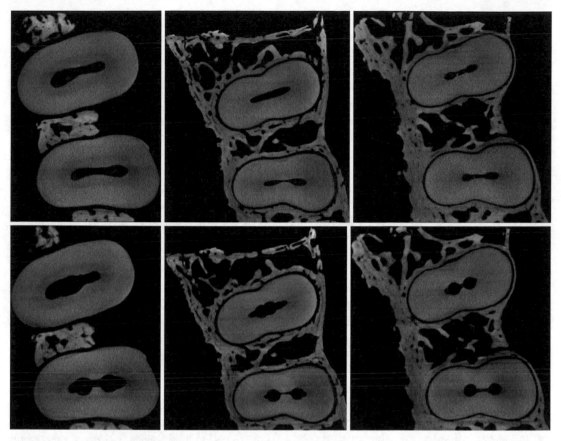

Fig. 4.12 Cross-sectional images of coronal, middle and apical thirds of roots of maxillary premolar teeth before and after root canal preparation

The issue takes place because the flutes of reciprocating instruments are designed to remove debris only in a single direction. In the framework of rotation, the forward movement continually removes dentinal debris coronally, and this is the potential reason why rotary files make a point in this regard. This means that, theoretically, movement kinematics itself may play a role in packing the debris into the irregularities of the root canal space and pushing them beyond the apex as a consequence of the backward movement (relief angle). The counter-argument says that more technical steps tend to extrude more debris and irrigants. This means that, at the end of canal shaping, conventional rotary multi-file systems will extract more undesired material than a single-file preparation.

Several studies have tried to shed some light on this topic [102–111], but the existing research conclusions remain inconclusive. A recent comprehensive review of the literature [59] concluded that there is no influence of the movement on the accumulation and extrusion of dentinal debris. Therefore, there is no robust evidence that reciprocating files extrude more debris, even if this motion is prone to push debris down. In vivo studies [103, 112] have evaluated the possible effects of debris extrusion by measuring the substances released by the human periodontal ligament and the inflammatory procedures created by different root canal preparation techniques. The first results pointed out that hand-file instrumentation created a significantly higher inflammatory response as compared to both WaveOne and Reciproc reciprocating techniques. Moreover, WaveOne instruments were more related to higher inflammation than Reciproc, possibly due to differences in the design between these files. WaveOne and Reciproc movements are quite the same, while the triangular design of WaveOne is probably less effective in removing debris, because its larger metal core reduces the depths of the blades and, consequently, the space to carry debris coronally [103]. The second study compared the expression of substance P and calcitonin gene-related peptide in healthy human periodontal ligaments from premolars after root canal preparation with Reciproc Blue, WaveOne Gold, XP-endo Shaper and hand files, and demonstrated lower neuropeptide release for reciprocating files when compared to both XP-endo Shaper and hand files instrumentation [112]. There are also other two in vivo studies that demonstrated that reciprocating instruments had similar impacts on the quality of life of patients in primary treatments when compared to rotary files [113], while reporting lower values of post-operative pain when compared to rotary files in retreatments [114].

Therefore, in a general manner, the interplay among several factors of reciprocating systems such as instrument design, improved alloy, fewer instruments, high cutting ability, and reciprocation kinematics can be used to support their clinical usage regarding the apically extruded debris issue [59]. Last but not least, the positive clinical results on post-operative pain restates that the amount of apically extruded debris is well controlled and, for sure, clinically tolerated.

Due to its previously described advantages, mainly due to excellent shaping performance plus a lower instrument fracture rate, associated with an absence of disadvantages when compared to continuous rotary kinematics, it is possible to affirm that reciprocating kinematics per se is today the most minimally invasive activation mode for NiTi canal preparation.

4.5 Apical Size and the Limits of Shaping

The presence of microorganisms inside the root canal system space has been widely documented as the major determining factor influencing the outcome of root canal treatment [115–117]. Thus, control of bacteria loads is the seminal goal of endodontics [118, 119]. Debridement and disinfection protocols search to optimize intracanal bacterial load reduction, as well as vital or necrotic pulp tissue removal, that may serve as substrate for pulp space bacterial recontamination [120, 121]. The complexity of the root canal system space is well reported and known [122, 123], representing the major challenge for root canal treatment protocols. The presence of hard-to-reach areas, such as isthmuses, irregularities, ramifications and accessory canals, root dilacerations and fusions, or even developmental anomalies, such as *dens invaginatus,* may lead to strong limitations in the clinical approach [124].

One of the most relevant areas when considering the necessity of mechanical debridement and disinfection is the apical area. The working length determination is a clinical step that is susceptible to being controlled by the clinician but difficult to be performed with precision. According to Grove [125], the working length should, ideally, have its apical limit at the cemento-dentinal junction, since this is the hard tissues landmark that best approaches the soft tissues zone, which corresponds to the transition of pulp to periodontal tissues. However, this perimeter of this anatomical area can be extensive and variable [126]. Thus, the apical constriction has been presented as the anatomic apical limit, where the root canal instrumentation and obturation should be finished [127]. Important histological studies on apical anatomy, developed in the second half of the past century [128], noticed that the anatomical apex, apical foramen and apical constriction were different morphologic landmarks with different locations among them. Moreover, the area of minor diameter, or apical constriction, usually near the cemento-dentinal junction, displayed an average distance to the centre of the apical foramen of 0.524 mm [128]. The distance between the anatomical apex and the apical constriction may vary from 0.07 mm to 2.69 mm, with an average distance of 0.89 mm [129]. However, recent robust micro-CT-based studies revealed that these differences might even be larger [130] and also different anatomic configurations of the apical constriction have also been described.

Considering the variations, emphasis was given in understanding this not only in the distance between the apical constriction and the anatomical apex but also in the apical typology. The exact location of the apical constriction is extremely difficult to establish in clinical practice. Today, there is no doubt about the superiority of electronic apex locators working length determination over the traditional radiographic method of determining the apical constriction [131, 132]. Actually, the combined method of using the electronic apex locator plus radiographic confirmation is the most reliable approach to determine the apical limit of instrumentation [132]. In the 1960s, Ingle [133] proposed the apical constriction as the apical limit of root canal instrumentation, which became a classic concept in endodontics. Since the narrow diameter position of the apical constriction does not match the radiographic apex, the author recommends that the working length determination should be performed 0.5–1.0 mm short with regard to the radiographic apex. Moreover, the shaping and filling procedures performed at the apical limit through the X-ray could be easily considered as over-instrumentation and overfilling. Ricucci and Langeland [127] have performed a histological evaluation of the periapical tissues in humans at several follow-up periods after root canal treatments. They noticed that, independently of the pulp diagnosis, the results were more favourable when root canal instrumentation and filling had their apical limit at the level or slightly short of apical constriction. Regardless of the symptoms, the inflammatory reaction was always observed when overfilling was present.

Two problems might be associated with the apical limit of the instrumentation: the complex morphology itself and the fact that this complex anatomy may harbour biofilm, which may dictate a poor root canal treatment outcome. Minimizing the impact of infection on treatment outcomes may be performed through careful apical chemo-mechanical instrumentation. Although the choice of the apical constriction might be more easily accepted by both clinical and scientific communities as the reference point for the apical limit of root canal preparation, the desirable size of the apical preparation still remains controversial. Taking into consideration the documented sizes of apical constriction [128], apical preparations to ISO sizes from 0.25 mm to 0.35 mm have been recommended [133–135]; however, this approach is easy questionable, considering the amount of unprepared intracanal surfaces left behind [136]. Weiger et al. [137] performed an in vitro assessment of the most appropriate apical enlargement for both maxillary and mandibular molars using 212 root canals. The authors concluded that enlarging to more than 0.40 mm above the original apical size in maxillary palatal and mandibular distal canals would lead to a complete circumferential preparation of the original apical morphology in 78% of cases, while the enlargement to more than 0.30 mm in maxillary buccal and mandibular mesial canals was able to completely instrument the apical morphology in 72% of cases. Moreover, the apical preparation to more than 0.60 mm above the original apical size would lead to 98% of cases with a complete circumferential preparation of the original apical anatomy. Globally, this represents 6–8 sizes above the first apical binding file. Although the authors have stated that root canals should be instrumented to larger sizes than normally recommended, it is also important to notice that this may be associated with a higher risk of iatrogenic errors, such as zips, ledges or perforations. These risks are much less common when using NiTi instruments [138]; however, they can still occur, especially in over-preparations, independently of the kinematic used [139].

Although the capacity to mechanically shape the apical portion of the root canal is of major clinical importance, infection control appears to be the seminal condition to trigger the healing process and determine the treatment outcome. Taking this into consideration, some authors addressed bacterial load reduction depending on the apical enlargement. Mickel et al. [140] performed the inoculation of 100 single-rooted teeth with *Enterococus faecalis*, followed by instrumentation to 1, 2 and 3 sizes above the first crown-down file to reach the apical limit. The authors concluded that there was a significant increase in the number of samples with negative cultures in the larger apical sizes. Rodrigues et al. [141] performed the apical preparation up to the first and third instrument of a rotary system, using saline or sodium hypochlorite irrigation, and concluded that the apical instrumentation up to the third instrument provided superior bacterial control, independently of the irrigation used, although superior results were noticed with sodium hypochlorite. Taking these results into consideration, larger apical preparations seem to be able to optimize bacterial control.

When deciding which apical preparation to choose for a particular clinical case, other factors such as smear layer removal, debris extrusion or post-operative pain are also to be considered. A scanning electron microscopic analysis of debris and smear layer present in the apical portion of the root canal after instrumentation with file sizes of 0.20 mm and 0.25 mm with both 4% and 6% tapers, respectively, has shown that, independently of the taper, debridement with the larger file size was superior with regard to smear layer elimination [142]. As for the apical extrusion of debris and bacteria, an in vitro study noticed that the debris extrusion was lower when performing instrumentation with crown-down techniques with smaller tapers as opposed to larger taper and full-length linear instrumentation [143]. Regarding the post-operative pain evaluated in randomized clinical trials, the maintenance of apical patency during apical preparation, apparently, does not influence post-operative pain [144], while contradictory information exists on the influence of apical foramen enlargement [145, 146]. The decision of performing or not performing apical patency during root canal instrumentation is not consensual. Some histological studies have noticed acute apical inflammatory responses [126, 127], while others suggest [17] that infected debris might be extruded during root canal treatment procedures when patency is included in the protocol. However, other evidence supports this technical aspect arguing the reduction in accumulation of soft tissue remnants in the apical region [147], which attests to

superior irrigation in the apical third [148] and, ultimately, superior bacterial elimination around the apical foramen [149]. Moreover, the apical patency step also minimizes the risk of iatrogenic errors, such as canal transportation, ledges, apical perforations or loss of working length [147, 150].

Although the decision on which apical size to choose should be based on several factors, it is also important to understand that some in vitro assessments are difficult to extrapolate to clinical practice. Understanding how all these variables are clinically combined in the resolution, or not, of clinical cases is also important. A long-term outcome study [151], with observation periods up to 5 years, concluded that apical preparation sizes between 0.20 mm and 0.40 mm and between 0.45 mm and 1.00 mm had exactly the same prognosis. Another retrospective study concluded that there was no difference in the clinical success rate with different apical preparation sizes, although a decrease of the success rate along with an increase of the apical size was also noticed [152]. A randomized controlled trial [153], which followed 167 patients over 12 months after root canal treatment of pulp necrosis cases, used five different groups in which the apical size was enlarged to 2, 3, 4, 5 and 6 sizes above the first apical binding file. The authors concluded that enlarging to 3 sizes larger than the first binding apical file was adequate, and further enlargement did not provide any benefit. This may be seen as a much more conservative approach.

Although preparation size seems to matter with regard to the root canal treatment prognosis, it is also important to balance the advantages of large apical sizes with the conservative approach of the smaller sizes. For these reasons, the authors have developed a clinical concept called "visual gauging" that aims to customize the apical preparation size on the specific canal that should be treated [154]. In this technique, the most important aspect to be evaluated from a clinical point of view to decide the final apical size of enlargement is the type of dentin debris cut that remains on the tip of the instrument. As a consequence, some different clinical conditions may happen depending on the characteristics of the dentin debris cut by mechanical files:

1. Presence of pulp remnants debris or "pink/red" dentin debris on the tip of the instrument used (in vital cases): pending that the correct working length has been chosen, the diameter of apical preparation is still insufficient and residual pulp is probably still present.
2. Very little dentin debris present inside the flutes of the apical 3–4 mm of the instrument used: the diameter of apical preparation is still insufficient to cut dentinal walls in the apical third.
3. Presence of "yellow/brown" dentin debris on the tip of the instrument used (in necrotic cases): even if probably the instrument is circumferentially cutting dentinal walls in the apical third, this is still contaminated dentin that requires further apical enlargement.
4. Presence of white clean dentin inside the flutes of the apical 1–2 mm of the instrument used: the instrument is cutting sound dentin in the apical third but probably not circumferentially.
5. Presence of white clean dentin inside the flutes of the apical 3–4 mm of the instrument used: presumably the instrument is cutting sound dentin circumferentially in the apical third and this may be the correct size of apical preparation. Results from a microbiological analysis of the different types of dentin that remained on the tip of the instrument described above seem to confirm that less bacteria were present in this last type of dentin cut with respect to the "brown-yellow" type described above (Plotino and Grande unpublished results).

Moreover, a micro-CT study has assessed possible microcrack formation after root canal instrumentation with two different reciprocating and a conventional full-sequence rotary system, with size 25 and after enlarging to size 40. No new cracks were noticed after the initial instrumentation or after the apical enlargement [95]. Thus, remaining minimally invasive in apical size diameters might not suggest superior outcomes from both a microbiological and biomechanical point of view.

4.6 Taper of Root Canal Instrumentation

The main objectives of mechanical instrumentation in endodontics are not only restricted to the removal of vital and necrotic tissues from the root canal system space but also in the creation of enough intracanal space to promote efficient intracanal irrigation and medication in order to control the root canal infection [155, 156]. It also aims to facilitate the root canal obturation procedures and preserve the location and integrity of the root canal apical morphology while avoiding iatrogenic damage of root and root canal anatomy. It should also avoid the aggression of periapical tissues, whether bone or periodontal ligament, while being able to preserve sound dentin in order to allow a good structural prognosis [150]. To achieve these mechanical instrumentation goals, Schilder [157] has idealized five root canal shape design objectives plus four biological objectives. As for the shaping design, it was advocated that the final root canal shape should be a continuous tapering funnel from the apex to the coronal canal opening, the canal cross-sectional diameter should be narrower at every point apically, the shaped canal should preserve the original morphology, the apical foramen should remain in the same position and the apical opening should remain as small as possible. As for the biological objectives of the mechanical preparation, it should be kept confined to the root canal system only, it should not force dentin debris with necrotic tissue beyond the foramen, it should be able to remove all tissues from the intracanal space and it should create enough space for intracanal disinfection [157]. Although intracanal infection is mainly controlled by irrigation, the mechanical instrumentation itself may also significantly reduce the bacterial count. A classic study from Byström and Sundqvist [158] was able to document a significant reduction of the bacterial count between 100- and 1000-fold on teeth with necrotic pulp and apical periodontitis by performing only mechanical instrumentation with saline irrigation. Although a strong reduction was noticed, no case became bacteria-free after the first appointment, and seven teeth out of a total of 15 became bacteria-free only after the fifth visit. Another study from Orstavik et al. [159] performed the mechanical shape of the root canals in 23 teeth using irrigation only with physiological saline, and concluded that only 13 cases became bacteria-free. Both studies concluded that although a significant bacterial load reduction was noticed after mechanical preparation, the results were clearly insufficient in reducing the bacterial load to a desired level. Another study from Siqueira et al. [160] performed an in vitro assessment on the efficacy of several instrumentation techniques with different regimens in reducing the intracanal bacterial load. After having the root canals inoculated with *Enterococcus faecalis*, they were shaped by using one of two mechanized methodologies and one of four root canal irrigation protocols. The four experimental groups were able to provide a bacterial load decrease between 78.4% (2.5% sodium hypochlorite with citric acid) and 60.3% (2.5% sodium hypochlorite alone) of the original microbial count. As for the control group with instrumentation assisted with saline solution irrigation, the mean bacterial reduction was 38.3%. The authors concluded that all groups reached significantly higher reductions of the microbial load when compared to the saline solution group. Therefore, the combination of mechanical instrumentation with root canal irrigation appears to be the most reliable method to guarantee effective root canal disinfection.

Theoretically, root canal instrumentation with large-tapered instruments would be able to clean more effectively a less tapered root canal. However, due to the complexity of the root canal system morphology, which presents fins, inner surface irregularities, isthmuses, transversal anastomoses or oval canal shapes, the concept of larger tapers has been proved as not having the expected practical relevance with several studies showing similar results in root canal cleanliness when comparing smaller with larger tapers [142, 161–163].

The percentage of untouched inner root canal area after mechanical instrumentation may be as high as 40–55%, according to micro-CT analysis [11, 164]. A minimally invasive treatment should aim to reduce the amount of untouched inner area not by increasing the instrumentation taper but by using complementary cleaning methods, avoiding unnecessary dentin removal from the middle and coronal portions of the root canal, which ultimately may lead to a lower resistance to root fracture [10]. A recent study has also demonstrated that using modern activation devices may guarantee optimal canal cleanliness in the middle and coronal thirds, even in root canals with a minimal preparation size of 0.20/taper 0.04 [142], but it must be underlined that an increase in the apical diameter of preparation is still needed to obtain cleaner canals in the apical third [59].

Thus, a root canal instrumentation procedure reaching an adequate diameter of apical enlargement while maintaining a reduced taper or a limited maximum coronal file diameter seems to best follow the tendency of modern endodontics, which aims to find a balance between a minimally invasive intervention to minimize unnecessary dental structure removal and the need to reach biological and microbiological objectives in cleaning the root canal space.

4.7 Concluding Remarks

In summary, the era of minimally invasive endodontics is yet in its first childhood depending on more consistent scientific support and improved technology to become a standard affordable class of treatment.

The rationale of this chapter follows from the fact that the current concerns around the so-called minimally invasive endodontics is indeed a pursuit for optimal balance between what should be taken and what should be preserved. In order words, a matter of size. The rationale is that, while an overall smaller size root canal treatment (from the crown to the apex) may better preserve the important PCD tissue and thus improve the long-term retention of the tooth, it may compromise proper disinfection, cleanliness and filling of the root canal space and thus compromise the healing process in infected cases. On the other hand, over-accessed and over-prepared root canals may not only render disinfection, cleanliness (especially in the coronal and mid-root areas where the majority of bacteria biofilm is present) and filling easier and more effective procedures but also increase teeth predisposition to VRF by a significant reduction of root structure.

Sooner or later, minimally invasive techniques and instruments will be better supported by the rigour of the scientific method. Nevertheless, in the meantime, caution with this topic is very necessary, as common-sense logic would lead to biased ways of thinking that superficial technical approaches such as "ninja accesses" or "non-shaped canals" can improve the long-term retention of teeth.

In its current status, minimally invasive endodontics is a bunch of very technically sensitive approaches strictly and fundamentally based on the operator's skills and experience. In this scenario, the operative microscope is restated as the backbone of contemporary endodontic practice, which is a strong positive aspect of this discussion. However, there is an important educational cost involved with minimally invasive endodontics that needs to be taken into consideration; therefore, it is key to scientifically test and define how operative procedures can indeed be meaningful in the improvement of the long-term retention of teeth.

References

1. Rivera EM, Walton RE. Longitudinal tooth cracks and fractures: an update and review. Endod Topics. 2015;33:14–42.
2. Arnold LH. Discussion. J Am Dent Assoc. 1931;18:483.
3. Touré B, Faye B, Kane AW, Lo CM, Niang B, Boucher Y. Analysis of reasons for extraction of endodontically treated teeth: a prospective study. J Endod. 2011;37:1512–5.
4. Currey JD. The design of mineralized hard tissues for their mechanical functions. J Exp Biol. 1999;202:3285–94.
5. Kinney JH, Habelitz S, Marshall SJ, Marshall GW. The importance of intrafibrillar mineralization of collagen on the mechanical properties of dentin. J Dent Res. 2003;82:957–61.
6. Missau T, De Carlo BM, Michelon C, et al. Influence of endodontic treatment and retreatment on the fatigue failure load, numbers of cycles for failure, and survival rates of human canine teeth. J Endod. 2017;43:2081–7.
7. Rundquist BD, Versluis A. How does canal taper affect root stresses? Int Endod J. 2006;39:226–37.
8. Eliasson S, Bergstrom J, Sanda A. Periodontal bone loss of teeth with metal posts: a radiographic study. J Clin Periodontol. 1995;22:850–3.
9. Tian SY, Bai W, Jiang WR, Liang YH. Fracture resistance of roots in mandibular premolars following root canal instrumentation of different sizes. Chin J Dent Res. 2019;22:197–202.
10. Krikeli E, Mikrogeorgis G, Lyroudia K. In vitro comparative study of the influence of instrument taper on the fracture resistance of endodontically treated teeth: an integrative approach-based analysis. J Endod. 2018;44:1407–11.
11. Paqué F, Balmer M, Attin T, Peters OA. Preparation of oval-shaped root canals in mandibular molars using nickel-titanium rotary instruments: a micro-computed tomography study. J Endod. 2010;36:703–7.
12. Paqué F, Peters OA. Micro-computed tomography evaluation of the preparation of long oval root canals in mandibular molars with the self-adjusting file. J Endod. 2011;37:517–21.
13. Versiani MA, Leoni GB, Steier L, et al. Micro-computed tomography study of oval-shaped canals prepared with the self-adjusting file, Reciproc, WaveOne and Pro-Taper Universal systems. J Endod. 2013;39:1060–6.
14. De-Deus G, Belladonna FG, Silva EJ, et al. Micro-CT evaluation of non-instrumented canal areas with different enlargements performed by NiTi systems. Braz Dent J. 2015;26:624–9.
15. Belladonna FG, Carvalho MS, Cavalcante DM, et al. Micro-computed tomography shaping ability assessment of the new blue thermal treated Reciproc instrument. J Endod. 2018;44:1146–50.
16. Silva AA, Belladonna FG, Rover G, et al. Does ultra-conservative access affect the efficacy of root canal treatment and the fracture resistance of two-rooted maxillary premolars? Int Endod J. 2020;53:265–75.
17. Siqueira JF Jr. Microbial causes of endodontic flare-ups. Int Endod J. 2003;36:453–63.
18. Waltimo T, Trope M, Haapasalo M, Ørstavik D. Clinical efficacy of treatment procedures in endodontic infection control and one year follow-up of periapical healing. J Endod. 2005;31:863–6.
19. Siqueira JF Jr, Roças IN. Clinical implications and microbiology of bacterial persistence after treatment procedures. J Endod. 2008;34:1291–301.
20. De-Deus G, Belladonna FG, Simões-Carvalho M, et al. Shaping efficiency as a function of time of a new heat-treated instrument. Int Endod J. 2019;52:337–42.
21. Rover G, Belladonna FG, Bortoluzzi EA, De-Deus G, Silva EJ, Teixeira CS. Influence of access cavity design on root canal detection, instrumentation effi-

cacy, and fracture resistance assessed in maxillary molars. J Endod. 2017;43:1657–62.

22. Zuolo ML, Zaia AA, Belladonna FG, et al. Micro-CT assessment of the shaping ability of four root canal instrumentation systems in oval-shaped canals. Int Endod J. 2018;51:564–71.

23. Kishen A. Mechanisms and risk factors for fracture predilection in endodontically treated teeth. Endod Topics. 2006;13:57–83.

24. Kessler JR, Peters DD, Lorton L. Comparison of the relative risk of molar root perforations using various endodontic instrumentation techniques. J Endod. 1983;9:439–47.

25. Isom TL, Marshall JG, Baumgartner JC. Evaluation of root thickness in curved canals after flaring. J Endod. 1995;21:368–71.

26. Wu MK, van der Sluis LW, Wesselink PR. The risk of furcal perforation in mandibular molars using gates-Glidden drills with anticurvature pressure. Oral Surg Oral Med Oral Pathol Oral Radiol Endod. 2005;99:378–82.

27. Ehrhardt IC, Zuolo ML, Cunha RS, et al. Assessment of the separation incidence of mtwo files used with preflaring: prospective clinical study. J Endod. 2012;38:1078–81.

28. Tan BT, Messer HH. The effect of instrument type and preflaring on apical file size determination. Int Endod J. 2002;35:752–8.

29. Reeh ES, Messer HH, Douglas WH. Reduction in tooth stiffness as a result of endodontic and restorative procedures. J Endod. 1989;15:512–6.

30. Clark D, Khademi J. Modern molar endodontic access and directed dentin conservation. Dent Clin N Am. 2010;54:249–73.

31. Estrela C, Decurcio DA, Rossi-Fedele G, Silva JA, Guedes OA, Borges ÁH. Root perforations: a review of diagnosis, prognosis and materials. Braz Dent J. 2018;18:e73.

32. Abou-Rass M, Frank AL, Glick D. The anticurvature filing method to prepare the curved root canal. J Am Dent Assoc. 1980;101:792–4.

33. Haapasalo M, Shen Y. Evolution of nickel-titanium instruments: from past to future. Endod Topics. 2013;29:3–17.

34. Pasqualini D, Alovisi M, Cemenasco A, et al. Micro-computed tomography evaluation of ProTaper Next and BioRace shaping outcomes in maxillary first molar curved canals. J Endod. 2015;41:1706–10.

35. You SY, Bae KS, Baek SH, Kum KY, Shon WJ, Lee W. Lifespan of one nickel-titanium rotary file with reciprocating motion in curved root canals. J Endod. 2010;36:1991–4.

36. De-Deus G, Moreira EJ, Lopes HP, Elias CN. Extended cyclic fatigue life of F2 ProTaper instruments used in reciprocating movement. Int Endod J. 2010;43:1063–8.

37. Buehler W, Gilfrich J, Wiley RC. Effects of low-temperature phase changes on the mechanical properties of alloys near composition TiNi. J Appl Phys. 1963;34:1475–7.

38. Andreasen GF, Morrow RE. Laboratory and clinical analyses of nitinol wire. Am J Orthod Dentofac Orthop. 1978;73:142–51.

39. Civjan S, Huget EF, DeSimon LB. Potential applications of certain nickel-titanium (nitinol) alloys. J Dent Res. 1975;54:89–96.

40. Walia HM, Brantley WA, Gerstein H. An initial investigation of the bending and torsional properties of Nitinol root canal files. J Endod. 1988;14:346–51.

41. Lopes HP, Gambarra-Soares T, Elias CN, et al. Comparison of the mechanical properties of rotary instruments made of conventional nickel-titanium, M-wire, or nickel-titanium alloy in R-phase. J Endod. 2013;39:516–20.

42. Zupanc J, Vahdat-Pajouh N, Schäfer E. New thermomechanically treated NiTi alloys—a review. Int Endod J. 2018;51:1088–103.

43. Zhou H, Peng B, Zheng YF. An overview of the mechanical properties of nickel-titanium endodontic instruments. Endod Topics. 2013;29:42–54.

44. Otsuka K, Wayman CM. Shape memory alloys. 1st ed. Cambridge: Cambridge University Press; 1998.

45. Alapati SB, Brantley WA, Iijima M, et al. Metallurgical characterization of a new nickel-titanium wire for rotary endodontic instruments. J Endod. 2009;35:1589–93.

46. Otsuka K, Ren X. Physical metallurgy of Ti-Ni based shape memory alloys. Prog Mater Sci. 2005;50:511–678.

47. Lee DH, Park B, Saxena A, Serene TP. Enhanced surface hardness by boron implantation in Nitinol alloy. J Endod. 1996;22:543–6.

48. Rapisarda E, Bonaccorso A, Tripi TR, Fragalk I, Condorelli GG. The effect of surface treatments of nickel-titanium files on wear and cutting efficiency. Oral Surg Oral Med Oral Pathol Oral Radiol Endod. 2000;89:363–8.

49. Rapisarda E, Bonaccorso A, Tripi TR, Condorelli GG, Torrisi L. Wear of nickel-titanium endodontic instruments evaluated by scanning electron microscopy: effect of ion implantation. J Endod. 2001;27:588–92.

50. Thompson SA. An overview of nickel-titanium alloys used in dentistry. Int Endod J. 2000;33:297–310.

51. Al-Hadlaq SM, Aljarbou FA, AlThumairy RI. Evaluation of cyclic flexural fatigue of M-wire nickel-titanium rotary instruments. J Endod. 2010;36:305–7.

52. Gao Y, Gutmann JL, Wilkinson K, Maxwell R, Ammon D. Evaluation of the impact of raw materials on the fatigue and mechanical properties of ProFile Vortex rotary instruments. J Endod. 2012;38:398–401.

53. Braga LC, Faria Silva AC, Buono VT, de Azevedo Bahia MG. Impact of heat treatments on the fatigue resistance of different rotary nickel–titanium instruments. J Endod. 2014;40:1494–7.

54. Plotino G, Testarelli L, Al-Sudani D, Pongione G, Grande NM, Gambarini G. Fatigue resistance of rotary instruments manufactured using differ-

ent nickel-titanium alloys: a comparative study. Odontology. 2014;102:31–5.

55. De-Deus G, Silva EJ, Vieira VT, et al. Blue thermomechanical treatment optimizes fatigue resistance and flexibility of the Reciproc files. J Endod. 2017;43:462–6.

56. Silva EJ, Vieira VT, Hecksher F, Dos Santos Oliveira MR, Dos Santos AH, Moreira EJL. Cyclic fatigue using severely curved canals and torsional resistance of thermally treated reciprocating instruments. Clin Oral Investig. 2018;22:2633–8.

57. Silva EJ, Giraldes JFN, de Lima CO, Vieira VTL, Elias CN, Antunes HS. Influence of heat treatment on torsional resistance and surface roughness of nickel-titanium instruments. Int Endod J. 2019;52:1645–51.

58. Bürklein S, Hinschitza K, Dammaschke T, Schäfer E. Shaping ability and cleaning effectiveness of two single-file systems in severely curved root canals of extracted teeth: Reciproc and WaveOne versus Mtwo and ProTaper. Int Endod J. 2012;45:449–61.

59. Plotino G, Ahmed HM, Grande NM, Cohen S, Bukiet F. Current assessment of reciprocation in endodontic preparation: a comprehensive review—part II: properties and effectiveness. J Endod. 2015;41:1939–50.

60. Zanesco C, Só MV, Schmidt S, Fontanella VR, Grazziotin-Soares R, Barletta FB. Apical transportation, centering ratio, and volume increase after manual, rotary, and reciprocating instrumentation in curved root canals: analysis by micro-computed tomographic and digital subtraction radiography. J Endod. 2017;43:486–90.

61. Bürklein S, Flüch S, Schäfer E. Shaping ability of reciprocating single-file systems in severely curved canals: WaveOne and Reciproc versus WaveOne Gold and Reciproc blue. Odontology. 2019;107:96–102.

62. Pedullà E, Lo Savio F, Boninelli S, et al. Torsional and cyclic fatigue resistance of a new nickel-titanium instrument manufactured by electrical discharge machining. J Endod. 2016;42:56–9.

63. Silva EJ, Hecksher F, Antunes HDS, De-Deus G, Elias CN, Vieira VTL. Torsional fatigue resistance of blue-treated reciprocating instruments. J Endod. 2018;44:1038–41.

64. Grande NM, Ahmed HM, Cohen S, Bukiet F, Plotino G. Current assessment of reciprocation in endodontic preparation: a comprehensive review-part I: historic perspectives and current applications. J Endod. 2015;41:1778–83.

65. Frank AL. An evaluation of the Giromatic endodontic handpiece. Oral Surg Oral Med Oral Pathol. 1967;24:419–21.

66. Klayman S, Brilliant J. A comparison of the efficacy of serial preparation versus Giromatic preparation. J Endod. 1974;1:334–7.

67. Turek T, Langeland K. A light microscopic study of the efficacy of the telescopic and the Giromatic preparation of root canals. J Endod. 1982;8:437–43.

68. Lehman JW, Gerstein H. An evaluation of a new mechanized endodontic device: the Endolift. Oral Surg Oral Med Oral Pathol. 1982;53:417–24.

69. Spyropoulos S, Eldeeb ME, Messer HH. The effect of Giromatic files on the preparation shape of severely curved canals. Int Endod J. 1987;20:133–42.

70. Ianno NR, Weine FS. Canal preparation using two mechanical handpieces: distortions, ledging, and potential solutions. Compendium. 1989;10:100–2, 104–5

71. Besse H, Normand B, Labarre P, Woda A. An evaluation of four methods of root canal preparation using 14C urea. J Endod. 1991;17:54–8.

72. Hennequin M, Andre JF, Botta G. Dentin removal efficiency of six endodontic systems: a quantitative comparison. J Endod. 1992;18:601–4.

73. Hülsmann M, Stryga F. Comparison of root canal preparation using different automated devices and hand instrumentation. J Endod. 1993;19:141–5.

74. Dautel-Morazin A, Vulcain JM, Guigand M, Bonnaure-Mallet M. An ultrastructural study of debris retention by endodontic reamers. J Endod. 1995;21:358–61.

75. Yared G. Canal preparation using only one Ni-Ti rotary instrument: preliminary observations. Int Endod J. 2008;41:339–44.

76. Gambarini G, Gergi R, Naaman A, et al. Cyclic fatigue analysis of twisted file rotary NiTi instruments used in reciprocating motion. Int Endod J. 2012;45:802–6.

77. Pedullà E, Grande NM, Plotino G, et al. Influence of continuous or reciprocating motion on cyclic fatigue resistance of 4 different nickel-titanium rotary instruments. J Endod. 2013;39:258–61.

78. Pérez-Higueras JJ, Arias A, de la Macorra JC. Cyclic fatigue resistance of K3, K3XF, and twisted file nickel-titanium files under continuous rotation or reciprocating motion. J Endod. 2013;39:1585–8.

79. Rodrigues E, De-Deus G, Souza E, Silva EJ. Safe mechanical preparation with reciprocation movement without glide path creation: result from a pool of 673 root canals. Braz Dent J. 2016;27:22–7.

80. Cunha RS, Junaid A, Ensinas P, Nudera W, Bueno CE. Assessment of the separation incidence of reciprocating WaveOne files: a prospective clinical study. J Endod. 2014;40:922–4.

81. Plotino G, Grande NM, Porciani PF. Deformation and fracture incidence of Reciproc instruments: a clinical evaluation. Int Endod J. 2015;48:199–205.

82. Bueno CSP, Oliveira DP, Pelegrine RA, Fontana CE, Rocha DGP, Bueno CEDS. Fracture incidence of WaveOne and Reciproc files during root canal preparation of up to 3 posterior teeth: a prospective clinical study. J Endod. 2017;43:705–8.

83. Giansiracusa Rubini A, Plotino G, Al-Sudani D, et al. A new device to test cutting efficiency of mechanical endodontic instruments. Med Sci Monit. 2014;20:374–8.

84. Gambarini G, Giansiracusa Rubini A, Sannino G, et al. Cutting efficiency of nickel-titanium rotary and reciprocating instruments after prolonged use. Odontology. 2016;104:77–81.

85. Pedullà E, Plotino G, Grande NM, et al. Shaping ability of two nickel-titanium instruments activated by continuous rotation or adaptive motion: a micro-computed tomography study. Clin Oral Investig. 2016;20:2227–33.

86. Franco V, Fabiani C, Taschieri S, Malentacca A, Bortolin M, Del Fabbro M. Investigation on the shaping ability of nickel-titanium files when used with a reciprocating motion. J Endod. 2011;37:1398–401.

87. Roane JB, Sabala CL, Duncanson MG Jr. The 'balanced force' concept for instrumentation of curved canals. J Endod. 1985;11:203–11.

88. Hin ES, Wu MK, Wesselink PR, Shemesh H. Effects of self-adjusting file, Mtwo, and ProTaper on the root canal wall. J Endod. 2013;39:262–4.

89. Liu R, Hou BX, Wesselink PR, Wu MK, Shemesh H. The incidence of root microcracks caused by 3 different single-file systems versus the ProTaper system. J Endod. 2013;39:1054–6.

90. Arias A, Lee YH, Peters CI, Gluskin AH, Peters OA. Comparison of 2 canal preparation techniques in the induction of microcracks: a pilot study with cadaver mandibles. J Endod. 2014;40:982–5.

91. Karatas E, Gunduz HA, Kırıcı DO, Arslan H. Incidence of dentinal cracks after root canal preparation with ProTaper Gold, Profile Vortex, F360, Reciproc and ProTaper Universal instruments. Int Endod J. 2016;49:905–10.

92. Saber SE, Schafer E. Incidence of dentinal defects after preparation of severely curved root canals using the Reciproc single-file system with and without prior creation of a glide path. Int Endod J. 2016;49:1057–64.

93. Bahrami P, Scott R, Galicia JC, Arias A, Peters OA. Detecting dentinal microcracks using different preparation techniques: an in situ study with cadaver mandibles. J Endod. 2017;43:2070–3.

94. Kfir A, Elkes D, Pawar A, Weissman A, Tsesis I. Incidence of microcracks in maxillary first premolars after instrumentation with three different mechanize file systems: a comparative ex vivo study. Clin Oral Investig. 2017;21:405–11.

95. De-Deus G, Silva EJ, Marins J, et al. Lack of causal relationship between dentinal microcracks and root canal preparation with reciprocation systems. J Endod. 2014;40:1447–50.

96. De-Deus G, Belladonna FG, Souza EM, et al. Microcomputed tomographic assessment on the effect of ProTaper Next and Twisted File Adaptive systems on dentinal cracks. J Endod. 2015;41:1116–9.

97. De-Deus G, Belladonna FG, Marins JR, et al. On the causality between dentinal defects and root canal preparation: a micro-CT assessment. Braz Dent J. 2016;27:664–9.

98. De-Deus G, Carvalhal JCA, Belladonna FG, et al. Dentinal microcrack development after canal preparation: a longitudinal in situ micro-computed tomography study using a cadaver model. J Endod. 2017;43:1553–8.

99. Bayram HM, Bayram E, Ocak M, Uzuner MB, Geneci F, Celik HH. Micro-computed tomographic evaluation of dentinal microcrack formation after using new heat-treated nickel-titanium systems. J Endod. 2017;43:1736–9.

100. Zuolo ML, De-Deus G, Belladonna FG, et al. Microcomputed tomography assessment of dentinal microcracks after root canal preparation with TRUShape and self-adjusting file systems. J Endod. 2017;43:619–22.

101. De-Deus G, Cavalcante DM, Belladonna FG, et al. Root dentinal microcracks: a post-extraction experimental phenomenon? Int Endod J. 2019;52:857–65.

102. Al-Omari MA, Dummer PM. Canal blockage and debris extrusion with eight preparation techniques. J Endod. 1995;21:154–8.

103. Caviedes-Bucheli J, Moreno JO, Carreno CP, et al. The effect of single-file reciprocating systems on Substance P and Calcitonin gene-related peptide expression in human periodontal ligament. Int Endod J. 2013;46:419–26.

104. Koçak S, Kocak MM, Saglam BC, et al. Apical extrusion of debris using selfadjusting file, reciprocating single-file, and 2 rotary instrumentation systems. J Endod. 2013;39:1278–80.

105. Ozsu D, Karatas E, Arslan H, Topcu MC. Quantitative evaluation of apically extruded debris during root canal instrumentation with ProTaper Universal, ProTaper Next, WaveOne, and self-adjusting file systems. Eur J Dent. 2014;8:504–8.

106. Silva EJ, Sa L, Belladonna FG, et al. Reciprocating versus rotary systems for root filling removal: assessment of the apically extruded material. J Endod. 2014;40:2077–80.

107. Surakanti JR, Venkata RC, Vemisetty HK, et al. Comparative evaluation of apically extruded debris during root canal preparation using ProTaper, Hyflex and Waveone rotary systems. J Conserv Dent. 2014;17:129–32.

108. Teixeira JM, Cunha FM, Jesus RO, et al. Influence of working length and apical preparation size on apical bacterial extrusion during reciprocating instrumentation. Int Endod J. 2014;48:648–53.

109. Tinoco JM, De-Deus G, Tinoco EM, et al. Apical extrusion of bacteria when using reciprocating single-file and rotary multifile instrumentation systems. Int Endod J. 2014;47:560–6.

110. Xavier F, Nevares G, Romeiro MK, et al. Apical extrusion of debris from root canals using reciprocating files associated with two irrigation systems. Int Endod J. 2014;48:661–5.

111. De-Deus G, Neves A, Silva EJ, et al. Apically extruded dentin debris by reciprocating single-

file and multi-file rotary system. Clin Oral Invest. 2015;19:357–61.

112. Caviedes-Bucheli J, Rios-Osorio N, Rey-Rojas M, et al. Substance P and Calcitonin gene-related peptide expression in human periodontal ligament after root canal preparation with Reciproc Blue, WaveOne Gold, XP EndoShaper and hand files. Int Endod J. 2018;51:1358–66.

113. Oliveira PS, da Costa KNB, Carvalho CN, Ferreira MC. Impact of root canal preparation performed by ProTaper Next or Reciproc on the quality of life of patients: a randomized clinical trial. Int Endod J. 2019;52:139–48.

114. Garcia-Font M, Durán-Sindreu F, Morelló S, et al. Postoperative pain after removal of gutta-percha from root canals in endodontic retreatment using rotary or reciprocating instruments: a prospective clinical study. Clin Oral Investig. 2018;22:2623–31.

115. Kakehashi S, Stanley HR, Fitzgerald RJ. The effects of surgical exposures of dental pulps in germ-free and conventional laboratory rats. Oral Surg Oral Med Oral Pathol. 1965;20:340–9.

116. Lin LM, Skribner JE, Gaengler P. Factors associated with endodontic treatment failures. J Endod. 1992;18:625–7.

117. Siqueira JF Jr. Aetiology of root canal treatment failure: why well-treated teeth can fail. Int Endod J. 2001;34:1–10.

118. Sjogren U, Figdor D, Persson S, Sundqvist G. Influence of infection at the time of root filling on the outcome of endodontic treatment of teeth with apical periodontitis. Int Endod J. 1997;30:297–306.

119. Molander A, Warfvinge J, Reit C, Kvist T. Clinical and radiographic evaluation of one- and two-visit endodontic treatment of asymptomatic necrotic teeth with apical periodontitis: a randomized clinical trial. J Endod. 2007;33:1145–8.

120. Haapasalo M, Zandi H, Coil J. Eradication of endodontic infection by instrumentation and irrigation solutions. Endod Topics. 2005;10:77–102.

121. Spangberg LS, Haapasalo M. Rationale and efficacy of root canal medicaments and root filling materials with emphasis on treatment outcome. Endod Topics. 2005;2:35–58.

122. Ordinola-Zapata R, Martins JNR, Bramante CM, Villas-Boas MH, Duarte MH, Versiani MA. Morphological evaluation of maxillary second molars with fused roots: a micro-CT study. Int Endod J. 2017;50:1192–200.

123. Ordinola-Zapata R, Martins JNR, Niemczyk S, Bramante CM. Apical root canal anatomy in the mesiobuccal root of maxillary first molars: influence of root apical shape and prevalence of apical foramina—a micro-CT study. Int Endod J. 2019;52:1218–27.

124. Chaniotis A, Guerreiro D, Kottoor J, et al. Managing complex root canal anatomies. In: Versiani M, Basrani B, Sousa-Neto MD, editors. The root canal anatomy in permanent dentition. Cham: Springer International Publishing; 2018. p. 343–74.

125. Grove C. Why canals should be filled to the dentino-cemental junction. J Am Dent Assoc. 1930;17:293–6.

126. Ricucci D. Apical limit of root canal instrumentation and obturation, part 1. Literature review. Int Endod J. 1999;31:384–93.

127. Ricucci D, Langeland K. Apical limit of root canal instrumentation and obturation, part 2. A histological study. Int Endod J. 1998;31:394–409.

128. Kuttler Y. Microscopic investigation of root apexes. J Am Dent Assoc. 1955;50:544–52.

129. Dummer PM, McGinn JH, Rees DG. The position and topography of the apical canal constriction and apical foramen. Int Endod J. 1984;17:192–8.

130. Versiani MA, Ahmed HM, Sousa-Neto MD, De-Deus G, Dummer PM. Unusual deviation of the main foramen from the root apex. Braz Dent J. 2016;27:589–91.

131. Vieyra JP, Acosta J. Comparison of working length determination with radiographs and four electronic apex locators. Int Endod J. 2011;44:510–8.

132. Martins JN, Marques D, Mata A, Carames J. Clinical efficacy of electronic apex locators: systematic review. J Endod. 2014;40:759–77.

133. Ingle JI. Endodontic cavity preparations. In: Ingle JI, Bakland L, editors. Endodontics. 5th ed. Hamilton: BC Decker Inc.; 2002. p. 405–570.

134. Grossman L, Oliet S, Del Rio C. Endodontic practice. 11th ed. Philadelphia: Lea&Febiger; 1988.

135. Torabinejad M. Passive step-back technique. Oral Surg Oral Med Oral Pathol. 1994;77:398–401.

136. Bolanos OR, Jensen JR. Scanning electron microscope comparisons of the efficacy of various methods of root canal preparation. J Endod. 1980;6:815–22.

137. Weiger R, Bartha T, Kalwitzki M, Lost C. A clinical method to determine the optimal apical preparation size. Part I. Oral Surg Oral Med Oral Pathol Oral Radiol Endod. 2006;102:686–91.

138. Sant'Anna Junior A, Cavenago BC, Ordinola-Zapata R, De-Deus G, Bramante CM, Duarte MA. The effect of larger apical preparations in the danger zone of lower molars prepared using the Mtwo and Reciproc systems. J Endod. 2014;40:1855–9.

139. Silva Santos AM, Portela F, Coelho MS, Fontana CE, De Martin AS. Foraminal deformation after foraminal enlargement with rotary and reciprocating kinematics: a scanning electronic microscopy study. J Endod. 2018;44:145–8.

140. Mickel AK, Chogle S, Liddle J, Huffaker K, Jones JJ. The role of apical size determination and enlargement in the reduction of intracanal bacteria. J Endod. 2007;33:21–3.

141. Rodrigues RCV, Zandi H, Kristoffersen AK, et al. Influence of the apical preparation size and the irrigant type on bacterial reduction in root canal-treated teeth with apical periodontitis. J Endod. 2017;43:1058–63.

142. Plotino G, Ozyurek T, Grande NM, Gundogar M. Influence of size and taper of basic root canal preparation on root canal cleanliness: a scanning electron microscopy study. Int Endod J. 2019;52:343–51.

143. Aksel H, Kucukkaya Eren S, Cakar A, Serper A, Ozkuyumcu C, Azim AA. Effect of instrumentation techniques and preparation taper on apical extrusion of bacteria. J Endod. 2017;43:1008–10.

144. Arora M, Sangwan P, Tewari S, Duhan J. Effect of maintaining apical patency on endodontic pain in posterior teeth with pulp necrosis and apical periodontitis: a randomized controlled trial. Int Endod J. 2016;49:317–24.

145. Silva EJ, Menaged K, Ajuz N, Monteiro MR, Coutinho-Filho TS. Postoperative pain after foraminal enlargement in anterior teeth with necrosis and apical periodontitis: a prospective and randomized clinical trial. J Endod. 2013;39:173–6.

146. Saini HR, Sangwan P, Sangwan A. Pain following foraminal enlargement in mandibular molars with necrosis and apical periodontitis: a randomized controlled trial. Int Endod J. 2016;49:1116–23.

147. Abdulrab S, Rodrigues JC, Al-Maweri SA, Halboub E, Alqutaibi AY, Alhadainy H. Effect of apical patency on postoperative pain: a meta-analysis. J Endod. 2018;44:1467–73.

148. Vera J, Hernandez EM, Romero M, Arias A, van der Sluis LW. Effect of maintaining apical patency on irrigant penetration into the apical two millimeters of large root canals: an in vivo study. J Endod. 2012;38:1340–3.

149. Siqueira JF Jr. Reaction of periapical tissues to root canal treatment: benefits and drawbacks. Endod Topics. 2005;10:123–47.

150. Hülsmann M, Peters OA, Dummer PM. Mechanical preparation of root canals: shaping goals, techniques and means. Endod Topics. 2005;10:30–76.

151. Kerekes K, Tronstad L. Long-term results of endodontic treatment performed with a standardized technique. J Endod. 1979;5:83–90.

152. Hoskinson SE, Ng YL, Hoskinson AE, Moles DR, Gulabivala K. A retrospective comparison of outcome of root canal treatment using two different protocols. Oral Surg Oral Med Oral Pathol Oral Radiol Endod. 2002;93:705–15.

153. Saini HR, Tewari S, Sangwan P, Duhan J, Gupta A. Effect of different apical preparation sizes on outcome of primary endodontic treatment: a randomized controlled trial. J Endod. 2012;38:1309–15.

154. Plotino G, Grande NM. Root canal shaping and debridement. ED. Piccin; 2020.

155. Sjögren U, Hagglund B, Sundqvist G, Wing K. Factors affecting the long-term results of endodontic treatment. J Endod. 1990;16:498–504.

156. Endal U, Shen Y, Knut A, Gao Y, Haapasalo M. A high-resolution computed tomographic study of changes in root canal isthmus area by instrumentation and root filling. J Endod. 2011;37:223–7.

157. Schilder H. Cleaning and shaping the root canal. Dent Clin N Am. 1974;18:269–96.

158. Byström A, Sundqvist G. Bacteriologic evaluation of the efficacy of mechanical root canal instrumentation in endodontic therapy. Scand J Dent Res. 1981;89:321–8.

159. Orstavik D, Kerekes K, Molven O. Effects of extensive apical reaming and calcium hydroxide dressing on bacterial infection during treatment of apical periodontitis: a pilot study. Int Endod J. 1991;24:1–7.

160. Siqueira JF Jr, Rocas IN, Santos SR, Lima KC, Magalhaes FA, de Uzeda M. Efficacy of instrumentation techniques and irrigation regimens in reducing the bacterial population within root canals. J Endod. 2002;28:181–4.

161. van der Sluis LW, Wu MK, Wesselink PR. The efficacy of ultrasonic irrigation to remove artificially placed dentine debris from human root canals prepared using instruments of varying taper. Int Endod J. 2005;38:764–8.

162. Arvaniti IS, Khabbaz MG. Influence of root canal taper on its cleanliness: a scanning electron microscopic study. J Endod. 2011;37:871–4.

163. Zarei M, Javidi M, Afkhami F, Tanbakuchi B, Zadeh MM, Mohammadi MM. Influence of root canal tapering on smear layer removal. N Y State Dent J. 2016;82:35–8.

164. Guimaraes LS, Gomes CC, Marceliano-Alves MF, Cunha RS, Provenzano JC, Siqueira JF Jr. Preparation of oval-shaped canals with TRUShape and Reciproc systems: a micro-computed tomography study using contralateral premolars. J Endod. 2017;43:1018–22.

Root Canal Debridement and Disinfection in Minimally Invasive Preparation

5

Ronald Ordinola-Zapata, Joseph T. Crepps, and Prasanna Neelakantan

Contents

5.1   Introduction

Mechanical and chemical cleaning has been the hallmark of pulp canal space debridement for several decades. Historically, access convenience form has been advocated in order to obtain improved visualization and direct access of the mechanical instruments to the apical third. These concepts have been redefined with the introduc-tion of operating microscopes, cone-beam computed tomography, and heat-treated nickel-titanium alloys. Access through magnification avoids the removal of unnecessary cervical tooth structure during endodontic procedures and super elastic alloys do not rely on straight-line access to shape root canal curvatures. Although these clinical advantages are intuitive, not all of them have been researched extensively from the basic science or the clinical research point of view. The aim of this chapter is to present the current information available in the literature on the irrigation of minimally invasive root canal preparations and to discuss the challenges of this concept to improve the prognosis of root canal treatment.

R. Ordinola-Zapata (✉) · J. T. Crepps
Division of Endodontics, University of Minnesota School of Dentistry, Minneapolis, MN, USA
e-mail: crepp003@umn.edu

P. Neelakantan
Division of Restorative Dental Sciences,
Faculty of Dentistry, The University of Hong Kong,
Hong Kong, Hong Kong

© Springer Nature Switzerland AG 2021
G. Plotino (ed.), *Minimally Invasive Approaches in Endodontic Practice*,
https://doi.org/10.1007/978-3-030-45866-9_5

5.2 Chemical Debridement of the Root Canal System

The goal of endodontic chemo-mechanical prep-aration is to remove the necrotic pulp, microor-ganisms, and the by-products and to generate proper conditions for the subsequent obturation [1, 2]. The ideal way to remove biofilms is by cut-ting and removing the affected dentin using an endodontic instrument; however, it has been demonstrated that a significant surface of the canal space is not accessible to the mechanical action of endodontic instruments due to the com-plex geometry of the root canal space [3–6] (Fig. 5.1). In order to improve the cleaning of these anatomical irregularities such as lateral canals, apical deltas, fins, isthmuses, and other non-instrumented areas, the original anatomy of the root canal space must be modified by increas-ing the natural taper of the main canal. This pro-cedure allows the placement of endodontic instruments into the apical third, improves the flowability of the antimicrobial solutions, and facilitates the placement of intracanal dressings and filling materials, subsequently creating the conditions for healing.

Endodontic infections are polymicrobial and include the presence of facultative and anaerobic bacteria arranged in several layers of cells; these bacterial communities are known as biofilms [7–9] (Fig. 5.2). Clinical studies have shown that the mechanical instrumentation process using dis-tilled water is able to remove the bulk of infected tissue without the use of antimicrobials in teeth with simple anatomy [10]; however, the proce-dure is not consistent requiring several visits. In addition, without the use of an antimicrobial medicament, bacteria can repopulate the root canal system in a matter of days or weeks. Due to these characteristics, nonspecific strong antimi-crobials are necessary. Irrigant solutions can have the ability to disrupt the biofilm architecture, remove or inactivate virulence factors, and dis-solve the necrotic pulp from the root canal space [11–14]. The main challenge for minimally inva-sive endodontic procedures is improving the debridement of the root canal space while decreasing the size of the access and the size of the preparation.

Endodontic irrigant solutions are critical for decontamination of the canal space. Sodium hypochlorite (NaOCl) is the most widely used

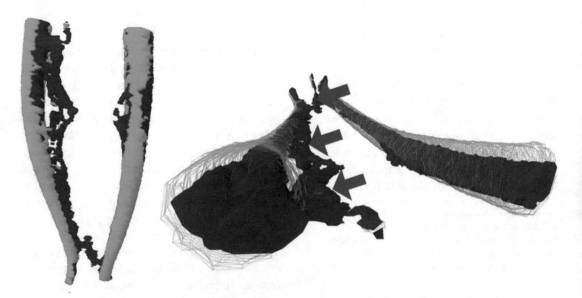

Fig. 5.1 Micro-computed tomography reconstruction of a mesial root of mandibular molar instrumented using nickel-titanium instruments. The pre-operative anatomy is highlighted in red and the removed dentin in green. Several non-instrumented areas can be observed (blue arrows). It can be also observed that the pre-operative anatomy dictates the amount of mechanical removal of the root canal dentine

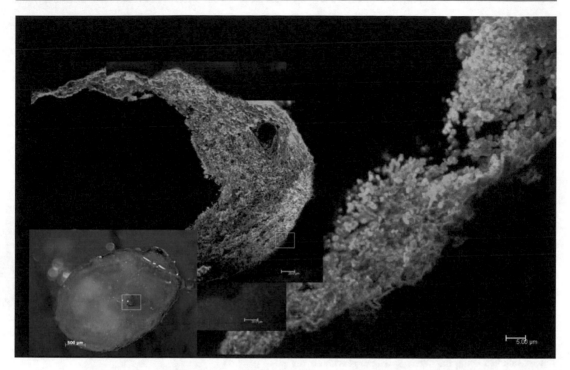

Fig. 5.2 Confocal laser scanning microscopy of a necrotic tooth root canal space (Syto 9 Propidium iodide staining). An organic layer attached to the root canal wall can be observed. A high magnification microphotograph shows a dense biofilm attached to the dentinal walls (right)

solution for root canal disinfection purposes [13]. Its properties include strong antimicrobial activity against both planktonic bacteria and biofilms and presents a unique ability to dissolve organic tissue and endotoxins from necrotic canals [12]. From a chemical point of view, the effectiveness of the NaOCl reaction depends on several factors such as concentration, exposure time, volume, temperature, refreshment rate, and ultrasonic activation among others [2, 15–17]. It is important to note that the root canal space can contain inactivators that are able to reduce the amount of available chlorine; these inactivators are dentin debris, bacterial cells, organic material as pulp tissue, blood, and inflammatory exudates [18]. One limitation of NaOCl has been recognized: it does not remove the smear layer, which allows the compaction of dentin debris against fins or isthmuses (Fig. 5.3). As mentioned before, dentin debris may physically limit the distribution of NaOCl into these areas, thereby inactivating its antimicrobial activity and consequently decreas-

ing its effectiveness [18, 19]. Thus, the use of ethylene-diamine-tetraacetic acid (EDTA) after the decontamination procedures is also recommended for the elimination of inorganic debris before the obturation step [20]. The combination of irrigants mentioned above enhances chemical debridement during endodontic treatment.

In a classic study, Baumgartner and Mader [21] observed that pulp remnants on non-instrumented canal walls of maxillary premolars were completely dissolved by chemical means using 2.5% NaOCl. In the same way, direct contact test experiments have proven that biofilm can be successfully decontaminated and removed from the dentin structure using this agent without the use of mechanical instruments; this effect was observed even using the 1% NaOCl concentration [2] (Fig. 5.4). These findings suggest that mechanical instrumentation can be avoided if an antimicrobial and proteolytic irrigant solution like NaOCl can be delivered and evacuated in an effective way throughout the root canal space.

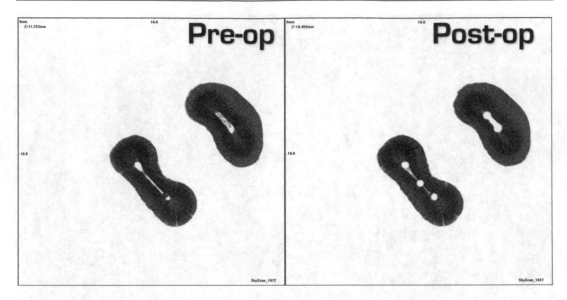

Fig. 5.3 Micro-computed tomography cross-sections at the mid-root level of an extracted mandibular molar with three canals in the mesial root before (left, pre-op) and after (right, post-op) the mechanical instrumentation of the root canals using only syringe irrigation without any activation. To note the accumulation of hard tissue debris in the isthmus and lateral communications among the three mesial root canals in the post-op cross-section. Courtesy of Gianluca Plotino, Rome, Italy

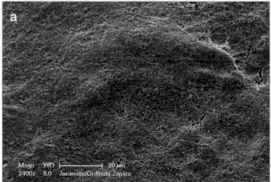 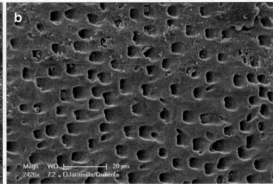

Fig. 5.4 Scanning electron microscope image of an intra-orally infected dentin. A dense contamination can be observed in (**a**). After 5 min of treatment with 5.25% sodium hypochlorite, detachment of the bacterial biofilm is observed, most of dentinal tubules are patent, and minimal amount of debris in the intertubular dentin is present (**b**)

However, several challenges are faced during the irrigation of a minimally shaped canal. Irrigant solutions present a chemical effect: the active compound of NaOCl is the free available chlorine (hypochlorite ions and hypochlorous acid) and those molecules are consumed as the solution reacts with the pulp and other intracanal organic substances, indicating that it has an instable and limited effect [18, 22]. In order to keep the concentration constant, a large volume of irrigant is used to refresh and maintain the effectiveness of the NaOCl solution. The action of irrigation also produces a mechanical effect and forces are applied by the irrigant's flowability capacity [23, 24]. The movement and subsequent cleaning produced by the NaOCl fluid can also be increased in the root canal system by sonic, ultrasonic, or laser-activated irrigation [17, 25]. These methods can create contact between active chlorine molecules and organic tissue or biofilms. To date, little information regarding the ideal taper to use these irrigation devices is found in the literature. Sodium hypochlorite is usually delivered by a syringe and a 30-gauge needle. It is accepted that irrigant exchange can happen at the apical third if the needle is placed at 1 mm from the working length [26]; due to the needle dimensions, the apical third needs to be enlarged until size 0.30 or 0.35 mm. From a technical perspective, minimally invasive endodontic procedures can restrict the flow of the irrigant solution to the apical third, and, therefore, other clinical factors need to be addressed before executing a minimally invasive preparation.

5.3 Clinical Factors and Minimally Invasive Cleaning and Shaping Procedures

Two systematic reviews have addressed the ideal master apical file size required for healing outcomes [27, 28]. The authors concluded that a large instrumentation size may be beneficial for the healing of apical pathosis in teeth with necrotic pulps and periradicular lesions. However, like many systematic reviews in endodontics, the authors stated that limited evidence was available. To date, it is not possible to define the "optimal" master apical size for teeth with vital or necrotic pulps. Several factors can affect the chemical and mechanical debridement of the root canal space and it is the clinician's decision to determine the taper and diameter necessary for the canal debridement in every particular case. Some factors are purely related to the anatomical characteristics of the tooth such as age, curvature, root canal diameter, presence of danger zones, presence of isthmuses, or the transversal cross-section of the root canal space. Other factors are related to the presence of infection or a pathological process, such as the presence of an infected pulp or the presence of internal or external root resorption.

Pulp changes can also be associated with the aging process; age-related changes such as a decrease in dentin permeability, a decrease in cell density, and the constant odontoblastic activity can lead to the presence of calcified pulp chambers. The decrease in the volume of the root canal space due to the increase in dentinal thickness can lead to the presence of calcified canals [29]. Taking this into account, it may be more difficult to debride a mandibular molar in a child or a young adult which may contain a large volume of necrotic tissue and a consistent amount of hard to reach areas compared to an elderly patient with a reduced amount of organic tissue, narrow and calcified canals, and less permeable dentin. On the other hand, irrigants may flow more efficiently in bigger canals and consequently reach inaccessible areas better compared to tight and constricted root canals.

The apical diameter is an important topic often discussed in the literature. The apical third is the critical area for therapeutic reasons; it is in close proximity to the periodontal ligament and the alveolar process. Additionally, it is the most challenging area to disinfect. A series of studies have highlighted the importance of proper apical enlargement for the decontamination of the root canal system [30, 31]. However, one limitation of the endodontic literature regarding this topic is that current studies on root canal apical diameters did not include the age variable in the study design. For example, the median of the apical diameter reported in mandibular incisors presenting a single canal is 0.36 mm [32]; however, the data was widespread distributed and apical diameters ranged approximately from 0.10 to 0.80 mm. In another study [33], the apical anatomy of 60 mandibular molars was measured, the apical analysis at the 1 mm level was reduced to only 19 samples due to the presence of large fins and isthmuses connecting the two mesial canals and the authors found that the average apical diameter was close to 0.35 mm with ranges of 0.20–0.70 mm. Although it is debatable whether these differences should be attributed to the root canal configuration or age, other studies have determined that the complexity of lateral anatomy, including the presence of isthmuses, decreases with age [34].

Curvatures also play a role during the apical diameter selection and subsequent instrumentation and irrigation. The role of root canal curvature and its association to instrument separation is not a common modern problem when compared to the literature found in the previous decades [35]. Nickel-titanium instruments, especially those that are heat-treated and reciprocating, have been demonstrated to present enough flexibility and fatigue resistance to manage difficult curvatures with rare occurrences of separation [35]. However, clinicians should be aware of the amount of dentin that is removed at the cervical level during the instrumentation of severely curved canals or "S"-shaped canals [36]. The delicate balance that exists between the shaping of the canal system and the decrease in dentinal thickness at the cervical level in teeth with severe curvatures needs to be addressed in the future.

The pathological conditions of the periapex and associated structures should also be considered. Several clinical signs can suggest the presence of a long-standing or an aggressive infection such as teeth with furcation involvement, lateral root lesions, and non-circumscribed radiolucencies. These signs could suggest an increase in the virulence of the microbiota of a root canal system, an immunocompromised patient, or a combination of both situations. Another inflammatory condition is internal apical resorption. This pathological process is associated with the presence of apical periodontitis [37]; in this scenario, the size of the last apical millimeters is modified by the pathological process increasing the diameter necessary for the debridement of this critical zone. This scenario is opposite to the presence of a necrotic tooth in an asymptomatic patient with minimal periapical changes and calcified canals. In both situations, clinical judgment is important to determine the dimensions necessary to obtain a proper irrigation and decontamination of the root canal space.

As already discussed in Chap. 3, anatomical evidence of root canal diameters in the apical third of both physiologic and pathologically resorbed situations suggests that anatomical

enlargement of the apical third should be performed to control infection and reduce the presence of debris and remnants in this area. Studies have demonstrated that apical enlargement is required to obtain cleaner root canals in the apical third, but enlargement is not needed to obtain clean canals in the middle and coronal thirds [38]. In fact, increasing the taper of the preparation does not appear to have further influence on canal cleanliness [39, 40]. On the other hand, when considering the middle and coronal third of the root, a recent study has demonstrated that, if a proper irrigation activation technique is used, root canals may be cleaned even in root canals instrumented using a minimal taper of preparation such as 20/0.04 or 25/0.04 [41].

As a consequence, a minimally invasive instrumentation that is respectful of pericervical dentin may be carried out in specific situations with low taper instrument while still allowing for cleaning in the coronal and middle thirds. Minimally invasive instrumentation can increase apical diameters of instrumentation as large as necessary to promote healing without increasing taper of the basic preparation.

5.4 Chemical Cleaning of the Pulp Chamber

One of the key clinical challenges in this context is the lack of definition of a conservative or ultra-conservative access. While it is well accepted that the main purpose of an access cavity is to gain straight-line access to the root canal system, it should also facilitate optimal debridement of the access cavity itself. This implies that the access design should not impede disinfection. The modern access cavity designs recommend preservation of coronal and pericervical tooth structure, without complete de-roofing of the pulp chamber, to enhance the structural integrity of the tooth [42]. One access cavity design where the chamber floor may be subject to compromised debridement is the orifice-directed dentin conservation access or the "truss" access. In this design, cavities are prepared to approach the mesial and distal canal systems in a mandibular molar while for maxillary molars, the mesio- and disto-buccal canals are approached through one cavity and the palatal canal through another [43].

A recent study [44] investigated the debridement of the pulp chamber, the mesial root canals, and the isthmus between the mesiobuccal and mesiolingual root canals of mandibular first molars after preparing access cavities of two designs: the traditional access and the "truss" access. Root canals were prepared to the same dimensions (30/0.06) in all the specimens, using 3% of sodium hypochlorite as the irrigating solution. The experiment was performed on vital molars extracted for periodontal reasons. Using a histological analysis, the percentage of remaining pulp tissue was calculated at the pulp chamber, coronal, middle, and apical thirds of the root canal, and the isthmus region. The pulp chambers were found to house significantly less remaining pulp tissue in the teeth where traditional accesses were prepared (Fig. 5.5). Interestingly, the isthmus and the root canals did not show any significant differences in the percentage of remaining pulp tissue with either access cavity design.

These results have a certain clinical implication such as the debridement of chamber canals and furcation canals have been described in the literature [45, 46]. These portals may serve as a source of continued nutrition to bacterial biofilms that remain within root canals, contributing to the persistence of post-treatment disease. Similarly, in an infected root canal system, egress of microbial biofilms and toxins into the furcal region can initiate periodontal breakdown secondary to endodontic disease. An important consideration in this work was that irrigation was performed only with a syringe and needle. Given the results obtained in vitro by different irrigant activating systems [47], it may be assumed that activated irrigation may result also in cleaner pulp chambers and root canal systems regardless of the access cavity design.

5.5 Minimally Instrumentation and Irrigation Procedures

In some cases, root canals of single-rooted teeth are naturally tapered; a good example is a tooth with an history of dental trauma and arrested tooth development and incomplete root wall formation. In this particular case, the disinfection strategy is supported by minimal instrumentation and the use of antimicrobial solutions and intracanal medicaments to reduce the microbial load. Current research has focused on answering the

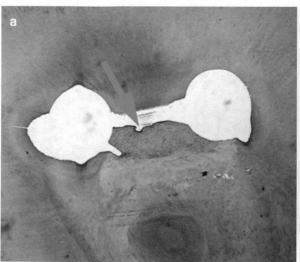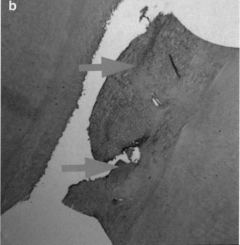

Fig. 5.5 Histological section of the pulp chamber of a mandibular molar after minimally invasive access and sodium hypochlorite syringe irrigation (**a, b**). Remaining organic tissue can be observed between the mesial canals (blue arrow)

question: Can minimally prepared access cavities and root canals be debrided to the same extent as conventional preparations? Few studies have attempted to address this question from a biological stand point (histological or microbiological).

To date, there is substantial evidence that instruments used for root canal preparation do not contact the walls completely and these walls retain pulp tissue or debris even after root canal preparation to sizes 25 or 40 with sodium hypochlorite irrigation using a syringe and needle. Several studies have addressed this important topic in the past in order to investigate the effect of root canal preparation sizes on several outcome measures including cleanliness [39, 48], microbial reduction [30, 49, 50], or healing outcome [51]. Rather surprisingly, all these studies were performed with only syringe-and-needle irrigation.

It has been shown that canals prepared to size 35, 0.04 taper with the SAF 2.0 instrument or size 30, 0.04 XP-Endo Shaper still had remnant pulp tissue (1.36% and 13.29%, respectively) in the apical third of root canals, while another instrument (TRUShape, Dentsply Sirona) with its size 30.06 preparation resulted in <0.5% residual tissue [52]. Three recent studies attempted to compare the histological cleanliness of root canals prepared to small sizes. Using a brush-based supplementary irrigant agitation technique (Finisher GF Brush, MedicNRG, Kibbutz Afikim, Israel), one study reported that oval root canals were significantly cleaner than those where the oval root canals were prepared to a size 25, 0.04 taper and irrigated with a syringe and needle [53]. In this study, root canals were prepared either with a core-less stainless-steel rotary instrument (Gentlefile, MedicNRG, Israel) or a rotary nickel-titanium instrument (EdgeFile X7, EdgeEndo, Albuquerque, New Mexico, USA). Another study [54] prepared root canals using the Reciproc R25 instrument and root canals were irrigated with sodium hypochlorite, which was then activated/agitated using ultrasonics, sonic, or manual dynamic methods. The authors concluded that ultrasonic activation resulted in significantly less pulp tissue remnants than the other methods.

The first study [55] to demonstrate the effect of activated irrigation on cleanliness of premolar canals prepared to small sizes showed that when sodium hypochlorite was ultrasonically activated the root canal cleanliness was not dependent on the apical preparation size (20 vs. 40/ 0.04 taper) (Fig. 5.6). However, when irrigated only with a syringe and a needle, root canals prepared to

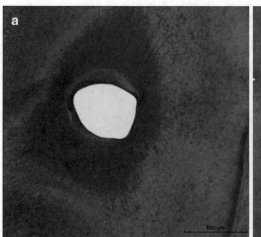 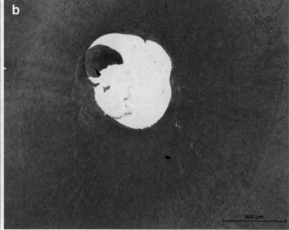

Fig. 5.6 Histological sections of the apical third of a minimally instrumented mandibular premolar (20/0.04) that was irrigated using ultrasonic activation (**a**); no remaining debris could be observed compared to the case that was irrigated without using ultrasonic activation (**b**)

larger sizes were cleaner, despite the fact that they housed substantial amounts of pulp tissue. Furthermore, these results were independent of the cross-sectional shape of the root canal (round vs. oval). The important caveat in this paper, as reported by the authors, was that 18 mL of 3% sodium hypochlorite was used per root canal. Despite this volume, root canals retained significant tissue remnants when irrigated with a syringe and a needle. Thus far, no study has investigated the ability of minimal preparations to debride infected root canals, especially in the apical third. Until such literature demonstrates positive findings, the current evidence suggests that minimal apical preparation of root canals should be eventually limited to vital teeth and with the mandatory use of activated irrigation. In fact, it must be considered the importance of the mechanical cleaning of the root canals, especially in the apical third, when an enlarged apical preparation is performed in infected teeth. In these cases, reduction of intracanal infection through the mechanical removal of infected dentin cannot be substituted by the chemical action of irrigants.

5.6 Adjunctive Systems to Clean Minimally Instrumented Root Canals

Despite the numerous advantages of sodium hypochlorite, its ability to disinfect the root canal environment in a predictable manner has not been consistent in studies [9, 11, 14, 56]. The efficacy of this solution depends not only on its chemical effect but also on the mechanical effectiveness of the irrigation technique and the interaction with intracanal content. Conventional positive apical needle irrigation has shown limitations to improve the delivery of the irrigant solution to the apical third. Nair et al. [57] observed this fact microscopically, demonstrating that residual biofilms can be present in the accessory anatomy of mandibular molars even after instrumentation and full-strength sodium hypochlorite irrigation. In order to improve the antimicrobial and cleaning ability of the irriga-

tion step, several supplemental irrigation techniques have been proposed.

The use of ultrasonic energy during the irrigation procedure is an accepted step to improve the cleaning and disinfection of the root canal space. Ultrasonic activation of the irrigant solution for 1 min using three cycles of 20 s appears to be an accepted time for the final irrigation step [58]. The effectiveness of the ultrasonic irrigation is determined by its capability to create "cavitation" and "acoustic streaming" [58]. Previous researchers have demonstrated that sodium hypochlorite activation enhances the effectiveness of organic tissue dissolution [59], improves the removal of calcium hydroxide medicament [60], increases the removal of hard tissue debris [25], and facilitates the final cleaning during retreatment procedures [61]. Most of these benefits have been confirmed in bench top studies, but at this time, ultrasonic irrigation has not been demonstrated to improve the healing rate of apical periodontitis [62] (Fig. 5.7).

In order to increase the effectiveness of chemical intracanal cleaning, several other systems have been introduced over the years. The EndoVac system (Discus Dental, Culver city, USA), for example, uses apical negative pressure to promote the flow of the irrigant solution placed into the pulp chamber to the apical third of the root canal where the tip of a microcannula is placed. Apical instrumentation to a minimum size of 0.35 mm must be achieved to ensure the microcannula tip (0.32 mm) reaches the apical third. Satisfactory cleaning efficacy at the apical third of extracted teeth with vital pulps in comparison to classic needle irrigation was observed using this system in teeth with simple and complex anatomy [63, 64]. Despite the different mechanism of action of passive ultrasonic irrigation and the EndoVac system, research has shown similar results for the elimination of hard tissue debris [65, 66] and ability to deliver the irrigant solution to the working length [67].

The Lussi's non-instrumentation technique [68, 69] probably represented the first attempt for an actual minimally invasive cleaning of the root canals system. The advantages of the non-instrumentation technique were published in

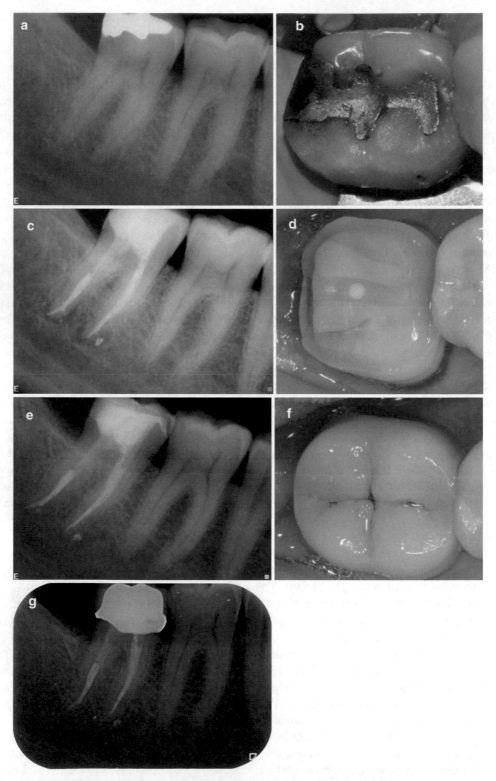

Fig. 5.7 Pre-operative radiograph (**a**) and image (**b**) of a lower right second molar with a caries penetrating the pulp chamber and periapical lesions in both the mesial and distal roots; post-operative radiograph (**c**) and image (**d**) after endodontic treatment and post reconstruction; 5-years radiographic (**e**) and clinical (**f**) control and 10-years radiographic control (**g**), showing the complete resolution of the periapical lesions. (Courtesy of Gianluca Plotino, Rome, Italy)

1993 [69], and, according to its developer, the system was able to create hydrodynamic turbulence and controlled cavitation (25 Hz). Exchange of the irrigant solution (NaOCl) was accomplished using a double tube model. Injection of the irrigant fluid was in the outer tube, while the reflux occurred in the inner tube. The tooth had to be isolated to achieve reduced pressure. This allowed cleaning of the canal system in 10 min independently of the number of root canals presented in the case. The non-instrumentation technique did not recommend the use of hand or rotary instruments. Despite its promising in vitro results, a clinical evaluation of 22 teeth treated by the non-instrumentation technique and extracted after the therapy showed a significant amount of organic debris at the middle and apical third [70].

Following some concepts of the Lussi technique, the GentleWave system (Sonendo, Orange, CA, USA) attempted to propose a novel irrigation system to clean the root canal system after a minimal instrumentation [71–74]. It is based on several principles that include degassing of the irrigant solution, the use of negative pressure, circulation of a fluid in a close circuit, the use of sound waves below and above the ultrasonic spectrum that can propagate the degassed fluid to reach remotes areas of the root canal space, and the use of tissue dissolving agents such as sodium hypochlorite and EDTA. The GWS is able to generate negative pressure [73] in part due to the "closed-loop" system created with a resin platform built by the clinician that serves as a gasket between the tooth and the handpiece. After platform creation, the system delivers high-speed streams of irrigants through a handpiece. The manufacturer of the GentleWave system recommends maximal preservation of the tooth structure so that the suggested dimension of the preparation is a size 20/0.06 taper. According to the manufacturer, contraindications to using the device are resorption, perforations, open apices, and roots adjacent to anatomical structures such as the maxillary sinus or the inferior alveolar nerve. These contraindications may be due to concerns about irrigant extrusion.

During the irrigation process of this system, the irrigant streams collide with a concave plate at the terminus of the handpiece, which is positioned 1 mm or more occlusal to the pulpal floor. After collision with the plate, the irrigants are deflected around the chamber and into the root canals producing a cavitation cloud. Fluid circulation helps replenish reactants and remove byproducts from the root canal system, thus increasing the tissue dissolution rate [71]. Additionally, refreshment is important since bubbles may form and stay at the chemical reaction site and may act as barriers impeding fresh reactants reaching areas such as isthmuses and fins. However, except for one report [72], no study has examined the efficacy of debridement using this system with a minimal instrumentation size. In this study, authors treated extracted human molars instrumented until a 15/0.04 apical size and the GentleWave protocol was compared to the conventional instrumentation and irrigation technique. The results showed that the minimal instrumentation technique was able to clean the canal space significantly better than the conventional irrigation group [72].

A recent debris removal analysis [74] using microCT imaging revealed that accumulated hard tissue debris removal was enhanced with the GentleWave when compared to continuous ultrasonic irrigation (ProUltra PiezoFlow, Dentsply Maillefer; Charlotte, NC); however, there was no difference between the GentleWave and intermittent, passive ultrasonic irrigation (Irrisafe wire, Satelec, Bordeaux, France). Although minimal evidence exists concerning the efficacy of the GentleWave, the device appears to have the ability to debride minimally prepared root canal systems (Fig. 5.8).

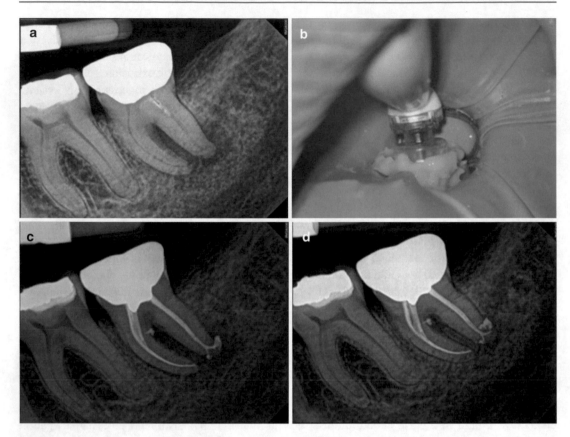

Fig. 5.8 (**a**) Mandibular second molar diagnosed with a previously initiated treatment and asymptomatic apical periodontitis. The root canal was minimally instrumented and irrigated with 500 mL of irrigant solution using the Gentlewave system; the resin platform for the use of the irrigation handpiece can observed in (**b**). Immediate obturation shows the presence of accessory anatomy at the furcation and apical level (**c**). A 3-month follow-up shows that the healing is in process (**d**)

5.7   Concluding Remarks

The disinfection of root canal systems has traditionally been achieved physically, through instrumentation and chemically, through the use of irrigating solutions. Achieving the goal of complete debridement within the root canal space while conserving tooth structure is a delicate balance. Enlarging root canal systems to improve mechanical and chemical debridement can reduce the microbial load present. On the other hand, this enlargement has the potential to structurally weaken teeth due to dentin removal. Modern endodontic research and technology in irrigation have allowed the specialty to explore the long-term preservation of teeth through minimally invasive approaches, or better defined "anatomically invasive approach." This concept means that clinicians can be minimally invasive when possible (i.e., maintain a low taper in the middle and coronal thirds when root canals are originally constricted and with no or minimal taper), while enlarging the canal when anatomy dictates (i.e., apical diameter of preparations needed to touch circumferentially the root canal walls in the apical third) and to activate irrigants and/or use innovative cleaning systems in minimally instrumented canals.

References

1. Peters OA. Current challenges and concepts in the preparation of root canal systems: a review. J Endod. 2004;30:559–67.
2. Ordinola-Zapata R, Bramante CM, Cavenago B, Graeff MS, Gomes de Moraes I, Marciano M, et al. Antimicrobial effect of endodontic solutions used as final irrigants on a dentine biofilm model. Int Endod J. 2012;45:162–8.
3. Paqué F, Balmer M, Attin T, Peters OA. Preparation of oval-shaped root canals in mandibular molars using nickel-titanium rotary instruments: a micro-computed tomography study. J Endod. 2010;36:703–7.
4. Paqué F, Peters OA. Micro-computed tomography evaluation of the preparation of long oval root canals in mandibular molars with the self-adjusting file. J Endod. 2011;37:517–21.
5. Peters OA, Schonenberger K, Laib A. Effects of four Ni-Ti preparation techniques on root canal geometry assessed by micro computed tomography. Int Endod J. 2001;34:221–30.
6. Peters OA, Peters CI, Schonenberger K, Barbakow F. ProTaper rotary root canal preparation: effects of canal anatomy on final shape analysed by micro CT. Int Endod J. 2003;36:86–92.
7. Ricucci D, Siqueira JF. Biofilms and apical periodontitis: study of prevalence and association with clinical and histopathologic findings. J Endod. 2010;36:1277–88.
8. Ricucci D, Loghin S, Siqueira JF. Exuberant biofilm infection in a lateral canal as the cause of short-term endodontic treatment failure: report of a case. J Endod. 2013;39:712–8.
9. Vera J, Siqueira JF, Ricucci D, Loghin S, Fernández N, Flores B, et al. One- versus two-visit endodontic treatment of teeth with apical periodontitis: a histobacteriologic study. J Endod. 2012;38:1040–52.
10. Byström A, Sundqvist G. Bacteriologic evaluation of the efficacy of mechanical root canal instrumentation in endodontic therapy. Scand J Dent Res. 1981;89:321–8.
11. Rodrigues RCV, Zandi H, Kristoffersen AK, Enersen M, Mdala I, Ørstavik D, et al. Influence of the apical preparation size and the irrigant type on bacterial reduction in root canal-treated teeth with apical periodontitis. J Endod. 2017;43:1058–63.
12. Neelakantan P, Herrera DR, Pecorari VGA, Gomes BPFA. Endotoxin levels after chemomechanical preparation of root canals with sodium hypochlorite or chlorhexidine: a systematic review of clinical trials and meta-analysis. Int Endod J. 2019;52:19–27.
13. Zehnder M. Root canal irrigants. J Endod. 2006;32:389–98.
14. Byström A, Sundqvist G. Bacteriologic evaluation of the effect of 0.5 percent sodium hypochlorite in endodontic therapy. Oral Surg Oral Med Oral Pathol. 1983;55:307–12.
15. Del Carpio-Perochena AE, Bramante CM, Duarte MA, Cavenago BC, Villas-Boas MH, Graeff MS, et al. Biofilm dissolution and cleaning ability of different irrigant solutions on intraorally infected dentin. J Endod. 2011;37:1134–8.
16. Ordinola-Zapata R, Bramante CM, Garcia RB, de Andrade FB, Bernardineli N, de Moraes IG, et al. The antimicrobial effect of new and conventional endodontic irrigants on intra-orally infected dentin. Acta Odontol Scand. 2013;71:424–31.
17. Ordinola-Zapata R, Bramante CM, Aprecio RM, Handysides R, Jaramillo DE. Biofilm removal by 6% sodium hypochlorite activated by different irrigation techniques. Int Endod J. 2014;47:659–66.
18. Arias-Moliz MT, Morago A, Ordinola-Zapata R, Ferrer-Luque CM, Ruiz-Linares M, Baca P. Effects of dentin debris on the antimicrobial properties of sodium hypochlorite and etidronic acid. J Endod. 2016;42:771–5.
19. Morago A, Ordinola-Zapata R, Ferrer-Luque CM, Baca P, Ruiz-Linares M, Arias-Moliz MT. Influence of smear layer on the antimicrobial activity of a sodium hypochlorite/etidronic acid irrigating solution in infected dentin. J Endod. 2016;42:1647–50.
20. Neelakantan P, Ounsi HF, Devaraj S, Cheung GSP, Grandini S. Effectiveness of irrigation strategies on the removal of the smear layer from root canal dentin. Odontology. 2019;107:142–9.
21. Baumgartner JC, Mader CL. A scanning electron microscopic evaluation of 4 root canal irrigation regimens. J Endod. 1987;13:147–57.
22. Estrela C, Estrela CR, Barbin EL, Spanó JC, Marchesan MA, Pécora JD. Mechanism of action of sodium hypochlorite. Braz Dent J. 2002;13:113–7.
23. Boutsioukis C, Lambrianidis T, Verhaagen B, Versluis M, Kastrinakis E, Wesselink PR, et al. The effect of needle-insertion depth on the irrigant flow in the root canal: evaluation using an unsteady computational fluid dynamics model. J Endod. 2010;36:1664–8.
24. Boutsioukis C, Gogos C, Verhaagen B, Versluis M, Kastrinakis E, Van der Sluis LW. The effect of apical preparation size on irrigant flow in root canals evaluated using an unsteady Computational Fluid Dynamics model. Int Endod J. 2010;43:874–81.
25. van der Sluis LW, Gambarini G, Wu MK, Wesselink PR. The influence of volume, type of irrigant and flushing method on removing artificially placed dentine debris from the apical root canal during passive ultrasonic irrigation. Int Endod J. 2006;39:472–6.
26. Chow TW. Mechanical effectiveness of root canal irrigation. J Endod. 1983;9:475–9.
27. Aminoshariae A, Kulild JC. Master apical file size—smaller or larger: a systematic review of healing outcomes. Int Endod J. 2015;48:639–47.
28. Aminoshariae A, Kulild J. Master apical file size—smaller or larger: a systematic review of microbial reduction. Int Endod J. 2015;48:1007–22.
29. Carvalho TS, Lussi A. Age-related morphological, histological and functional changes in teeth. J Oral Rehabil. 2017;44:291–8.
30. Card SJ, Sigurdsson A, Orstavik D, Trope M. The effectiveness of increased apical enlargement in reducing intracanal bacteria. J Endod. 2002;28:779–83.

31. Dalton BC, Orstavik D, Phillips C, Pettiette M, Trope M. Bacterial reduction with nickel-titanium rotary instrumentation. J Endod. 1998;24:763–7.
32. Milanezi de Almeida M, Bernardineli N, Ordinola-Zapata R, Villas-Bôas MH, Amoroso-Silva PA, Brandão CG, et al. Micro-computed tomography analysis of the root canal anatomy and prevalence of oval canals in mandibular incisors. J Endod. 2013;39:1529–33.
33. Villas-Bôas MH, Bernardineli N, Cavenago BC, Marciano M, Del Carpio-Perochena A, de Moraes IG, et al. Micro-computed tomography study of the internal anatomy of mesial root canals of mandibular molars. J Endod. 2011;37:1682–6.
34. Peiris HR, Pitakotuwage TN, Takahashi M, Sasaki K, Kanazawa E. Root canal morphology of mandibular permanent molars at different ages. Int Endod J. 2008;41:828–35.
35. Cunha RS, Junaid A, Ensinas P, Nudera W, Bueno CE. Assessment of the separation incidence of reciprocating WaveOne files: a prospective clinical study. J Endod. 2014;40:922–4.
36. Ordinola-Zapata R, Bramante CM, Duarte MA, Cavenago BC, Jaramillo D, Versiani MA. Shaping ability of reciproc and TF adaptive systems in severely curved canals of rapid microCT-based prototyping molar replicas. J Appl Oral Sci. 2014;22:509–15.
37. Vier FV, Figueiredo JA. Internal apical resorption and its correlation with the type of apical lesion. Int Endod J. 2004;37:730–7.
38. Plotino G, Grande NM, Tocci L, Testarelli L, Gambarini G. Influence of different apical preparations on root canal cleanliness in human molars: a SEM study. J Oral Maxillofac Res. 2014;5:e4.
39. Usman N, Baumgartner JC, Marshall JG. Influence of instrument size on root canal debridement. J Endod. 2004;30:110–2.
40. Arvaniti IS, Khabbaz MG. Influence of root canal taper on its cleanliness: a scanning electron microscopic study. J Endod. 2011;37:871–4.
41. Plotino G, Özyürek T, Grande NM, Gündoğar M. Influence of size and taper of basic root canal preparation on root canal cleanliness: a scanning electron microscopy study. Int Endod J. 2019;52:343–51.
42. Clark D, Khademi JA. Case studies in modern molar endodontic access and directed dentin conservation. Dent Clin N Am. 2010;54:275–89.
43. Narayana P. Access cavity preparation. In: Publishing Q, editor. Best practices in endodontics. 1st ed. Chicago, IL: Quintessene Publishing; 2015. p. 89–104.
44. Neelakantan P, Khan K, Hei Ng GP, Yip CY, Zhang C, Pan Cheung GS. Does the orifice-directed dentin conservation access design debride pulp chamber and mesial root canal systems of mandibular molars similar to a traditional access design? J Endod. 2018;44:274–9.
45. Vertucci FJ, Williams RG. Furcation canals in the human mandibular first molar. Oral Surg Oral Med Oral Pathol. 1974;38:308–14.
46. Gutmann JL. Prevalence, location, and patency of accessory canals in the furcation region of permanent molars. J Periodontol. 1978;49:21–6.
47. Plotino G, Cortese T, Grande NM, Leonardi DP, Di Giorgio G, Testarelli L, et al. New technologies to improve root canal disinfection. Braz Dent J. 2016;27:3–8.
48. Fornari VJ, Silva-Sousa YT, Vanni JR, Pecora JD, Versiani MA, Sousa-Neto MD. Histological evaluation of the effectiveness of increased apical enlargement for cleaning the apical third of curved canals. Int Endod J. 2010;43:988–94.
49. Coldero LG, McHugh S, MacKenzie D, Saunders WP. Reduction in intracanal bacteria during root canal preparation with and without apical enlargement. Int Endod J. 2002;35:437–46.
50. Orstavik D, Kerekes K, Molven O. Effects of extensive apical reaming and calcium hydroxide dressing on bacterial infection during treatment of apical periodontitis: a pilot study. Int Endod J. 1991;24:1–7.
51. Azim AA, Griggs JA, Huang GT. The Tennessee study: factors affecting treatment outcome and healing time following nonsurgical root canal treatment. Int Endod J. 2016;49:6–16.
52. Lacerda MFLS, Marceliano-Alves MF, Pérez AR, Provenzano JC, Neves MAS, Pires FR, et al. Cleaning and shaping oval canals with 3 instrumentation systems: a correlative micro-computed tomographic and histologic study. J Endod. 2017;43:1878–84.
53. Neelakantan P, Khan K, Li KY, Shetty H, Xi W. Effectiveness of supplementary irrigant agitation with the Finisher GF Brush on the debridement of oval root canals instrumented with the Gentlefile or nickel titanium rotary instruments. Int Endod J. 2018;51:800–7.
54. Varela P, Souza E, de Deus G, Duran-Sindreu F, Mercadé M. Effectiveness of complementary irrigation routines in debriding pulp tissue from root canals instrumented with a single reciprocating file. Int Endod J. 2019;52:475–83.
55. Lee OYS, Khan K, Li KY, Shetty H, Abiad RS, Cheung GSP, et al. Influence of apical preparation size and irrigation technique on root canal debridement: a histological analysis of round and oval root canals. Int Endod J. 2019;52:1366–76.
56. Bystrom A, Sundqvist G. The antibacterial action of sodium hypochlorite and EDTA in 60 cases of endodontic therapy. Int Endod J. 1985;18:35–40.
57. Nair PN, Henry S, Cano V, Vera J. Microbial status of apical root canal system of human mandibular first molars with primary apical periodontitis after "one-visit" endodontic treatment. Oral Surg Oral Med Oral Pathol Oral Radiol Endod. 2005;99:231–52.
58. van der Sluis LWM, Versluis M, Wu MK, Wesselink PR. Passive ultrasonic irrigation of the root canal: a review of the literature. Int Endod J. 2007;40:415–26.
59. Conde AJ, Estevez R, Loroño G, Valencia de Pablo Ó, Rossi-Fedele G, Cisneros R. Effect of sonic and ultra-

sonic activation on organic tissue dissolution from simulated grooves in root canals using sodium hypochlorite and EDTA. Int Endod J. 2017;50:976–82.

60. van der Sluis LW, Wu MK, Wesselink PR. The evaluation of removal of calcium hydroxide paste from an artificial standardized groove in the apical root canal using different irrigation methodologies. Int Endod J. 2007;40:52–7.

61. Cavenago BC, Ordinola-Zapata R, Duarte MA, del Carpio-Perochena AE, Villas-Bôas MH, Marciano MA, et al. Efficacy of xylene and passive ultrasonic irrigation on remaining root filling material during retreatment of anatomically complex teeth. Int Endod J. 2014;47:1078–83.

62. Liang YH, Jiang LM, Jiang L, Chen XB, Liu YY, Tian FC, et al. Radiographic healing after a root canal treatment performed in single-rooted teeth with and without ultrasonic activation of the irrigant: a randomized controlled trial. J Endod. 2013;39:1218–25.

63. Nielsen BA, Craig BJ. Comparison of the EndoVac system to needle irrigation of root canals. J Endod. 2007;33:611–5.

64. Susin L, Liu Y, Yoon JC, Parente JM, Loushine RJ, Ricucci D, et al. Canal and isthmus debridement efficacies of two irrigant agitation techniques in a closed system. Int Endod J. 2010;43:1077–90.

65. Silva EJNL, Carvalho CR, Belladonna FG, Prado MC, Lopes RT, De-Deus G, et al. Micro-CT evaluation of different final irrigation protocols on the removal of hard-tissue debris from isthmus-containing mesial root of mandibular molars. Clin Oral Investig. 2019;23:681–7.

66. Freire LG, Iglecias EF, Cunha RS, Dos Santos M, Gavini G. Micro-computed tomographic evaluation of hard tissue debris removal after different irrigation methods and its influence on the filling of curved canals. J Endod. 2015;41:1660–6.

67. Munoz HR, Camacho-Cuadra K. In vivo efficacy of three different endodontic irrigation systems for irrigant delivery to working length of mesial canals of mandibular molars. J Endod. 2012;38:445–8.

68. Lussi A, Portmann P, Nussbächer U, Imwinkelried S, Grosrey J. Comparison of two devices for root canal cleansing by the noninstrumentation technology. J Endod. 1999;25:9–13.

69. Lussi A, Nussbächer U, Grosrey J. A novel noninstrumented technique for cleansing the root canal system. J Endod. 1993;19:549–53.

70. Attin T, Buchalla W, Zirkel C, Lussi A. Clinical evaluation of the cleansing properties of the noninstrumental technique for cleaning root canals. Int Endod J. 2002;35:929–33.

71. Haapasalo M, Wang Z, Shen Y, Curtis A, Patel P, Khakpour M. Tissue dissolution by a novel multisonic ultracleaning system and sodium hypochlorite. J Endod. 2014;40:1178–81.

72. Molina B, Glickman G, Vandrangi P, Khakpour M. Evaluation of root canal debridement of human molars using the GentleWave system. J Endod. 2015;41:1701–5.

73. Charara K, Friedman S, Sherman A, Kishen A, Malkhassian G, Khakpour M, et al. Assessment of apical extrusion during root canal irrigation with the novel GentleWave system in a simulated apical environment. J Endod. 2016;42:135–9.

74. Chan R, Versiani MA, Friedman S, Malkhassian G, Sousa-Neto MD, Leoni GB, et al. Efficacy of 3 supplementary irrigation protocols in the removal of hard tissue debris from the mesial root canal system of mandibular molars. J Endod. 2019;45:923–9.

Filling of Root Canals After Minimally Invasive Preparation

6

Gilberto Debelian and Gianluca Plotino

Contents

6.1 Introduction

Instrumentation creates space for canal irrigation, disinfection and root filling. All of these phases have an impact on the method and size of instrumentation, depending on the philosophy of the dentist and the limitations and requirements set by the equipment used in each phase,

G. Debelian
Private Practice, Endo Inn Endodontic Training Center, Oslo, Norway

G. Plotino (✉)
Private Practice, Grancde Plotino and Torsello - Studio di Odontoiatria, Rome, Italy
e-mail: endo@gianlucaplotino.com

© Springer Nature Switzerland AG 2021
G. Plotino (ed.), *Minimally Invasive Approaches in Endodontic Practice*,
https://doi.org/10.1007/978-3-030-45866-9_6

especially in root filling. Optimal root filling has many requirements which have been difficult if not impossible to fulfil. Gutta-percha has been and still is the core material of choice in root fillings, but it requires the use of a sealer in order to obtain better short- and long-term seal. Thermoplastic obturation methods and warm vertical condensation techniques have been introduced in the 70s to overcome the vulnerability of the most popular endodontic sealer materials which undergo shrinkage and wash out upon setting. In order to apply such obturation techniques there is a need for an access cavity with a large tapered preparation on the coronal part of the root canals to allow a hydraulic condensation of a soften gutta-percha, minimizing the layer of such sealers. The use of large tapered instruments has been shown to weaken the tooth potentially leaving the root unnecessarily susceptible to fracture [1, 2].

With the introduction of the operative microscope almost 3 decades ago, the concept of minimally invasive endodontics has gradually been introduced and taught to specialists and general practitioners (Fig. 6.1a, b). The use of operative microscope with high magnification provides a high-precision clinical work preventing unnecessary removal of tooth structure that is imperative for successful treatment, thus reducing tooth weakening, non-restorable cases, micro-cracks and coronal leakage.

This chapter presents a panorama of presently available material and methods suggested for root canal filling to adapt to the minimally invasive preparation concept.

6.2   Terminology

The term obturation is what most people use to describe the third stage of root canal therapy after root canal instrumentation and irrigation. Obturation by definition is to "close off a space", but makes no requirement for filling that space [3–7]. In fact, the term obturation is more appropriate for a retro-filling in apicoectomy procedures, since the root canal space is closed off but the contents of the root canal are not disturbed. Root canal filling is a much more appropriate description of what clinicians are attempting and thus a better term to use.

6.3   Rational for Root Canal Filling

Root canal filling is performed as the third phase of root canal therapy after microbial control through mechanical shaping and chemical cleaning, where microbes are prevented from re-entering the root canal space (vital teeth) following their removal by instrumentation and irrigation (infected necrotic teeth). The aim of root canal filling is to maintain the low microbial load left within the root canal system below the threshold for clinical and radiographic success (Fig. 6.2), limiting the intra-canal infection found in the main canal and dentinal tubules communicating with the peri-radicular tissues (Fig. 6.3).

It also assumes that a coronal filling of sufficient quality will be placed as soon as possible after the canal/s are filled. At the present time, it is also assumed that it is not possible to sterilize the root canal and physically remove all biofilms from

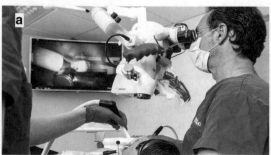
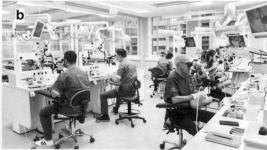

Fig. 6.1 (**a**) The use of operative microscope in the endodontic specialty practice; (**b**) systematic teaching to general practitioners on the use of operative microscope

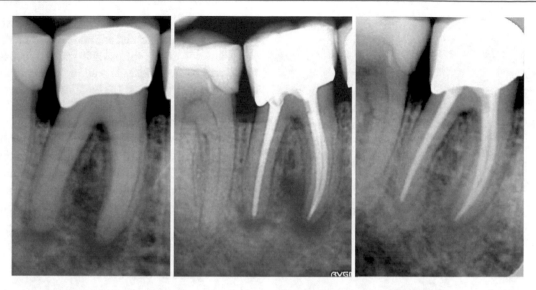

Fig. 6.2 Endodontic therapy on a non-vital case with an apical periodontitis. With an adequate treatment protocol to control intra-canal infection, the root filling will main- tain the low microbial load below the threshold for clini- cal and radiographic success

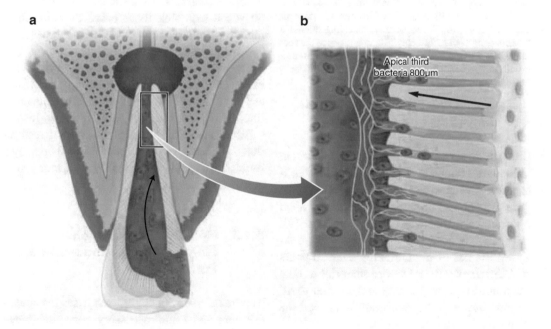

Fig. 6.3 Illustration demonstrating the intra-canal infection in the main canal (**a**) and in the dentinal tubules (**b**)

its complex anatomy. Thus, there are three basic requirements from a root canal filling [8] (Fig. 6.4):

(a) Guarantee a tight apical seal to prevent influx of periapical fluids, which may nourish sur- viving microbes in the root canal.

(b) Isolate surviving microbes in the root canal space so that they cannot multiply and/or communicate with the peri-radicular tissues.

(c) Stop coronal leakage after the root canal and crown is filled.

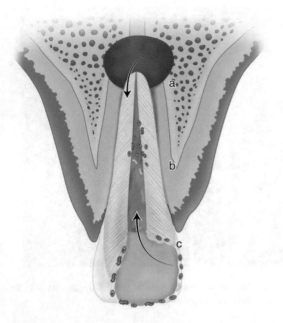

Fig. 6.4 Three basic requirements from a root canal filling: (**a**) Guarantee a tight apical seal to prevent influx of periapical fluids, which may nourish surviving microbes in the root canal; (**b**) Isolate surviving microbes in the root canal space so that they cannot multiply and/or communicate with the peri-radicular tissues; (**c**) Stop coronal leakage after the root canal and crown is filled

6.4 Materials and Techniques

Filling the root canal requires the development of adequate materials and techniques to maximize the properties of those materials. Figure 6.5 reports the list of Grossman's ideal properties of a root canal filling material [9]. Not much has changed since Grossman constructed his list of requirements over 70 years ago. Clinicians still use a core material to take up as much space as possible and a sealer to fill the voids between the core material(s) and the dentin.

6.4.1 Core Materials

Gutta-percha (GP) and silver points have been the most used core materials over the last 100 years [10–12]. In 2017, a position statement

from the American Association of Endodontists [13] recommended to discontinue the use of silver points due to: (1) corrosion in the presence of blood and tissue fluids; (2) staining of the tooth and surrounding tissues; (3) inability to perform post and cores after root filling and (4) difficulty to remove in apical surgery retrograde preparations. Thus, GP is the primary core material in use today. Cones of GP contain approximately 20% GP and 80% fillers used for colouring and radiographic contrast [14]. GP comes in its natural form (alpha phase) or manufactured form (beta phase) [14–17].

6.4.2 Types of Sealers

As mentioned, sealers are the most important factor for the quality of the seal in root filling. Many different sealers have been used over the last 50 years, including those based on chloroform mixed with GP, zinc oxide–eugenol, calcium hydroxide, silicon, glass-ionomer cement and epoxy or methacrylate resins [14, 17, 18]. All are mixed and introduced in the canal in a fluid form and have enough working time to allow the practitioner to place the root canal filling to his/her satisfaction before placing the coronal restoration. It is then assumed they will then harden by a setting reaction in a reasonable time after placement into the canal.

6.4.3 How Well Do Traditional Filling Materials and Methods Perform?

The traditional root filling comprises a standard GP core and round accessory cones combined with a sealer to fill the space between the GP points themselves and the GP and the dentinal walls. The GP core material acts only as a filler and does not seal the canal. In fact, when tested in an in vitro model microbes are able to travel throughout the length of the canal in 2 h if only gutta-percha is present in the canal without sealer

[19]. The leakage can be delayed for up to 30 days with the use of a sealer [4] (Fig. 6.6).

Despite sealers are the materials in root filling that actually provide resistance to leakage, traditional sealers have serious shortcomings in that they generally shrink on setting and wash out in the presence of tissue fluids [4, 14, 20–27] (Fig. 6.7).

In addition sealers do not bond to the gutta-percha core material, leaving gaps (Fig. 6.8) with potential for microbial leakage (Fig. 6.9) when the sealer shrinks on setting [28].

Thus, in order to maximize the sealing ability of sealers, but minimize their shortcomings, the sealer used in traditional root canal filling techniques needed to be as thin as possible. Since the GP core is generally produced in a cone shape with a round diameter, it is very difficult to keep the sealer thin in most root canals as they are generally irregular in shape and may have many communications.

Many in vitro, in vivo animal studies and clinical outcome studies on the traditional methods of

Fig. 6.5 Grossman's ideal properties of a root canal filling material

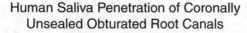

- Introduced **easily** in to the root canal
- It should **impervious** to moisture
- It should **seal** the canal laterally as well as apically
- It should **not shrink** after being inserted
- It should be **bacteriostatic** or least should discourage growth
- It should be **radiopaque**
- It should not **stain** tooth structure
- It should **not irritate** periapical tissue
- It should be **easily removed** from the root canal it necessary
- It should be **sterile** or easily and quickly sterilised immediately **before** insertion

Grossman, 1936

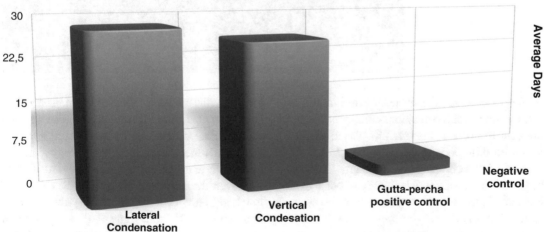

Fig. 6.6 In vitro evaluation of saliva penetration of root canals. Note that the seal achieved with GP alone is indistinguishable from the negative control. (From Khayat et al. [4])

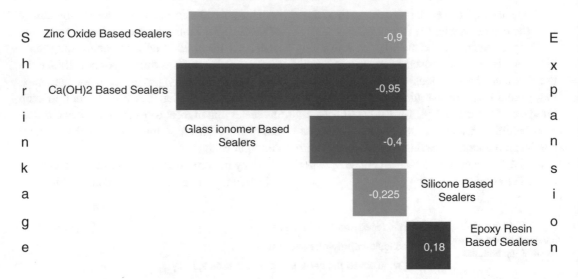

Fig. 6.7 Table showing expansion/contraction of popular sealers. Silicone and epoxy resin-based sealers expand slightly before shrinking [14]

Fig. 6.8 SEM image of the cut surface of a root filled with gutta-percha and a resin-based sealer. Note the gap between the GP and sealer (courtesy of Dr. Eldeniz [28])

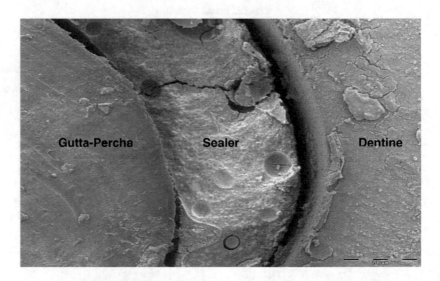

single-cone or lateral condensation techniques uniformly show that the traditional filling materials do not seal the root canal [27, 28]. Sabeti et al. [4] found no difference in the outcome when a canal was root filled compared to left empty. This study emphasizes the susceptible quality of our root filling techniques and the importance of the coronal restoration for root canal success [4–18, 20–27].

A review and meta-analysis showed no differences in the clinical outcome of root canal obturation by warm GP or cold lateral condensation, except in overextension that was more likely to occur in the warm GP obturation group in comparison with the lateral condensation group [29]. Friedman et al. in outcome studies also showed no statistical differences in the obturation methods used (lateral and vertical condensation) on teeth with and without apical periodontitis [30]. However, the recall rate of these studies was very low and below 20%. In the latest publication of these studies [31], Chevigny et al. discussed that obturation techniques appeared as a significant outcome predictor for teeth with apical periodontitis, but it should be important to confirm these data with properly designed randomized controlled trials [30].

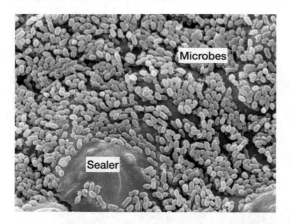

Fig. 6.9 SEM picture with microbial leakage when a resin-based sealer shrinks on setting (courtesy of Dr. Ørstavik [25])

6.5   Attempts to Improve Root Canal Fillings

The most influential attempt to improve the performance of root canal filling was by Herbert Schilder in the 1960s [32, 33]. Schilder recognized that one of the problems in filling was that the round gutta-percha core materials were unable to keep the sealer in a thin layer because the canals themselves were mostly oval. Thus, in too many areas the sealer was thick and vulnerable to shrinkage and wash out. Schilder heated gutta-percha in order to make it pliable and able to be moved into these non-round areas and keeping the sealer as thin as possible. Additionally, the hydraulic nature of the technique resulted in many accessory canals being visualized on the radiograph due to the sealer and/or gutta-percha being forced into these small spaces, creating a detailed picture on the radiograph with the impression that a superior "3D" filling had been placed (Fig. 6.10). This is the well-known warm vertical compaction technique by Schilder [34].

The logic behind this technique was comprehensive and the outstanding radiographic results were universally accepted as a technique for specialists or "advanced" generalists. The technique has been improved on the following years after its introduction and was named as continuous wave compaction technique by Buchanan [35].

This technique has several phases and requires a selection of instruments and devices: (1) selection of a greater taper GP corresponding to the last instrument; (2) selection of a plugger to be pre-fitted 4–5 mm from the working length; (3) the canal is coated with a thin layer of root canal sealer; (4) the primary GP cone is inserted at the working length (WL) minus 0.5 mm; (5) compaction heat carrier-plugger instrument is activated and stopped to the reference point (4–5 mm from WL); (6) the apical GP is now lightly condensed with selected hand pluggers; (7) a layer of sealer may be re-applied on the coronal part of the apical GP plug; (8) the back-filling of the coronal part is done by using a GP gun; (9) the coronal part now is condensed with large pluggers.

However, this technique can be technically sensitive, and it may do little to overcome the weak points of the original single-cone or lateral condensation techniques [30]. Once the heated gutta-percha cools, it may shrink even more than the sealer does on setting [36, 37]. In addition, the shrinkage of the GP and sealer (instead of sealer only) may result in a larger gap between the gutta-percha and sealer [28], exaggerating the weakness of no bond between the two. Furthermore, many points on the root canal wall force the sealer out, resulting in gutta-percha filling the canal without any sealer in that particular area of the root [38].

Even if the warm GP techniques may leave less voids and obtain a better 3D compaction of the filling materials [39, 40], other studies have shown no benefit in sealing the root canal with the heated vertical condensation technique compared to the traditional lateral condensation technique [38].

A recently identified complication of the warm compaction technique is the need for a larger taper to be used to instrument the mid-coronal portion of the canal, in order to place a heated plugger within 4 mm of the working length. The use of large tapered instruments (NiTi orifice openers or Gates-Glidden burs) has recently been shown to produce micro-fractures in the root [41–45]. Additionally, the thinning of the root dentin proportionally weakens the tooth

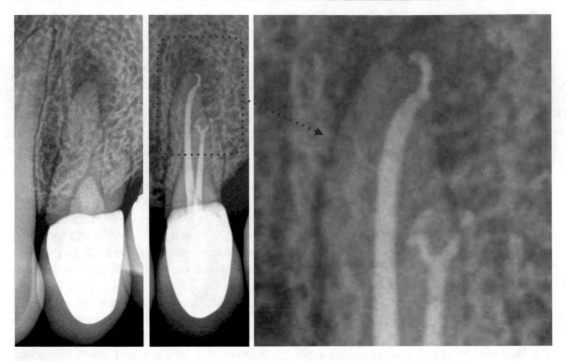

Fig. 6.10 Upper premolar root filled with the well-known warm vertical compaction technique

potentially leaving the root unnecessarily susceptible to fracture [42, 44–46].

This may be the main limitation to adopt this technique in particularly conservative root canal preparation and access cavity: in most of these cases the clinician may have difficulties to keep the heat carrier-plugger to 4–5 mm from the working length to properly execute the warm compaction of the apical GP. If it will remain more coronal than 5 mm from the working length, GP master point will be not modified by the heat in its last millimetres and the consequence may be presumably the presence of a single cone surrounded (covered) by sealer in the apical third of the canal.

To overcome the several and sensitive steps on the continuous wave compaction technique, a carried-based GP material and technique has been developed [47]. Thermafill (Dentsply-Sirona Endodontics, Baillagues, Switzerland) has been the most popular of these carried-based GP materials. Pirani et al. [48] have recently shown on a 5-year retrospective study that the survival and healing rates after root canal treatment with Thermafil were comparable to those

previously reported for conventional root filling techniques. The major disadvantage of a carrier-based technique in minimally invasive endodontic procedures may be the technical difficulty to insert the obturator through small coronal spaces without a straight-line access. This may increase the possibility to bend the obturator in an unnatural way, to detach the GP from the carrier, to cover the orifices of the other root canals of multi-rooted teeth with excess of GP flowing coronally and to fill undercuts in conservative access cavities with stocky sealers and GP, being very difficult to be cleaned after filling procedures.

Another attempt to improve root filling performance was the introduction of a methacrylate core-sealer resin [49]. The idea behind of this newly introduced material was to effectively bond to the resin core material (monoblock), thus eliminating one gap consistently present in the other techniques. The methacrylate resin was also aimed to chemically bond to clean dentin on the root walls. The use of these materials did not require large tapered canal preparation and warm vertical condensation techniques to minimize the layer of the sealer used which fits perfectly on the minimally invasive endodontic preparations.

While in vitro and in vivo studies results for this material were generally positive compared to traditional techniques [50–55], Strange et al. [56] have recently demonstrated on a low recall rate (21.6%) study, a statistically poorer clinical outcome for this material (Resilon) and technique compared to traditional gutta-percha/AH Plus. Thus, methacrylate-based sealers demonstrated the same shortcomings of the traditional sealers (shrinkage and wash out) and are also extremely technique-sensitive materials. In routine root canal instrumentation techniques, where sodium hypochlorite is used, the oxygen that is produced made the sealer particularly difficult to use and resulted in many cases where the sealer failed to set or disintegrate [57].

6.6 Bioceramic Materials

Bioceramics (BC) are ceramic materials specifically designed for medical and dental use. During the 1960s and 1970s, these materials were developed for use in the human body such as joint replacement, bone plates, bone cement, artificial ligaments and tendons, blood vessel prostheses, heart valves, skin repair devices (artificial tissue), cochlear replacements and contact lenses [58]. Bioceramics are inorganic, non-metallic, biocompatible materials that include alumina and zirconia, bioactive glass, coatings and composites, hydroxyapatite and resorbable calcium phosphates and radiotherapy glasses [59–61]. They are chemically stable, non-corrosive and interact well with organic tissue.

Bioceramics are classified as:

- Bioinert: non-interactive with biologic systems.
- Bioactive: durable in tissues that can undergo interfacial interactions with surrounding tissue.
- Biodegradable, soluble or resorbable: eventually replace or are incorporated into tissues.

There are numerous bioceramics currently in use in dentistry and medicine [62]. Alumina and

zirconia are bioinert ceramics used in prosthetics. Bioactive glass and glass ceramics are available for use in dentistry under various trade names. In addition, porous ceramics such as calcium phosphate-based materials have been used for filling bone defects. Some calcium-silicate-based materials (MTA—mineral trioxide aggregate, ProRoot® MTA Root Repair; DENTSPLY-Tulsa Dental Specialties, Tulsa, US) and bioaggregates (DiaRoot® BioAggregate; DiaDent, Almere, The Netherlands) have also been used in dentistry as materials for root repair and for apical root filling.

6.6.1 Bioceramics in Endodontics

Calcium-silicate-based materials used in endodontics are generally wide known as Bioceramics or Bioactive Endodontic Cements (BECs) [63, 64], but due to the wide range of materials undergoing this definition, materials for endodontic use should be better defined as "hydraulic cements", in both their version as root canal sealer (RCS) or repair/root-end material (RRM), as they are all based on the same active ingredient: tricalcium silicate [65].

These materials used in endodontics can be categorized by composition, setting mechanism and consistency [28, 58, 66]. There are sealers and pastes, developed for use with gutta-percha and putties, designed for use as the sole material, comparable to MTA [66]. Some are powder/liquid systems that require manual mixing. The mixing and handling characteristics of the powder/liquid systems may be technique sensitive and produce waste. Pre-mixed bioceramics require moisture from the surrounding tissues to set. The pre-mixed sealer, paste and putty have the advantage of uniform consistency and lack of waste. These pre-mixed bioceramics are all hydrophilic [66].

6.6.2 Available Hydraulic Endodontic Cements
(Tables 6.1–6.3)

Few clinicians realize that original MTA is a classic hydraulic cement with the addition of some heavy metals [62]. MTA is one of the most extensively researched materials in the dental field [67–74]. It has the properties of all bioceramics, i.e. high pH when unset, biocompatible and bioactive when set and provides an excellent seal over time [72]. However, it has some disadvantages. The initial setting time might be long, it requires mixing, it is not easy to manipulate and it is hard to remove [67]. Clinically both grey and white MTA may stain dentin, presumably due to the heavy metal content of the material or the inclusion of blood pigment while setting [75]. Finally, MTA is hard to apply in narrow canals, making the material poorly suited for use as a sealer, even if clinical techniques have been suggested [76]. Efforts have been made to overcome these shortcomings with new compositions of MTA or with additives to make it more fluid. However, these formulations affect its physical and mechanical characteristics, consequently affecting its performance [77, 78].

Biodentine (Septodont, Saint-Maur-des-Fosses, France) is considered a second generation of endodontic bioactive materials, which has similar properties to MTA and thus can be used for all the applications set out above for MTA [79, 80]. Its advantages over MTA are it has a shorter setting time (approximately 12–15 min) and has a compressive strength similar to dentin [81]. A major disadvantage is that it is triturated for 30 s in a preset quantity (capsule), making waste inevitable in the vast majority of cases, since only a small amount is usually required. BioRoot RCS (Septodont) is a new mixable powder/liquid calcium-silicate-based material, which has a fluid consistency to be used as root filling sealer [82].

In 2007, a Canadian research and product development company (Innovative BioCeramix, Inc., Vancouver, Canada) developed a pre-mixed, ready-to-use calcium silicate-based material, iRoot® SP injectable root canal sealer (iRoot® SP) [66]. Since 2008 these endodontic pre-mixed bioceramic products are available in North America from Brasseler USA as EndoSequence® BC Sealer™, RRM™ (Root Repair Material™, a syringable paste) and RRM-Fast Set Putty™.

Recently, these materials have also been marketed as Totalfill® BC Sealer™ [28]. In the last years several companies have developed pre-mixed bioceramic materials, which are today available on the market [62].

Both forms (sealer and putty) of these pre-mixed hydraulic cements are similar in chemical composition (calcium silicates, zirconium oxide, tantalum oxide, calcium phosphate monobasic and fillers) and have excellent mechanical and biological properties and good handling properties [83–116]. They are hydrophilic, insoluble, radiopaque, aluminium-free and with high pH and sealability properties [83–116].

6.6.3 Hydraulic Endodontic Cements for Root Filling

Hydraulic endodontic cements are not sensitive to moisture and blood contamination and therefore are less technique sensitive [66]. They are dimensionally stable and expand slightly on setting, making them one of the best sealing materials in dentistry [66, 84, 117–119]. When set they are hard and insoluble consequently ensuring a superior long-term seal [66]. The pH at setting is above 12, which is due to the hydration reaction forming calcium hydroxide and later dissociation into calcium and hydroxyl ions [66, 67, 110, 117] (Fig. 6.11a, b). When unset the material has antibacterial properties [82, 84]. When fully set it is biocompatible and even bioactive [84–95]. When hydraulic cements come in contact with tissue fluids, they release calcium hydroxide, which interact with phosphates in the tissue fluids, to form hydroxyapatite [66] (Fig. 6.11c). This latter property may also explain some of the tissue-inductive properties of the material [66]. For the reasons above, these materials are now the material of choice for pulp capping, pulpotomy, perforation repair, root-end filling and obturation of immature teeth with open apices, and given their properties, they are becoming more and more popular as sealers for root canal filling of mature teeth with closed apices [58, 62, 66].

Table 6.1 MTA materials commercially available

Name	Manufacturer	Composition	Setting time
ProRoot mineral trioxide aggregate (grey)	Dentsply Tulsa dental specialties, Johnson City, TN, USA	Tricalcium silicate, dicalcium silicate, bismuth oxide, tricalcium aluminate, calcium sulphate dihydrate (gypsum) and calcium aluminoferrite liquid: distilled water	Initial setting time has been reported from 70 to 74 min, while the final setting time is 210–320 min
Tooth-coloured ProRoot mineral trioxide aggregate (white)	Dentsply Tulsa dental specialties, Johnson City, TN, USA	Tricalcium silicate, dicalcium silicate, bismuth oxide, tricalcium aluminate, calcium sulphate dihydrate or gypsum liquid: distilled water	4 h
Angelus MTA (grey and white)	Angelus, Londrina, Brazil	Tricalcium silicate, dicalcium silicate, bismuth oxide, tricalcium aluminate, calcium oxide, aluminium oxide, silicon dioxide liquid: distilled water	The initial setting time of white angelus MTA has been reported to be about 8.5 ± 2.4 min; however, other studies reported 130–230 min as the setting time for angelus MTA
PD MTA white	Produits Dentaires SA, Vevey, Switzerland	SiO_2, K_2O, Al_2O_3, Na_2O, Fe_2O_3, SO_3, CaO, Bi_2O_3, MgO Insoluble residues of CaO, KSO_4, $NaSO_4$ and crystalline silica. To mix with distilled water	The material starts setting after approximately 10 min and the final setting time is 15 min. It is not necessary to wait for the final setting to continue the treatment procedure
Endocem MTA	Maruchi, Wonju, Korea	CaO, Al_2O_3, SiO_2, MgO, Fe_2O_3, SO_3, TiO_2, H_2O/CO_2, bismuth oxide	4.5–15 min
MicroMega MTA	MicroMega, Besancon, France	Tricalcium silicate, dicalcium silicate, tricalcium aluminate, bismuth oxide, calcium sulphate dehydrate and magnesium oxide	The manufacturer has claimed that the MicroMega MTA setting time is 20 min; however, there are reports that announced MM MTA has a setting time of 120–150 min
MTA bio	Angelus; Londrina, or angelus Solucoes Odontologicas, PR, Brazil	Portland cement and bismuth oxide	The initial setting time of MTA bio is 11 min. The final setting time of the material is 23.22 min
MTA plus (white)	Avalon biomed Inc., Bradenton, FL, USA	Tricalcium silicate, $2CaOSiO_2$, Bi_2O_3, $3CaOAl_2O_3$ and $CaSO_4$	MTA plus setting time is 128 ± 8 min. In contact with moisture the material needs longer time to set
MTA plus (grey)	Avalon biomed Inc., Bradenton, FL, USA	Tricalcium silicate, dicalcium silicate, bismuth oxide, tricalcium aluminium oxide, calcium sulphate and $Ca_2(Al,Fe)_2O_5$	Initial setting time at 37 °C: ~15 min when thickly mixed with gel; otherwise longer for sealer (~3 h)
OrthoMTA	BioMTA, Seoul, Korea	Tricalcium silicate, dicalcium silicate, tricalcium aluminate, tetracalcium aluminoferrite, free calcium oxide and bismuth oxide	324.0 ± 2.1 min
RetroMTA	BioMTA, Seoul, Korea	Calcium carbonate, silicon oxide, aluminium oxide and hydraulic calcium zirconia complex; liquid: water	Initial setting time of 150–180 s and final setting time of 360 min
Aureoseal MTA	Giovanni Ogna and Figli, Muggio, Milano, Italy	The powder consists of Portland cement, bismuth oxide, setting-time controllers, plastifying agents and radiopaque substances. The liquid is distilled water	No setting time has been reported for the material
CPM MTA	EGEO SRL, Buenos Aires, Argentina	MTA, calcium chloride, calcium carbonate, sodium citrate, propylene glycol alginate and propylene glycol	The initial setting time of end-CPM is 6–15 min, while the material's final setting time is 22–27 min

Table 6.2 Hydraulic endodontic cements for root repair

Name	Manufacturer	Composition	Setting time
BioAggregate	Innovative BioCeramix, Vancouver, BC, Canada	Tricalcium silicate, dicalcium silicate, calcium phosphate monobasic, amorphous silicon oxide and tantalum pentoxides liquid: deionized water	Based on the manufacturer data sheet, BioAggregate has a setting time of 240 min
Biodentine	Septodont, Saint-Maur-desFosses Cedex, France	Tricalcium silicate, dicalcium silicate, calcium carbonate, zirconium oxide, calcium oxide, iron oxide liquid: Calcium chloride, a hydrosoluble polymer and water	The setting time of biodentine has been reported as 6.5–45 min
Calcium-enriched mixture (CEM) cement	BioniqueDent, Tehran, Iran	Calcium oxide, silicon dioxide, Al_2O_3, MgO, SO_3, P_2O_5, Na_2O, Cl and H&C Liquid: water-based solution	50 min
EndoBinder	Binderware, Sao Carlos, Brazil	Al_2O_3 and CaO	60 min
Endocem Zr	Maruchi, Wonju, Korea	Calcium oxide, silicon dioxide, aluminium oxide, magnesium oxide, ferrous oxide, zirconium oxide	–
EndoSequence, RRM, RRP	Brasseler, Savannah, GA, USA	Zirconium oxide, calcium silicates, tantalum oxide, calcium phosphate monobasic and filling and thickening agents	The setting time of EndoSequence putty is 61.1 ± 2.5 min and the final setting time is 208 ± 10 min
TotallFill, RRM, RRP	FKG Dentaire, La-Chaux-De-Fonds, Switzerland	Zirconium oxide, calcium silicates, tantalum oxide, calcium phosphate monobasic and filling and thickening agents	The setting time of EndoSequence putty is 61.1 ± 2.5 min and the final setting time is 208 ± 10 min
NeoMTA plus	Avalon biomed Inc., Bradenton, FL, USA	Tricalcium silicate, dicalcium silicate, tantalite, calcium sulphate and silica	NeoMTA plus has had a 50- to 60-min setting time when prepared with putty consistency; otherwise, when used as a root canal sealer with loose consistency, it may take 5 h to set
Quick-set	Avalon biomed Inc., Bradenton, FL, USA, patent pending	Monocalcium aluminate powder that contains bismuth oxide (as a radiopacifier) and hydroxyapatite	12 min
iRoot FS (fast setting), iRoot BP (injectable) and iRoot BP plus (putty)	Innovative BioCeramix Inc., Vancouver, Canada	iRoot FS: Calcium silicates, zirconium oxide, tantalum oxide and calcium phosphate monobasic iRoot BP (BioCeramix Inc.) and EndoSequence BC sealer (Brasseler USA) have had the same formula including zirconium oxide, calcium silicates, tantalum oxide, calcium phosphate monobasic, and filler and thickening agents	iRoot FS showed setting after 1 h, iRoot BP and iRoot BP plus became solid after 5–7 days
Tech biosealer capping, tech biosealer root end, tech biosealer apex	Isasan, Como, Italy	Mixture of white CEM, calcium sulphate, calcium chloride, bismuth oxide, montmorillonite	The final setting time of various types of tech biosealer differ from each other. Tech biosealer capping has a final setting time of 55 min

Table 6.3 Hydraulic endodontic cements for root canal filling

Name	Manufacturer	Composition	Setting time
BioRoot RCS (root canal sealer)	Septodont, Saint-Maur-desFosses Cedex, France	Tricalcium silicate, zirconium oxide (opacifier) and excipients in its powder form, and calcium chloride and excipients as an aqueous liquid	Less than 4 h
Endosequence BC (bioceramic) sealer	Brasseler, Savannah, GA, USA	Zirconium oxide, calcium silicates, calcium phosphate monobasic, calcium hydroxide, filler and thickening agents	Setting time is 4 h measured according to ISO 6876:2001. However, in very dry root canals, the setting time can be more than 10 h
TotallFill (bioceramic sealer)	FKG Dentaire, La-Chaux-De-Fonds, Switzerland	Zirconium oxide, calcium silicates, calcium phosphate monobasic, calcium hydroxide, filler and thickening agents	Setting time is 4 h measured according to ISO 6876:2001. However, in very dry root canals, the setting time can be more than 10 h
iRoot SP (sealer)	Innovative BioCeramix Inc., Vancouver, Canada	iRoot SP:Zirconium oxide, calcium silicates, calcium phosphate, calcium hydroxide, filler and thickening agents	4 h
Tech biosealer Endo	Isasan, Como, Italy	Mixture of white CEM, calcium sulphate, calcium chloride, bismuth oxide, montmorillonite	Tech biosealer Endo has a final setting time of 77 min
EndoSeal MTA	Maruchi, Wonju, Korea	Calcium silicates, calcium aluminates, calcium aluminoferrite, calcium sulphates, radiopacifier and a thickening agent	12.31 min
MTA Fillapex	Angelus Industria de Produtos Odontologicos S/A, Londrina, Brazil	A MTA root canal sealer with nanoparticles of silica	The material's setting time is 19.3 min. In dry conditions, the material fails to set
TheraCal LC (light cured)	Bisco Inc., Schaumburg, IL, USA	CaO, Sr glass, fumed silica, barium sulphate, barium zirconate, Portland cement type III and resin containing Bis-GMA (bisphenol A-glycidyl methacrylate) and PEGDMA (polyethylene glycol-dimethacrylate)	The setting time has been reported to be 0.3 min because of the use of light cure technology

Fig. 6.11 (**a, b**) Hydration reaction of bioceramic material in contact with water with the release of $Ca(OH)_2$; (**c**) precipitation reaction of the bioceramic which releases calcium hydroxide and interacts with phosphates in the tissue fluids forming hydroxyapatite

• Hydration Reactions (a, b)

$$2[3CaO \cdot SiO_2] + 6H_2O \rightarrow 3CaO \cdot 2SiO_2 \cdot 3H_2O + 3Ca(OH)_2 \quad \textbf{(a)}$$

$$2[2CaO \cdot SiO_2] + 4H_2O \rightarrow 3CaO \cdot 2SiO_2 \cdot 3H_2O + Ca(OH)_2 \quad \textbf{(b)}$$

• Precipitation Reaction

$$7Ca(OH)_2 + 3Ca(H_2PO_4)_2 \rightarrow Ca_{10}(PO_4)_6(OH)_2 + 12H_2O \quad \textbf{(c)}$$

6.6.4 Properties of Hydraulic Endodontic Cements

To date, more than 90 studies have been performed on calcium-silicate hydraulic endodontic cements [83–119]. The vast majority of these studies have shown that the properties conform to those expected of a bioceramic material and are similar to MTA.

6.6.4.1 Biocompatibility and Cytotoxicity

Several in vitro studies report that BC materials display biocompatibility and cytotoxicity that are similar to MTA [83–94]. Cells required for wound healing attach to the BC materials and produce replacement tissue [84]. In comparison to AH Plus® (Dentsply-Maillefer) and Tubli-Seal™ (Kerr Endodontics), BC Sealer showed a lower cytotoxicity [83, 84]. On the other hand, one study concluded that BC Sealer remained moderately cytotoxic over the 6-week period [94] and osteoblast-like cells had reduced bioactivity and alkaline phosphatase activity compared to MTA and Geristore® (DenMat) [95]. A recent study comparing the results of apicoectomies done with MTA or bioceramic putty on dogs showed the bioceramic putty to be slightly better than the MTA, presumably due to its superior handling properties [96].

6.6.4.2 pH and Antibacterial Properties

BC materials have a pH of 12.7 while setting, similar to calcium hydroxide, resulting in antibacterial effects [97]. BC Sealer was shown to exhibit a significantly higher pH than AH Plus for a longer duration [98]. Alkaline pH promotes elimination of bacteria such as *E. faecalis*. In vitro studies reported EndoSequence paste produced a lower pH than white MTA in simulated root resorption defects [97] and EndoSequence paste, putty and MTA had similar antibacterial efficacy against clinical strains of *E. faecalis* [98].

6.6.4.3 Bioactivity

Exposure of MTA and EndoSequence Putty to phosphate-buffered saline (PBS) resulted in pre-cipitation of apatite crystalline structures that increased over time, suggesting that the materials are bioactive [99, 100]. iRoot SP exhibited significantly lower cytotoxicity and a higher level of cell attachment than MTA Fillapex, a salicylate resin-based, MTA particles containing root canal sealer [100]. EndoSequence Sealer had higher pH and greater Ca2+ release than AH Plus [98] and was shown to release fewer calcium ions than BioDentine® and White MTA [100].

6.6.4.4 Bond Strength

One study reported that iRoot SP and AH Plus performed similarly and better than EndoREZ® (Ultradent) and Sealapex™ (Kerr Endodontics) [101]. Another study found that iRoot SP displayed the highest bond strength to root dentin compared to AH Plus, Epiphany® and MTA Fillapex, irrespective of moisture conditions [102]. In a push-out test, it was similar to AH Plus and greater than MTA Fillapex [103]. When iRoot SP was used with a self-adhesive resin cement, the bond strength of fibre posts was not adversely affected [104]. Smear layer removal had no effect on bond strengths of EndoSequence Sealer and AH Plus, which had similar values [105]. The presence of phosphate-buffered saline (PBS) within the root canals increased the bond strength of EndoSequence Sealer/gutta-percha at 1 week, but no difference was found at 2 months [106]. Because of the low bond values in these studies, it is doubtful that any of these findings are clinically significant.

6.6.4.5 Resistance to Fracture

iRoot SP was shown in vitro to increase resistance to the fracture of endodontically treated roots, particularly when used with bioceramic impregnated and coated gutta-percha cones [107]. Fracture resistance was increased in simulated immature roots in teeth with iRoot SP and in mature roots with AH Plus, EndoSequence Sealer and MTA Fillapex [108]. Similar results were reported for EndoSequence Sealer and AH Plus Jet sealer in root-filled single-rooted premolar teeth [109].

6.6.4.6 Microleakage

Microleakage was reported to be equivalent in canals obturated with iRoot SP with a single-cone technique or continuous wave condensation and in canals filled with AH Plus sealer with continuous wave condensation [110]. A recent study showed a superior sealability of EndoSequence putty compared with grey MTA [111].

6.6.4.7 Solubility

High levels of Ca2+ release were reported from iRoot SP, MTA Fillapex, Sealapex, and MTA-Angelus, but not AH Plus. Release of Ca2+ ions is thought to result in higher solubility and surface changes [112]. However, the study tested the materials following ANSI/ADA spec. No. 57, which is not designed for pre-mixed materials that require only the presence of moisture to set. This could be the reason for the difference in findings in this study and in vivo observations.

6.6.4.8 Retreatment

Removal of EndoSequence Sealer and AH Plus were comparable in a study comparing hand instruments and ProTaper Universal retreatment instruments [113]. However, none of the filling materials could be removed completely from the root canals [114] and none of the retreatment techniques completely removed the gutta-percha/iRootSP sealer from oval canals [115].

6.6.5 Hydraulic Endodontic Cements: An Ideal Core-Sealer System for Filling Minimally Invasive Preparation?

The present trend to reduce coronal taper of root canal preparation to help maintenance of coronal tooth structure at the level of the peri-cervical dentin 4 mm above and below the cemento-enamel junction makes subsequent phases of the root canal treatment most difficult to be performed from a technical point of view [1, 2]. Despite present irrigant activation techniques seems to adequately clean middle and coronal thirds of the root even in minimally invasive root canal preparation with minimal taper [120], the root canal filling procedures for warm obturation techniques may be impaired by this modified shape of instrumentation. A high root canal taper

has been traditionally advocated to adequately perform the classic vertical compaction [121] or the modified continuous wave of compaction techniques [35] to permit the heat-carrier/plugger to reach 4–5 mm from the working length and exert the correct apical-lateral condensation forces. Conservative access cavities and minimally instrumented canals in terms of taper, while maintaining an adequate apical enlargement to permit debridement and disinfection of the most delicate apical area, may limit the heat carriers/pluggers currently available to reach the apical third, thus reducing the efficiency of the warm compaction techniques. For the same reasons, even a carrier-based technique may suffer of the same clinical limitations in these clinical conditions, being a limited coronal space an important limitation in practically executing this technique.

Hydraulic endodontic cements for filling root canals have some properties that may potentially change the root filling techniques in general and in minimally invasive instrumentation procedures in particular:

1. The hydraulic cements for root canal filling are highly hydrophilic and thus the natural moisture in the canal and tubules is an advantage, as they set in the presence of humidity, unlike most other sealers, specially the hydrophobic resin-based sealer, where moisture is detrimental to their performance.
2. When unset, the hydraulic cements have a pH of above 12. Thus, its antibacterial properties are similar to calcium hydroxide. Setting is dependent on physiologic moisture in the canal; therefore, it will set at different rates in different environments, but since they have a high pH, any delay in setting can be argued as a benefit, pending they will set properly.
3. These sealers do not shrink but expand slightly and are insoluble in tissue fluids.
4. Hydraulic endodontic cements are generally used in conjunction with a GP point that may be impregnated and coated on the surface with a nano-particle layer of bioceramic, which may reduce the gap between the sealer and the core and has shown to improve the seal of the filling.

5. Contrarily to the classic warm compaction techniques using GP and traditional sealers, in which compaction forces aim to reduce as much as possible the film thickness of the sealer, hydraulic calcium-silicate-based endodontic cements for root canal filling should be left undisturbed at a certain thickness in contact with the root canal walls and especially in the apical third, to act as the effective sealing part of the obturation materials. For this reason, high and deep condensation forces and high temperatures are not needed for these new filling materials.

The properties listed above, particularly in the presence of a sealer that does not shrink and is insoluble in tissue fluids, should change the long held rule that in root filings the core material should take up as much space as possible in order to mask the shortcomings of the sealer and by keeping the sealer as thin as possible. In fact, if it was possible to fill the root canal in a homogeneous way, ideally the need for a core material may be questionable. As it stands, the GP is only used to deliver the hydraulic cement through a hydraulic condensation and now the sealer can be the main component of the root filling.

6.6.6 Root Filling Technique with the Hydraulic Endodontic Cements

The single-cone technique [122] has been suggested to be used in conjunction with the use of hydraulic cements and has gained more and more popularity, if applied together with these materials in order to leave the sealer enough thickness to act as the main filling material. More importantly, the requirement to gain space for a plugger 4 mm from the working length is no longer required, allowing the practitioner a much more conservative antimicrobial instrumentation protocol for root canal treatment and leaving a thicker and stronger root. Interestingly when the taper is not excessive and the gutta-percha point is used primarily as a plugger to move the sealer into the canal irregularities and accessory canals,

a radiographic picture similar to the classical warm vertical condensation technique is often seen (Figs. 6.12, 6.13, 6.14). In this way these kinds of sealers are ideal to be used combined with the minimally invasive endodontic techniques (Fig. 6.15).

In any case, given the irregular shape of the root canals especially in the coronal and middle thirds and the fact that a deep compaction is no more required with hydraulic cements, a "mild

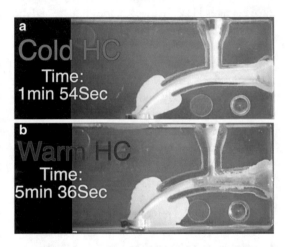

Fig. 6.12 Clinical demonstration of the cold hydraulic condensation (HC) on a simulated canal (**a**), compared to the warm vertical HC (**b**). Note that cold HC (**a**) is almost 400% less time consuming compared to (**b**) (courtesy by Dr. Allen Ali Nasseh)

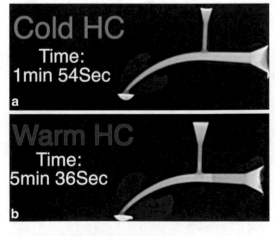

Fig. 6.13 Radiographic radiopacity of a simulated using the cold HC technique (**a**) compared to the warm HC technique (**b**). No differences are shown between these techniques (courtesy of Dr. Allen Ali Nasseh)

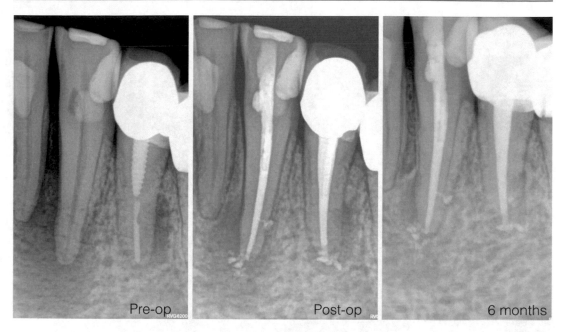

Fig. 6.14 Clinical case showing the radiographic aspect of a root filled with the cold hydraulic condensation technique

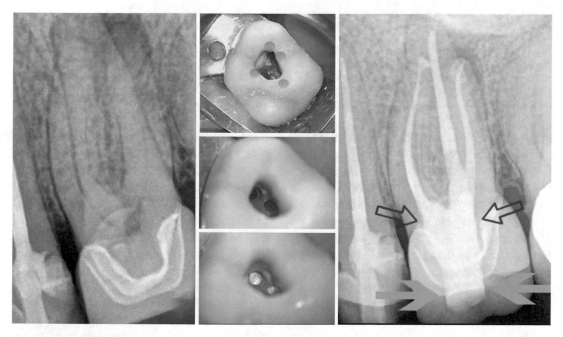

Fig. 6.15 Endodontic case root filled with the hydraulic endodontic cements. This type of sealers and technique are ideal to be used combined with the minimally invasive endodontic techniques

warm compaction technique" may also be suggested to be used with these sealers to unify the advantages of a warm compaction in filling the lateral irregular spaces, without impairing their thickness and their properties with the application of high and deep heat and compaction forces especially in the most delicate apical third of the root (Figs. 6.16 and 6.17). This clinical tech-

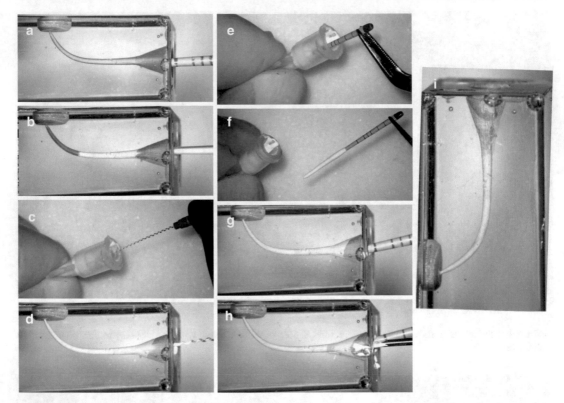

Fig. 6.16 Demonstration of the use of the hydraulic endodontic cements on a simulated canal in a transparent resin block. (**a**) Selection of a gutta-percha point to the correct working length; (**b**) application of the hydraulic cement using a transparent tip; (**c**) use of the tip as a depot for the sealer; (**d**) distribution of the sealer by a lentulo spiral; (**e, f**) coating the tip of the GP point; (**g**) placing the GP point inside the canal to the working length; (**h**) searing off the coronal part of the GP point with a heat plugger; (**i**) final case

nique aims to use the smallest electric heat plugger at the lowest temperature possible for the shortest time possible to compact the materials at half-length of the root or maximum 7–8 mm from the working length (Fig. 6.18). This aims to obtain what we can call a "champagne cork" effect, mechanically pushing the sealer through the cold cone in the apical third to increase the filling of lateral spaces without impairing sealer properties as the heat applied through the GP point so coronally will not be transferred to the sealer in the apical third. This technique may be easily applied in minimally invasive access cavity and root canal preparations, as it requires bringing the plugger only in the middle third of the root.

The amount of sealer introduced into the canal should be controlled so that only a modest amount is used and the surplus is not introduced in the periapical tissues. The syringe delivery system should not be positioned deeper than the interface of the coronal and middle third of the root canal (Figs. 6.16b and 6.17a). The bioceramic sealer flows easier than conventional resin-based sealers due to its particle size (<2 μ) and this mandates a degree of practice. A gutta-percha cone (ideally nano-coated with bioceramic particles) is matched to the root canal preparation (Fig 6.16a). Unlike traditional compaction techniques where the volume of gutta-percha needs to minimize the volume of sealer, the GP cone is used primarily to deliver the hydraulic cement to the apical seat without heat or pressure (GP act as a deliver device/plugger). It will allow hydraulic movement of the sealer into the irregularities of the root canal and

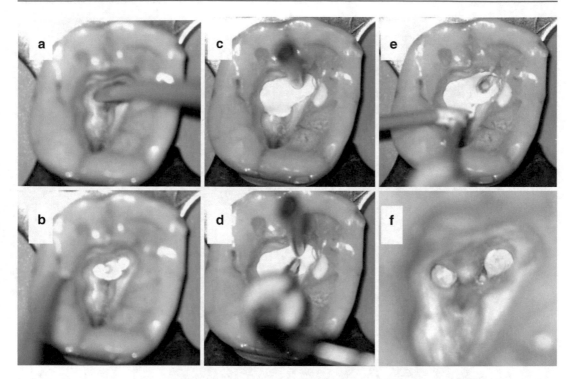

Fig. 6.17 Demonstration of the use of the hydraulic endodontic cement on the upper first molar. (**a**, **b**) Application of the hydraulic cement using a transparent tip; (**c**) placing the GP point inside the canal to the working length; (**d**, **e**) searing off the coronal part of the GP point with a heat plugger; (**f**) final image

accessory canals, thus reducing possible voids formation related to the injection of the sealer only; the bioceramic being bioactive and adherent to the interfacial dentin creates a true impervious apical seal. In addition, the GP will act as a pathway for post preparation and retreatment.

Depending on the shape of the apical region (circular or ovoid) and the intimacy of fit of the master GP cone, the master file used to apically gauge and size can be coated with sealer and introduced in a counterclockwise manner to deposit the sealer at the apical terminus. The master cone coated with a thin layer of sealer is then slowly introduced to the apical seat to avoid trapping air or excess sealer and preventing it seating fully (figure). The gutta-percha handle is cut with heat at the orifice or below for a canal footing or a post-space (Figs. 6.16h and 6.17d).

All variables in an equation are interdependent. In the case of endodontic success, each procedural event is accountable for the posi-

tive treatment outcome; however, regardless of its importance, if a concomitant event does not provide a suitable biologic conclusion, failure ensues. The shrinkage and instability of root canal sealers has mandated their use in thin layers and necessitated techniques to ensure this requirement. Bio-minimalism in canal space preparation requires a filling material that replicates the internal anatomy of the root canal space, adheres to interfacial dentin and creates an impervious, irreversible seal at all portals of exit.

Some drawbacks should be pointed out when using the hydraulic endodontic cements: as discussed previously, unlike traditional sealers, the setting reaction of bioceramic sealers is initiated by moisture (hydrophilic) in the canal; therefore drying the canal with solvents or alcohol are not recommended [123, 124]. Also, the high temperature by the heat pluggers exciding 200 °C might dry out the liquid sealer and turn in on charcoal-like material losing all its advantageous

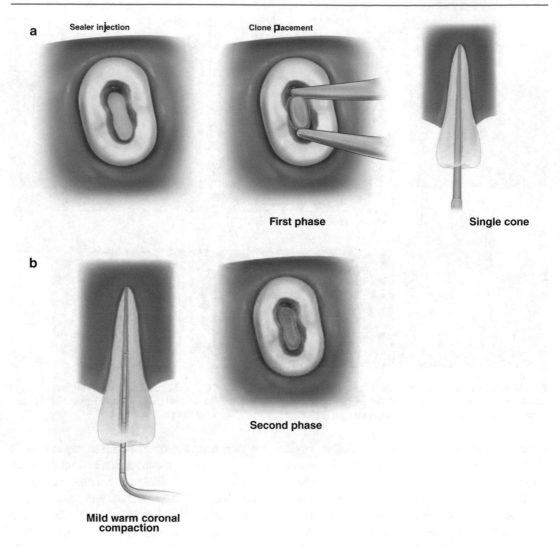

a Sealer injection   Clone placement

First phase   Single cone

b

Second phase

Mild warm coronal
compaction

Fig. 6.18 Representative drawings of the "mild warm compaction technique". (**a**) In the first phase the hydraulic cement is injected in the root canal and the máster GP cone is inserted at the working length; (**b**) in the second phase a mild warm compaction to mid-root is performed

properties [125, 126]. Therefore, a single-cone technique with the searing off the coronal part of the GP or the modified "mild warm compaction" technique described above is recommended.

For this reason, a new version of the sealer optimized for root filling techniques using high temperatures has been developed (BC Sealer HiFlow™, Brasseler). The intention is to lower the material's viscosity when heated over 200 °C. Even if scientific literature is still lacking to report on the characteristics and behaviour of this material, clinically it can be observed that the material doesn't dry out when using hot pluggers.

6.7   Use of Dental Operating Microscope During the Root Filling Phase on Minimally Invasive Canal Preparation

In all areas, from exposure of the access cavity and preparation to three-dimensional obturation, the operating microscope provides major advantages over working without appropriate magnification (Fig. 6.19).

Today clinicians have a number of methods, materials and technologically advanced instruments at their disposal to achieve their goals. Poor obturation quality as judged by radiographs has been associated with non-healing in 65% of retreatment cases. The use of the operative microscope will clinically access areas that are imperative for successful treatment and obturation.

All these high-precision work can be done also through micro-mirrors and micro-inva-sively, avoiding the removal of unnecessary tooth structure that are also imperative for successful treatment, preventing in this way tooth fracture, micro-cracks and coronal leakage (Fig. 6.20).

During the root filling phase the clinicians are able with the microscopic techniques to avoid obturation errors often as a result of inadequate cleaning and shaping (ledges, perforations, inaccurate working lengths and underprepared or overprepared canals), control the apical terminus without excessive material overextending into periapical tissues, control isthmus and irregular areas inside the root canals space condensing the sealers and core material in these areas, and adequately filling the root canal system in three-dimensions and, if inadequate obturation is not a result of an instrumentation error, the clinician should recognize this reversible procedural error and remedy this event.

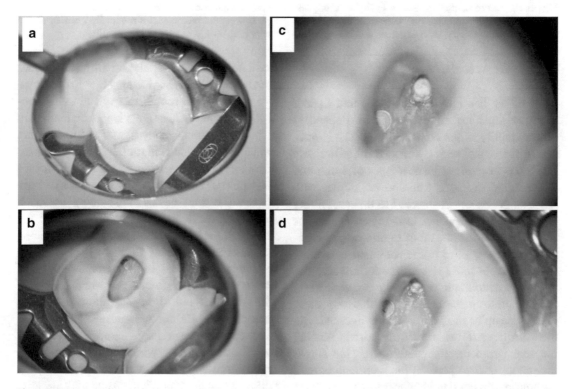

Fig. 6.19 A clinical case showing the minimally invasive access cavity (**a, b**) and root canal preparation with the aid of an operating microscope (**c, d**)

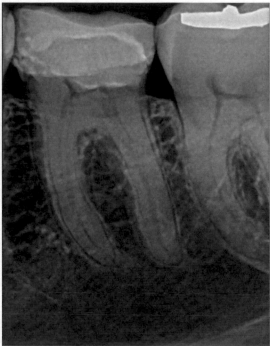
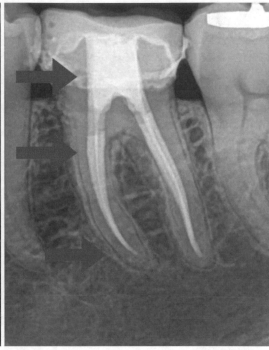

Fig. 6.20 Micro-invasively access cavity opening and root canal preparation has the advantage to avoid the removal of unnecessary tooth structure that is imperative to prevent tooth fracture, micro-cracks and coronal leakage. Lower first molar with a minimally invasive access cavity preparation, shaping and root filling

6.8 Conclusions

Root filling has long been a weak link in root treatment, making the endodontist too dependent on the quality of the coronal filling. The shrinkage of root canal sealers and instability in tissue fluids has necessitated a thin layer of sealer and has resulted in instrumentation techniques with large tapers primarily directed to this root filling techniques requirements. In many cases this has led to excessive removal of dentin on the coronal and middle third of the root canals, making the entire root more susceptible to fracture. The hydraulic endodontic cements do not shrink and are insoluble in tissue fluids. In this way these materials can be the primary filling material with the core material used only to assist in moving the sealer into canal irregularities. This allows the practitioner to perform the microbial control without removing dentin unnecessarily and leaving a stronger root for restorative reconstruction.

Combining these materials and filling techniques with low taper NiTi conforming files to conservatively prepare the root canals will fit to the concept of minimally invasive endodontic treatment.

In conclusion, many good techniques are available to the clinician for the root filling phase of root canal treatment. It seems that the use of low taper NiTi conforming files to conservatively prepare the root canals maintaining as much sound peri-cervical dentin as possible and the new calcium-silicate-based hydraulic endodontic cements can predictably fill the root canal space on a more biological and conservative settings. Excess of root filling material can be controlled with high magnification and allow the placement of a deep filling underneath the root canal entrance with a bacterial tight and permanent filling. The combination with a biological root filling material and an optimal tight coronal filling will lead to a more predictable and high successful endodontic therapy.

References

1. Gluskin AD, Peters CI, Peters OA. Minimally invasive endodontics: challenging prevailing paradigms. British Dent J. 2014;216:347–53.
2. Clark D, Khademi JA. Case studies in modern molar endodontic access and directed dentin conservation. Dent Clin N Am. 2010;54:249–73.
3. Sabeti M, Nekofar M, Motahhary P, Ghandi M, Simon J. Healing of apical periodontitis after endodontic treatment with and without obturation in dogs. J Endod. 2006;32:628–33.
4. Khayat A, Lee SJ, Torabinejad M. Human saliva penetration of coronally unsealed obturated root canals. J Endod. 1993;19:458–61.
5. Saunders WP, Saunders EM. Coronal leakage as a cause of failure in root canal therapy: a review. Endod Dent Traumatol. 1994;10:105–8.
6. Torabinejad M, Ung B, Kettering JD. In vitro bacterial penetration of coronally unsealed endodontically treated teeth. J Endod. 1990;16:566–9.
7. Gutmann JL. Clinical, radiographic, and histologic perspectives on success and failure in endodontics. Dent Clin N Am. 1992;36:379–81.
8. Sundqvist G, Figdor D. Endodontic treatment of apical periodontitis. In: Ørstavik D, Pitt Ford TR, editors. Essential endodontology. Prevention and treatment of apical periodontitis. Oxford: Blackwell; 1998. p. 242–77.
9. Grossman LI. Obturation of the radicular space. In: Grossman LI, editor. Grossmans endodontic practice. 12th ed. Philadelphia: William & Wilkins; 2010. p. 278–309.
10. Jasper EA. Root canal therapy in modern dentistry. Dental Cosmos. 1933;75:823–9.
11. Seltzer S, Green DB, Weiner N, De Renzis F. A scanning electron microscope examination of silver cones removed from endodontically treated teeth. Oral Surg Oral Med Oral Pathol. 1972;33:589–605.
12. Brady JM, del Rio CE. Corrosion of endodontic silver cones in humans: a scanning electron microscope and X-ray microprobe study. J Endod. 1975;1:205–10.
13. AAE Position Statement. Use of silver points. https://f3f142zs0k2w1kg84k5p9i1o-wpengine.netdna-ssl.com/specialty/wp-content/uploads/sites/2/2017/06/silverpointsstatement.pdf
14. Ørstavik D, Nordahl I, Tibbals JE. Dimensional change following setting of root canal sealer materials. Dent Mater. 2001;17:512–9.
15. Bunn CW. Molecular structure and rubber-like elasticity. Part I. The crystal structures of beta guttapercha, rubber and polychloroprene. Proc R Soc Lond A Math Phys Eng Sci. 1942;180:40–66.
16. Goodman A, Schilder H, Aldrich W. The thermomechanical properties of gutta percha. II. The history and molecular chemistry of gutta percha. Oral Surg Oral Med Oral Pathol. 1974;37:954–61.
17. Langeland K. Root canal sealants and pastes. Dent Clin North Amer. 1974;18:309–27.
18. Langeland K, Guttuso J, Langeland L, Tobon G. Methods in the study of biologic response to endodontic materials. Tissue response to N2. Oral Surg Oral Med Oral Pathol. 1969;27:522–42.
19. Kim S, Baek S. The microscope and endodontics. Dent Clin N Am. 2004;48:11–8.
20. Geurtsen W, Leyhausen G. Biological aspects of root canal filling materials—histocompatibility, cytotoxicity, and mutagenicity. Clin Oral Investig. 1997;1:5–11.
21. Ørstavik D. Antibacterial properties of root canal sealers, cements and pastes. Int Endod J. 1981;14:125–33.
22. Ørstavik D, Hongslo JK. Mutagenicity of endodontic sealers. Biomaterials. 1985;6:129–32.
23. Marin-Bauza GA, Silva-Sousa YT, da Cunha SA, Rached-Junior FJ, Bonetti-Filho I, Sousa-Neto MD, Miranda CE. Physicochemical properties of endodontic sealers of different bases. J Appl Oral Sci. 2012;20:455–61.
24. Barros J, Silva MG, Rodrigues MA, Alves FR, Lopes MA, Pina-Vaz I, Siqueira JF Jr. Antibacterial, physicochemical and mechanical properties of endodontic sealers containing quaternary ammonium polyethylenimine nanoparticles. Int Endod J. 2014;47:725–34.
25. Ørstavik D. Endodontic filling materials. Endod Topics. 2014;31:53–67.
26. Mutal L, Gani O. Presence of pores and vacuoles in set endodontic sealers. Int Endod J. 2005;38:690–6.
27. Ray HA, Trope M. Periapical status of endodontically treated teeth inrelation to the technical quality of the root filling and the coronal restoration. Int Endod J. 1995;28:12–8.
28. Trope M, Bunes A, Debelian G. Root filling materials and techniques: bioceramics a new hope? Endod Top. 2015;32:86–96.
29. Peng L, Ye L, Tan H, Zhou X. Outcome of root canal obturation by warm gutta-percha versus cold lateral condensation: a meta-analysis. J Endod. 2007;33:106–9.
30. Friedman S, Abitbol S, Lawrence HP. Treatment outcome in endodontics: the Toronto study. Phase I: initial treatment. J Endod. 2003;29:787–93.
31. Chevigny C, Dao TT, Basrani B, Marquis V, Farzaneh M, Abitbol S, Friedman S. Treatment outcome in endodontics: the TorontoStudy—phase 4: initial treatment. J Endod. 2008;34:258–63.
32. Schilder H. Endodontic therapy. In: Goldman H, editor. Current therapy in dentistry. St. Louis: The CV Mosby Co.; 1964.
33. Yee F, Marlin J, Krakow A, Gron P. Three dimensional obturation of the root canal using injected molded thermoplasticized dental gutta percha. J Endod. 1977;3:168–74.

34. Castelucci A, editor. Endodontics. Il Tridente Edizioni; 2002.
35. Buchanan LS. The continuous wave of obturation technique: 'centered' condensation of warm gutta percha in 12 seconds. Dent Today. 1996;15:60–7.
36. Tsukada G, Tanaka T, Torii M, Inoue K. Shear modulus and thermal properties of gutta percha for root canal filling. J Oral Rehab. 2004;31:1139–44.
37. Lee CQ, Chang Y, Robinson S, Hellmuth E. Dimensional stability of thermosensitive gutta percha. J Endod. 1997;23:579–82.
38. Siqueira J, Roças I, Favieiri A, Abad E, Castro A, Gahyva S. Bacterial leakage in coronally unsealed root canals obturated with 3 different techniques. Oral Surg Oral Med Oral Pathol Oral Radiol Endod. 2000;90:647–50.
39. Keles A, Alcin H, Kamalak A, Versiani MA. Micro-CT evaluation of root filling quality in oval-shaped canals. Int Endod J. 2014;47:1177–84.
40. Robberecht L, Colard T, Anne Claisse-Crinquette A. Qualitative evaluation of two endodontic obturation techniques: tapered single-cone method versus warm vertical condensation and injection system: an in vitro study. J Oral Sci. 2012;54:99–104.
41. Adorno CG, Yoshioka T, Suda H. The effect of working length and root canal preparation technique on crack development in the apical root canal wall. Int Endod J. 2010;43:321–7.
42. Zandbiglari T, Davids H, Schäfer E. Influence of instrument taper on the resistance to fracture of endodontically treated roots. Oral Surg Oral Med Oral Pathol Oral Radiol Endod. 2006;101:126–31.
43. Wilcox L, Roskelly C, Sutton T. The relationship of root canal enlargement to finger spreader induced vertical root fracture. J Endod. 1997;23:533–4.
44. Sathorn C, Palamara J, Messer H. A comparison of the effects of two canal preparation techniques on root fracture susceptibility and fracture pattern. J Endod. 2005;31:283–7.
45. Rundquist BD, Versluis A. How does canal taper affect root stresses? Int Endod J. 2006;39:226–37.
46. Ng YL, Mann V, Gulabivala K. A prospective study of the factors affecting outcomes of nonsurgical root canal treatment: part 1: periapical health. Int Endod J. 2011;44:583–609.
47. Pirani C, Friedman S, Gatto MR, Iacono F, Tinarelli V, Gandolfi MG, Pratti C. Survival and periapical health after root canal treatment with carrier-based root fillings: five-year retrospective assessment. Int Endod J. 2018;51:178–88.
48. Teixeira F, Teixeira E, Thompson J, Trope M. Fracture resistance of roots endodontically treated with a new resin filling material. J Am Dent Assoc. 2004;135:646–52.
49. Silva LA, Barnett F, Pumarola-Sunde J, Cañadas PS, Nelson-Filho P, Silva RA. Sealapex Xpress and Real-Seal XT feature tissue compatibility in vivo. J Endod. 2014;40:1424–8.
50. Nawal RR, Parande M, Sehgal R, Naik A, Rao NR. A comparative evaluation of antimicrobial efficacy and flow properties for Epiphany, Guttaflow and AH-Plus sealer. Int Endod J. 2011;44:307–13.
51. Gesi A, Raffaelli O, Goracci C, Pashley DH, Tay FR, Ferrari M. Interfacial strength of Resilon and gutta-percha to intraradicular dentin. J Endod. 2005;31:809–13.
52. Pameijer CH, Zmener O. Resin materials for root canal obturation. Dent Clin N Am. 2010;54:325–44.
53. Food and Drug Administration, K102163. Access data FDA. 2010. http://www.accessdata.fda.gov/cdrh_docs/pdf10/K102163.pdf.
54. Wong JG, Caputo AA, Li P, White SN. Microleakage of adhesive resinous materials in root canals. J Conserv Dent. 2013;16:213–8.
55. Strange KA, Tawil PZ, Phillips C, Walia HD, Fouad AF. Long-term outcomes of endodontic treatment performed with resilon/epiphany. J Endod. 2019;45:507–12.
56. Lotfi M, Ghasemi N, Rahimi S, Vosoughhosseini S, Saghiri MA, Shahidi A. Resilon: a comprehensive literature review. J Dent Res Dent Clin Dent Prospects. 2013;7:119–30.
57. Ree M, Schwartz R. Clinical applications of bioceramics materials in endodontics. Endod Prac. 2014;7:32–40.
58. Best SM, Porter AE, Thian ES, Huang J. Bioceramics: past, present and for the future. J Eur Ceram Soc. 2008;28:1319–27.
59. Dubok VA. Bioceramics: yesterday, today, tomorrow. Powder Metall Metal Ceram. 2000;39:381–94.
60. Hench LL. Bioceramics: from concept to clinic. J Am Ceram Soc. 1991;74:1487–510.
61. Staffoli S, Plotino G, Torrijos BGN, Grande NM, Bossù M, Gambarini G, Polimeni A. Regenerative endodontic procedures using contemporary endodontic materials. Materials. 2019;12:1–28.
62. Torabinejad M, Parirokh M, Dummer PMH. Mineral trioxide aggregate and other bioactive endodontic cements: an updated overview - part II: other clinical applications and complications. Int Endod J. 2018;3:284–317.
63. Parirokh M, Torabinejad M, Dummer PMH. Mineral trioxide aggregate and other bioactive endodontic cements: an updated overview - part I: vital pulp therapy. Int Endod J. 2018;2:177–205.
64. Wang Z. Bioceramic materials in endodontics. Endod Top. 2015;32:3–30.
65. Richardson IG. The calcium silicate hydrates. Cem Conc Res. 2008;38:137–215.
66. Debelian G, Trope M. The use of premixed bioceramics in endodontics. G Ital Endod. 2016;10:1–12.
67. Abedi HR, Ingle JI. Mineral trioxide aggregate: a review of a new cement. J Calif Dent Assoc. 1995;23:36–9.

68. Torabinejad M, Hong CU, McDonald F, Pitt Ford TR. Physical and chemical properties of a new rootend filling material. J Endod. 1995;21: 349–53.

69. Torabinejad M, White DJ. Tooth filling material and use. US Patent 5,769,638; 1995.

70. Torabinejad M, Chivian N. Clinical applications of mineral trioxide aggregate. J Endod. 1999;25:197–205.

71. Islam I, Chng HK, Yap AU. Comparison of the physical and mechanical properties of MTA and Portland cement. J Endod. 2006;32:193–7.

72. Funteas UR, Wallace JA, Fochtman EW. A comparative analysis of Mineral Trioxide Aggregate and Portland cement. Aust Endod J. 2003;29: 43–4.

73. Bozeman TB, Lemon RR, Eleazer PD. Elemental analysis of crystal precipitate from gray and white MTA. J Endod. 2006;32:425–8.

74. Parirokh M, Torabinejad M. Mineral trioxide aggregate: a comprehensive literature review—part III: clinical applications, drawbacks, and mechanism of action. J Endod. 2010;36:400–13.

75. Giovarruscio M, Uccioli U, Malentacca A, Koller G, Foschi F, Mannocci F. A technique for placement of apical MTA plugs using modified Thermafil carriers for the filling of canals with wide apices. Int Endod J. 2013;46:88–97.

76. Guven EP, Yalvac ME, Kayahan MB, Sunay H, Sahın F, Bayirli G. Human tooth germ stem cell response to calcium-silicate based endodontic cements. J Appl Oral Sci. 2013;21:351–7.

77. Topcuoglu HS, Tuncay O, Karatas E, Arslan H, Yeter K. In vitro fracture resistance of roots obturated with epoxy resin-based, mineral trioxide aggregate-based, and bioceramic root canal sealers. J Endod. 2013;39:1630–3.

78. Koubi G, Colon P, Franquin JC, Hartmann A, Richard G, Faure MO, Lambert G. Clinical evaluation of the performance and safety of a new dentine substitute, Biodentine, in the restoration of posterior teeth —a prospective study. Clin Oral Invest. 2013;17:243–9.

79. Camilleri J, Sorrentino F, Damidot D. Investigation of the hydration and bioactivity of radiopacified tricalcium silicate cement, Biodentine and MTA Angelus. Dent Mater. 2013;29:580–93.

80. Poggio C, Riva P, Chiesa M, Colombo M, Pietrocola G. Comparative cytotoxicity evaluation of eight root canal sealers. J Clin Exp Dent. 2017;9:574–8.

81. Candeiro GT, Correia FC, Duarte MA, Ribeiro-Siqueira DC, Gavini G. Evaluation of radiopacity, pH, release of calcium ions, and flow of a bioceramic root canal sealer. J Endod. 2012;38:842–5.

82. Kaur M, Singh H, Dhillon JS, Batra M, Saini M. MTA versus Biodentine: review of literature with a comparative analysis. J Clin Diagn Res. 2017;11:ZG01–5.

83. Zhang W, Li Z, Peng B. Ex vivo cytotoxicity of a new calcium silicate-based canal filling material. Int Endod J. 2010;43:769–74.

84. Zoufan K, Jiang J, Komabayashi T, Wang YH, Safavi KE, Zhu Q. Cytotoxicity evaluation of gutta flow and endo sequence BC Sealers. Oral Surg Oral Med Oral Pathol Oral Radiol Endod. 2011;112:657–61.

85. Ma J, Shen Y, Stojicic S, Haapasalo M. Biocompatibility of two novel root repair materials. J Endod. 2011;37:793–8.

86. Ciasca M, Aminoshariae A, Jin G, Montagnese T, Mickel A. A comparison of the cytotoxicity and pro-inflammatory cytokine production of EndoSequence root repair material and ProRoot mineral trioxide aggregate in human osteoblast cell culture using reverse-transcriptase polymerase chain reaction. J Endod. 2012;38:486–9.

87. Hirschman WR, Wheater MA, Bringas JS, Hoen MM. Cytotoxicity comparison of three current direct pulp-capping agents with a new bioceramic root repair putty. J Endod. 2012;38:385–8.

88. Willershausen I, Callaway A, Briseno B, Willershausen B. In vitro analysis of the cytotoxicity and the antimicrobial effect of four endodontic sealers. Head Face Med. 2011;7:15.

89. Damas BA, Wheater MA, Bringas JS, Hoen MM. Cytotoxicity comparison of mineral trioxide aggregates and EndoSequence bioceramic root repair materials. J Endod. 2011;37:372–5.

90. Mukhtar-Fayyad D. Cytocompatibility of new bioceramic-based materials on human fibroblast cells (MRC-5). Oral Surg Oral Med Oral Pathol Oral Radiol Endod. 2011;112:e137–42.

91. De-Deus G, Canabarro A, Alves GG, Marins JR, Linhares AB, Granjeiro JM. Cytocompatibility of the ready-to-use bioceramic putty repair cement iRoot BP Plus with primary human osteoblasts. Int Endod J. 2012;45:508–13.

92. Willershausen I, Wolf T, Kasaj A, Weyer V, Willershausen B, Marroquin BB. Influence of a bioceramic root end material and mineral trioxide aggregates on fibroblasts and osteoblasts. Arch Oral Biol. 2013;58:1232–7.

93. Modareszadeh MR, Di Fiore PM, Tipton DA, Salamat N. Cytotoxicity and alkaline phosphatase activity of EndoSequence root repair material. J Endod. 2012;38:1101–5.

94. Chen I, Bekir K, Wang C, Wang HG, Koyama E, Koli MR, et al. Healing after root-end microsurgery by using mineral trioxide aggregate and a new calcium silicate-based bioceramic material as root-end filling materials in dogs. J Endod. 2015;41: 390–9.

95. Zhou HM, Shen Y, Zheng W, Li L, Zheng YF, Haapasalo M. Physical properties of 5 root canal sealers. J Endod. 2013;39:1281–6.

96. Hansen SW, Marshall JG, Sedgley CM. Comparison of intracanal EndoSequence root repair material and

ProRoot MTA to induce pH changes in simulated root resorption defects over 4 weeks in matched pairs of human teeth. J Endod. 2011;37:502–6.

97. Lovato KF, Sedgley CM. Antibacterial activity of EndoSequence root repair material and ProRoot MTA against clinical isolates of Enterococcus faecalis. J Endod. 2011;37:1542–6.

98. Shokouhinejad N, Nekoofar MH, Razmi H, Sajadi S, Davies TE, Saghiri MA, et al. Bioactivity of EndoSequence root repair material and bioaggregate. Int Endod J. 2012;45:1127–34.

99. Guven EP, Yalvaç ME, Kayahan MB, Sunay H, Şahın F, Bayirli G. Human tooth germ stem cell response to calcium-silicate based endodontic cements. J Appl Oral Sci. 2013;21:351–7.

100. Han L, Okiji T. Bioactivity evaluation of three calcium silicatebased endodontic materials. Int Endod J. 2013;46:808–14.

101. Ersahan S, Aydin C. Dislocation resistance of iRoot SP, a calcium silicate based sealer, from radicular dentine. J Endod. 2010;36:2000–2.

102. Nagas E, Uyanik MO, Eymirli A, Cehreli ZC, Vallittu PK, Lassila LV, et al. Dentin moisture conditions affect the adhesion of root canal sealers. J Endod. 2012;38:240–4.

103. Sagsen B, Ustün Y, Demirbuga S, Pala K. Push-out bond strength of two new calcium silicate-based endodontic sealers to root canal dentine. Int Endod J. 2011;44:1088–91.

104. Özcan E, Çapar İD, Çetin AR, Tunçdemir AR, Aydınbelge HA. The effect of calcium silicate-based sealer on the push-out bond strength of fibre posts. Aust Dent J. 2012;57:166–70.

105. Shokouhinejad N, Gorjestani II, Nasseh AA, Hoscini A, Mohammadi M, Shamshiri AR. Push-out bond strength of gutta-percha with a new bioceramic sealer in the presence or absence of smear layer. Aust Endod J. 2013;39:102–6.

106. Shokouhinejad N, Hoseini A, Gorjestani H, Raoof M, Assadian H, Shamshiri AR. Effect of phosphate-buffered saline on push-out bond strength of a new bioceramic sealer to root canal dentin. Dent Res J (Isfahan). 2012;9:595–959.

107. Ghoneim AG, Lutfy RA, Sabet NE, Fayyad DM. Resistance to fracture of roots obturated with novel canal-filling systems. J Endod. 2011;37:1590–2.

108. Ulusoy OI, Nayır Y, Darendeliler-Yaman S. Effect of different root canal sealers on fracture strength of simulated immature roots. Oral Surg Oral Med Oral Pathol Oral Radiol Endod. 2011;112:544–7.

109. Topçuoğlu HS, Tuncay Ö, Karataş E, Arslan H, Yeter K. In vitro fracture resistance of roots obturated with epoxy resin-based, mineral trioxide aggregate-based, and bioceramic root canal sealers. J Endod. 2013;39:1630–3.

110. Zhang W, Li Z, Peng B. Assessment of a new root canal sealer's apical sealing ability. Oral Surg Oral Med Oral Pathol Oral Radiol Endod. 2009;107:79–82.

111. Antunes HS, Gominho LF, Andrade-Junior CV, Dessaune-Neto N, Alves FRF, Rocas IN, et al. Sealing ability of two root-end filling materials in a bacterial nutrient leakage model. Int End J. 2015;12:30–7.

112. Borges RP, Sousa-Neto MD, Versiani MA, Rached-Júnior FA, De-Deus G, Miranda CE, et al. Changes in the surface of four calcium silicate-containing endodontic materials and an epoxy resin based sealer after a solubility test. Int Endod J. 2012;45:419–42.

113. Hess D, Solomon E, Spears R, He J. Retreatability of a bioceramic root canal sealing material. J Endod. 2011;37:1547.

114. Ersev H, Yilmaz B, Dincol ME, Daglaroglu R. The efficacy of ProTaper University rotary retreatment instrumentation to remove single gutta-percha cones cemented with several endodontic sealers. Int Endod J. 2012;45:756–62.

115. Ma J, Al-Ashaw AJ, Shen Y, Gao Y, Yang Y, Zhang C, et al. Efficacy of ProTaper universal rotary retreatment system for gutta-percha removal from oval root canals: a micro-computed tomography study. J Endod. 2012;38:1516–20.

116. Azimi S, Fazlyab M, Sadri D, Saghiri MA, Khosravanifard B, Asgary S. Comparison of pulp response to mineral trioxide aggregate and a bioceramic paste in partial pulpotomy of sound human premolars: a randomized controlled trial. Int Endod J. 2014;47:873–81.

117. Jefferies S. Bioactive and biomimetic restorative mate- rials: a comprehensive review. Part II. J Esthet Restor Dent. 2014;26:27–39.

118. Loushine BA, Bryan TE, Looney SW, Gillen BM, Loushine RJ, Weller RN, Pashley DH, Tay FR. Setting properties and cytotoxicity evaluation of a pre-mixed bioceramic root canal sealer. J Endod. 2011;37:673–7.

119. Gandolfi MG, Iacono F, Agee K, Siboni F, Tay F, Pashley DH, Prati C. Setting time and expansion in different soaking media of experimental accelerated calcium-silicate cements and ProRoot MTA. Oral Surg Oral Med Oral Pathol Oral Radiol Endod. 2009;108:e39–45.

120. Plotino G, Özyürek T, Grande NM, Gündoğar M. Influence of size and taper of basic root canal preparation on root canal cleanliness: a scanning electron microscopy study. Int Endod J. 2019;52:343–51.

121. Schilder H. Filling root canals in three dimensions. 1967. J Endod. 2006;32:281–90.

122. Chybowski EA, Glickman GN, Patel Y, Fleury A, Solomon E, He J. Clinical outcome of nonsurgical root canal treatment using a single-cone technique with Endosequence bioceramic sealer: a retrospective analysis. J Endod. 2018;44:941–5.

123. Lee JK, Kwak SW, Ha JH, Lee W, Kim HC. Physicochemical properties of epoxy resin-based and bioceramic-based root canal sealers. Bioinorg Chem Appl. 2017;2017:2582849.

124. Colombo M, Poggio C, Dagna A, Meravini MV, Riva P, Trovati F, Pietrocola G. Biological and physicochemical properties of new root canal sealers. J Clin Exp Dent. 2018;10:e120–6.

125. Camilleri J. Sealers and warm gutta-percha obturation techniques. J Endod. 2015;41:72–8.

126. Qu W, Bai W, Liang YH, Gao XJ. Influence of warm vertical compaction technique on physical properties of root canal sealers. J Endod. 2016;42:1829–33.

Minimally Invasive Approach to Endodontic Retreatment and Surgical Endodontics

7

Mario Zuolo and Leandro Pereira

Contents

M. Zuolo (✉)
Endodontics, Faculdade de Odontologia da APCD –
FAOA, São Paulo, SP, Brazil

L. Pereira
Endodontics, Blantus Endodontic Center,
Campinas, SP, Brazil

7.1 Endodontic Retreatment

The concept of minimally invasive retreatment suggests conflict, because after all, how can it be minimally invasive when there is a need of a second intervention on the same tooth?

© Springer Nature Switzerland AG 2021
G. Plotino (ed.), *Minimally Invasive Approaches in Endodontic Practice*,
https://doi.org/10.1007/978-3-030-45866-9_7

In this chapter, we shall discuss clinical strategies to increase the success rate in cases of conventional gutta-percha retreatment (excluding mishaps and procedural errors) as well as cases recommended for endodontic surgery, keeping in mind the balance between preserving maximum possible healthy dental structure and the need to promote the removal of the etiologic agent responsible for failure of initial treatment.

Practice protocols will be described based on dental anatomy and its three-dimensional interpretation during clinical procedures based on clinical and scientific evidence and incorporating the most important technological advances within the specialty.

7.2 Conventional Retreatment of Gutta-Percha

7.2.1 Case Planning

In most endodontic retreatment cases gutta-percha and sealer must be removed before further

repreparation and refilling can be performed. The effectiveness of removing the filling material depends on its position, extent, and adaptation to the canal walls [1]. Therefore, proper planning must be done for each clinical case based on digital radiographic images and also high-resolution CT scan.

Cone-beam computed tomography (CBCT) has been increasingly used in endodontics and represents an important technological resource in retreatment cases not only for the proper diagnosis of each case but also for the planning of clinical actions to be adopted.

What to look for:

- Presence of lesion and its relationship with roots and adjacent dental structures (Fig. 7.1).
- Presence of root resorptions or procedural errors (Fig. 7.2).
- Position and extent of filling in each canal and its relation with the anatomy (Fig. 7.3).
- Presence of missed canals and other anatomic variables (Fig. 7.4).

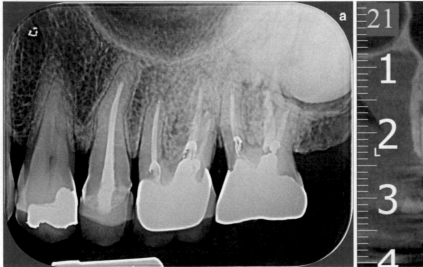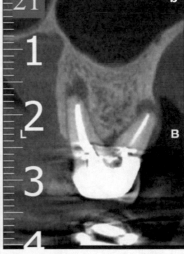

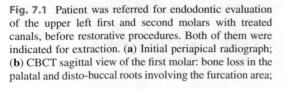

Fig. 7.1 Patient was referred for endodontic evaluation of the upper left first and second molars with treated canals, before restorative procedures. Both of them were indicated for extraction. (**a**) Initial periapical radiograph; (**b**) CBCT sagittal view of the first molar: bone loss in the palatal and disto-buccal roots involving the furcation area; (**c**) CBCT sagittal view of the second molar: despite the bone loss in the apical area, the roots contact a retained third molar; (**d**) CBCT cross-sectional view: the extension of the bone loss in the middle third of the second molar with fenestration of the palatal cortical plate

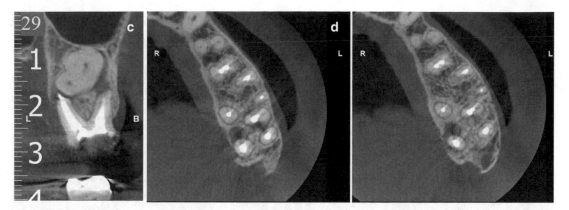

Fig. 7.1 (continued)

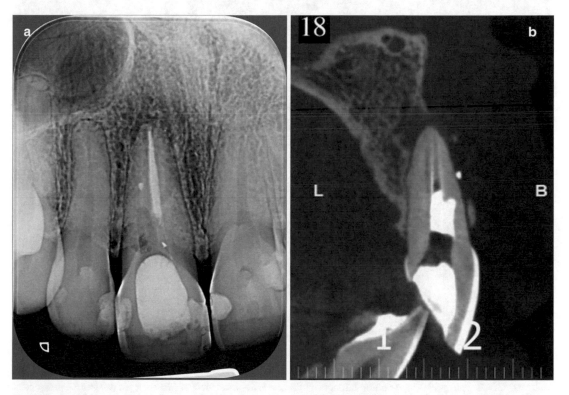

Fig. 7.2 Tooth 11 scheduled for retreatment after an unsuccessful attempt of gutta-percha removal by the referring dentist. (**a**) Initial radiograph showing a small periapical lesion and a suspect of canal deviation; (**b**) CBCT sagittal view showing buccal canal deviation with-out perforation and extensive bone loss with fenestration of the cortical plate; (**c**) Presence of an external root resorption in the cervical area with canal communication in the CBCT cross-sectional view

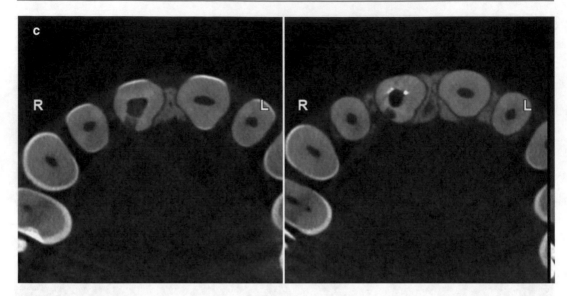

Fig. 7.2 (continued)

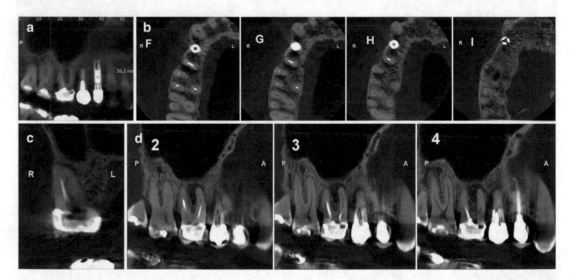

Fig. 7.3 Despite the artifacts given by the root filling material, CBCT can guide the operator throughout the anatomy of the canals and previous filling. CBCT navigation on tooth 16 referred for retreatment. (**a**) Initial image; (**b**) cross-sections at 3, 2, 1, and 0 mm from the apex; (**c**) Mesio-distal view of MB root; please note the presence of a MB2 canal with separated foramina. (**d**) Buccal-palatal view of the buccal roots

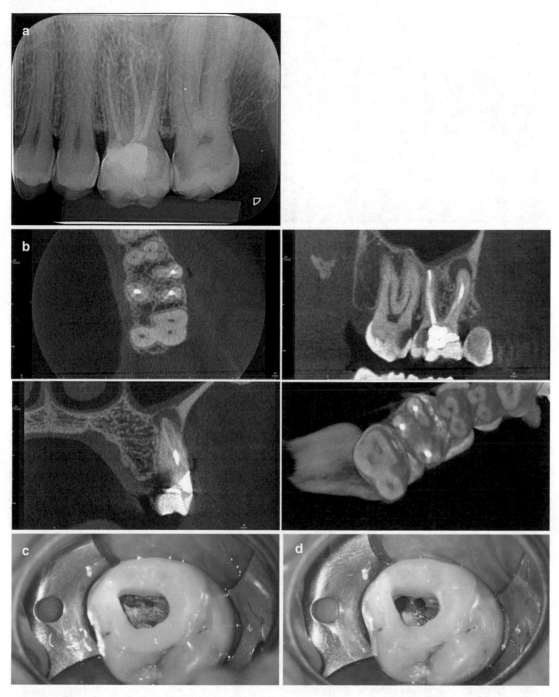

Fig. 7.4 An upper left first molar with a missed canal in the mesio-buccal root was referred for retreatment. (**a**) Initial radiograph; (**b**) CBCT images showing the presence of the MB2 canal and a periapical bone lesion; (**c**) access cavity after location of the MB canal; (**d**) MB1 and MB2 canals just before obturation; (**e**) final radiograph with all canals treated; (**f**) 3-year follow-up radiograph

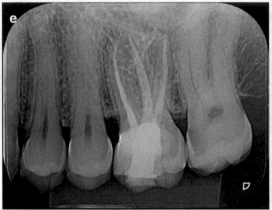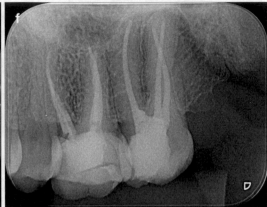

Fig. 7.4 (continued)

7.2.2 Endodontic Retreatment Access

In cases of endodontic retreatment, the size of the access cavity should not be an important consideration, as this procedure will always be performed on teeth with coronary anatomy modified by previous restorations, cavities or the presence of a wide range of prosthetic crowns. In addition, most of the posterior teeth indicated for retreatment should be restored with cusp coverage or full crown. However, the refinement of the access cavity with the use of magnification and illumination of the operation field together with the use of ultrasound inserts provides naturally smaller cavities, but without interference that could jeopardize the proper repreparation of the canals.

Some further considerations should be addressed as follows:

– Removal of previous restorations. The ideal scenario is to remove the previous restorations, all decayed tissue and inspect for fracture lines in the sound enamel and dentin. The presence of fracture lines in the crown is very frequent and may negatively influence the prognosis of the cases. In addition, proper mapping of these fracture lines will directly influence the type of final restoration indicated for each specific case [2] (Fig. 7.5).

– Missed canals. In cases of retreatment, the presence of missed canals is very frequent. Knowledge of the internal and external anatomy will provide the location of all canals present in a dental element and, of course, the use of CBCT will assist in the diagnosis and localization of these canals.

– Calcified canals: Calcified canals are also frequent findings in retreatment (Fig. 7.6). Again, knowledge of anatomical features coupled with technology can be of great value for locating these canals. However, the success of the procedure is closely linked to the position and extent of canal calcification. Clinically we can observe three types of situations: partial or total pulp chamber obliterations, canal entrance obliterations, and root canal obliterations from the cervical third to the apical third.

7.2.3 Retreatment Protocol

7.2.3.1 Gutta-Percha Removal

A large number of techniques and instruments have been indicated for the removal of gutta-percha and sealer from the interior of the canals, among which some can be emphasized [1].

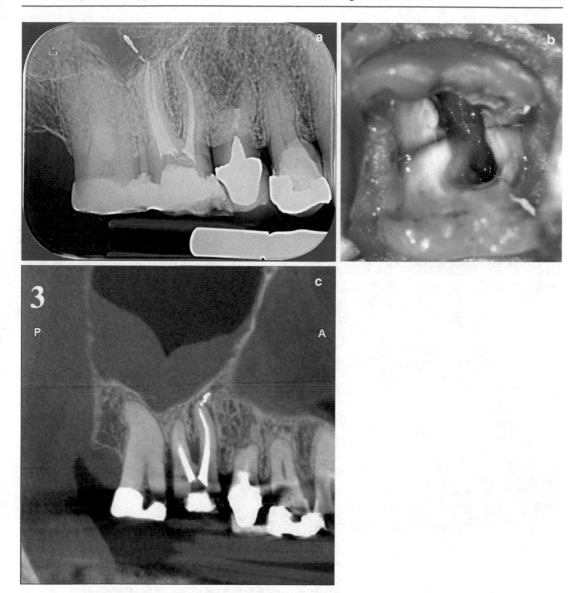

Fig. 7.5 Patient referred with pain when chewing after initial endodontic treatment executed 2 months before. (**a**) Initial radiograph showing good obturation of three canals; (**b**) after complete removal of the restoration, a coronal fracture could be observed; (**c**) CBCT showing severe bone loss located at furcal and distal area associated to the fracture lines

– Drills: Gates-Glidden and Peeso drills are very popular to initiate removal procedures, but nowadays they are not used very often because they promote inadequate removal of intra-root dentin especially in medial-distal flattened canals. In addition, the use of these drills tends to divert the canal in the same direction as the previous treatment.

– Solvents: Used for the purpose of facilitating the introduction of files into the filling material, its use is widely disseminated within the practice. However, its use results in a soft-

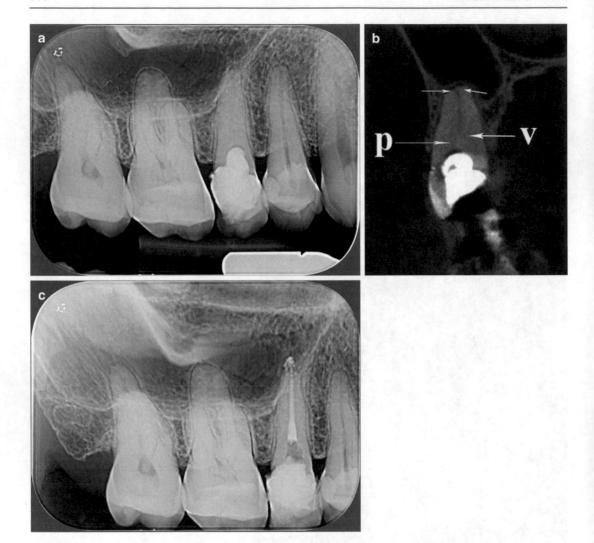

Fig. 7.6 Patient referred for endodontic treatment after an initial attempt to locate the canals of a maxillary right second premolar. (**a**) Initial radiograph showing destructive access and calcified canals; (**b**) CBCT sagittal cut in which the position of the two palatal (p) and buccal (v) canals may be imagine, joining each other in the middle third of the root and ending into just one foramen. (**c**) Final radiograph after canal location and treatment

ened mass that is constantly forced against the canal walls, so much dirtier dentin walls can be expected when using solvents [1]. Therefore, the use of solvents should be avoided during endodontic retreatment. Its use when necessary should be confined to removal of gutta-percha in the apical portion of the canal.

– Ultrasonics: Ultrasonic-specific inserts have been shown to be very useful in cases of gutta-percha and sealer removal from the canals,

leaving them cleaner and free of debris (Fig. 7.7).

– Endodontic instruments: A wide variety of files, made with different alloys used manually or driven with electric micro-motors, have been proposed to increase the effectiveness of gutta-percha removal during filling removal procedures. The use of reciprocating instruments for removal of filling material was initially reported by Zuolo et al. [3]. In this study, the effectiveness of reciprocating instruments (Reciproc

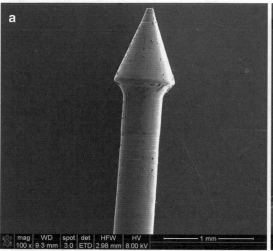

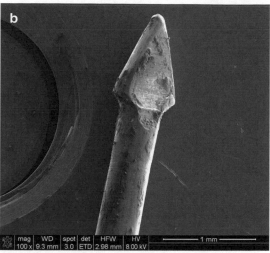

Fig. 7.7 A wide variety of inserts are available on the market ranging from straight types to those with angulated curves. The inserts also vary in relation to thickness and length. They can be smooth or diamond-coated and there are inserts specially designed for removing gutta-percha from the canals such as in (**a**) Clearsonic™ and (**b**) Flatsonic™ (courtesy of Helse—Brasil)

System) was compared to a manual and a rotary technique (M*two* System) for removal of filling material. The results showed that the technique that used reciprocating instruments was faster and more effective in producing clean walls when compared to the manual and rotary techniques. Several other studies have evaluated the behavior of reciprocating systems in retreatment and generally show that reciprocating motion is safe and effective for gutta-percha and sealer removal during the endodontic retreatment protocol [4–8].

7.2.3.2 Determining Working Length— Location of the Foramen or Apical Limit of the New Preparation

The vertical extent of instrumentation and filling in retreatment cases is one of the most controversial topics in the practice, generating still much discussion between different treatment philosophies and schools. The anatomical complexity of the apical region and the evaluation of the periradicular tissue response to the inflammatory and infectious process in this region of the canal may

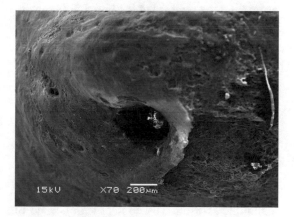

Fig. 7.8 Scanning electron microscope image of a file positioned just close to the apical foramen (courtesy of the Discipline of Endodontics, FOP-UNICAMP)

be pointed out as the factors responsible for generating confusion among specialists. In cases of apical periodontitis, where the presence of bacteria and biofilm can be observed in all thirds of the canals including the apical portion [9], it seems logical that the vertical extent of the new preparation should be positioned near the apical foramen (Fig. 7.8). A group of researchers and practitioners advocate zero foramen preparation with or without foramen enlargement and filling positioned less than 1 or 2 mm from the instrumentation limit [10, 11].

Currently, the use of state-of-the-art apex locators that work by impedance difference makes the correct location of the apical foramen viable, enabling the practitioner to respect the anatomical and morphological limits of the canal, providing greater predictability to endodontic treatment [12]. It is noteworthy that the repreparation and refilling procedure should always be limited to the interior of the canal, avoiding damage to the periapical tissues, favoring the healing and tissue repair process [1].

7.2.3.3 New Canal Preparation and Final Repreparation Diameter

The use of the crown-down preparation concept, promoting the removal of the initial filling material and the enlargement of the cervical and middle thirds before the apical third preparation, is the one that best achieves the repreparation objectives in cases of retreatment.

Wilcox and Van Surksum [13] and Wilcox and Swift [14] studied in vitro the effects of repreparation on straight and curved canals in human teeth using the step-back technique and pointed out that reinstrumented canals are generally widened in the same direction of initial preparation when the same instrumentation technique is used. The clinical significance of this finding is that, ideally, the repreparation should be conducted with adequate three-dimensional planning and directed efforts so that instruments and irrigant solutions can reach canal spaces not previously touched by the previous treatment.

Maintaining root canal anatomy during endodontic retreatment is a very important factor to be evaluated. Recent studies show the safety of the use of instruments in reciprocating kinematics during root canal system repreparation in cases of endodontic retreatment. The use of

reciprocating motion has resulted in low incidence of accidents such as perforations and ledges and little apical deviation even in severely curved canals [15, 16].

Regarding the final diameter of the preparation it should be considered that the final instrumentation file is related to the diameter and anatomical shape of the foramen and the presence of bacteria in the apical region. Baugh and Wallace [17] attested that larger apical preparations produce a greater reduction in bacteria and debris when compared to more conservative apical preparations, especially if we consider that the foramen's initial diameters vary widely between dental groups. In cases of retreatment, where the presence of apical lesion is a constant, use of the concept of large apical preparations seems to promote adequate cleaning and disinfection of the apical portion of the canals. The positive relationship between apical diameter increase and disinfection is well documented in the endodontic literature [18–22] (Fig. 7.9).

7.2.4 Clinical Protocol

The literature fully states that no retreatment protocol is effective in removing all prior filling material from the interior of the canals; therefore efforts should be made to combine techniques and materials in order to eliminate as much filling material as possible from the canal, thus qualifying the cleaning and disinfection procedures [23]

A retreatment protocol will be described as a general rule. The following materials and instruments are used: K-type manual files, a reciprocating system, ultrasonic inserts, magnification and illumination in the operation field, NaOCl, EDTA, and saline irrigating solutions, and sonic or ultrasonic apparatus for agitation of the irrigants.

1. After accessing and locating the canals, start removing gutta-percha and sealer

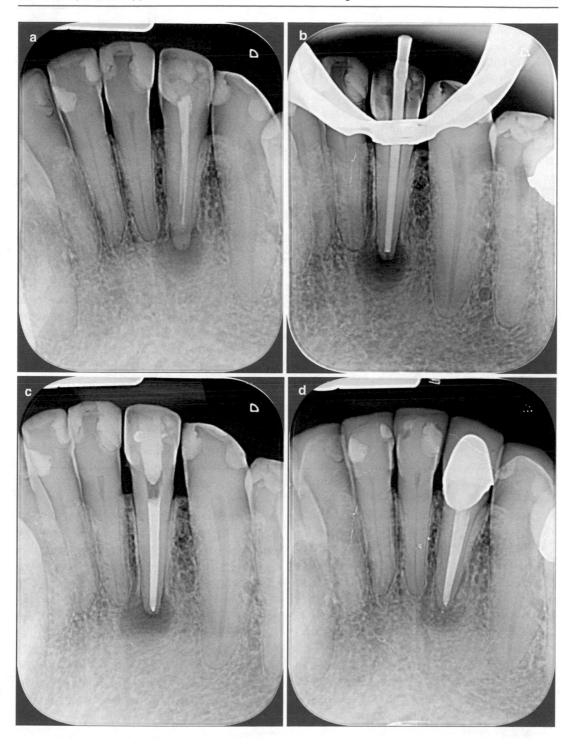

Fig. 7.9 (a) Initial radiograph of mandibular left lateral incisor showing poorly treated canal and a periapical lesion; (b) after removal of old filling material and canal repreparation the cone fit showed a large apical prepara-tion; (c) final radiograph; (d) 4-year follow-up radiograph showing bone repair and normal periodontal ligament space

within the first 2–3 mm below the canal entrance with an ultrasound insert compatible with the anatomy of the canals.

2. Alternate NaOCl and EDTA irrigation solutions agitated sonically or ultrasonically favoring the removal of debris. This irrigation protocol should be performed throughout the procedure always after the use of files or inserts in the canals.

3. Following the removal of gutta-percha in the cervical third, the objective is now to penetrate the filling using a reciprocating mechanical single-file that not requires glide path and which has a high cutting efficiency to better penetrate the filling material and high flexibility to follow the root canal curvatures. Small increments of maximum 3 mm of extent apically up to 1–2 from the estimated apical extent of the old root canal filling should be performed. After each use, the instrument should be cleaned and the canal irrigated as described above. Brushing movements should be performed sparingly avoiding the areas of lower intra-root dentin thickness.

4. The apical third should be explored with K-type size 0.10 or 0.15 manual files initially, without solvent. If resistance is present, a drop of solvent must be used to facilitate the exploration of the canal in the apical third, preventing the risk of deviations and perforations. After using the solvent, irrigate and dry the canals to eliminate softened gutta-percha from the walls and establish working length with an apex locator.

5. Saline solution irrigation can be performed at any time for mechanical debris removal. After irrigation and agitation, the canal can be dried with thin suction tips for observation of the canals with a microscope. Observe areas of isthmus and untouched walls. After drying use the irrigation protocol again and always work with instruments in a humid field.

6. With manual instruments size 10 and 15 perform glide path at specified working length.

7. Bring the mechanical reciprocating instrument used before to working length with gentle apical movements without forcing the instrument. In case of resistance return to glide path instrument.

8. Apical enlargement based on canal anatomy and initial instrument that cuts dentin in the apical portion. Enlarge the canal with at least three instruments with larger diameter than the initial instrument or using the visual gauging concept described in the Chap. 3.

9. After apical preparation, final irrigation should be performed and the solutions must be sonically or ultrasonically agitated.

10. Complete canal drying with thin suction tips and paper points.

In selected clinical cases, where it is possible to observe through CBCT that the presence of apical lesion occurs in only one of the roots, retreatment of the affected root only can be considered [24], especially in cases where a post is present and its removal may result in risks of fractures or other procedural accidents (Fig. 7.10).

7.3　Making Invasive Procedures During Nonsurgical Endodontic Retreatment Less Invasive

As previously anticipated, using the term minimally invasive when speaking about nonsurgical endodontic retreatment seems quite contradictory, but this philosophy may be followed during all the phases of an endodontic retreatment to avoid adding new stress on a tooth that has already been stressed from several previous treatments.

With this concept in mind, clinicians should attempt a retreatment using all the technologies, techniques, materials, and devices possible to be as much minimally invasive as possible in all the various retreatment procedures, such as disassembling of bridges, crowns, and posts (Fig. 7.11), searching for a missed or calcified root canal, and attempting the removal of a fractured file fragments (Fig. 7.12) or the repair of a perforation (Fig. 7.13) and/or of an open/resorbed apex (Fig. 7.14).

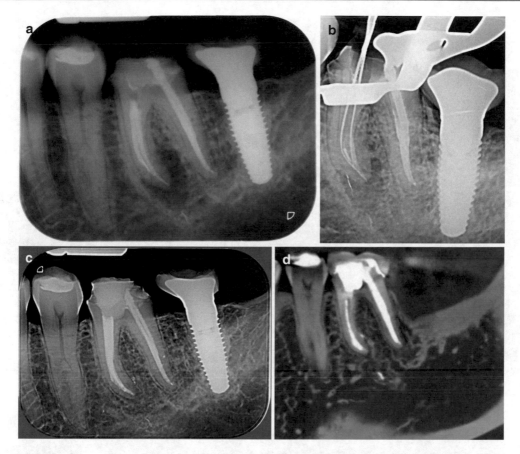

Fig. 7.10 Selective retreatment of the mesial canals of the mandibular left first molar since the distal root presented a large pre-fabricated post and no lesion. (**a**) Initial radiograph showing periradicular lesion in the mesial root; (**b**) working length radiograph; (**c**) 1-year follow-up showing complete healing; (**d**) CBCT at 1 year follow-up

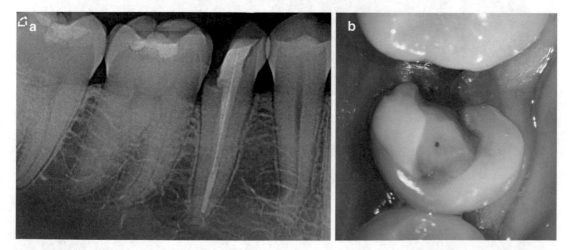

Fig. 7.11 Fiber post removal. (**a**) Initial radiograph showing a fiber post reaching the apical third of the root. (**b**) Clinical view of the fractured crown; (**c**) clinical view after core removal; (**d**) clinical view after post removal; (**e**) same as (**d**) with higher magnification (×20), note the untouched canal walls; (**f**) final radiograph

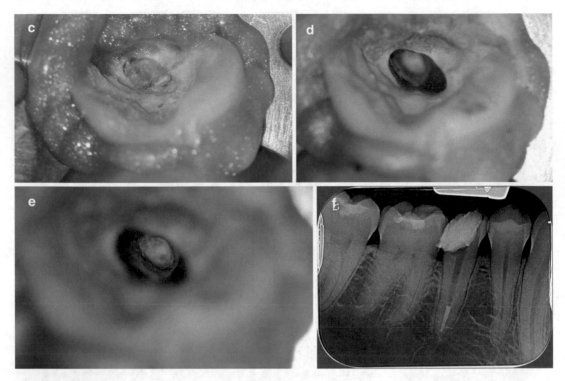

Fig. 7.11 (continued)

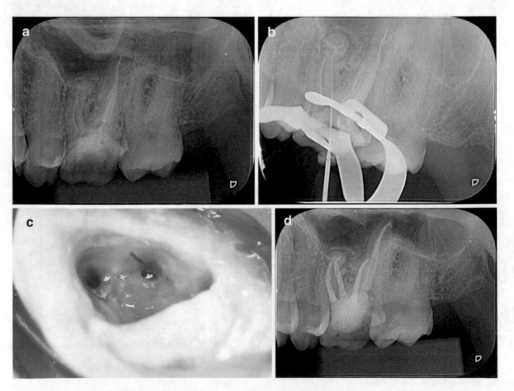

Fig. 7.12 Broken file by-pass and removal. (**a**) Initial radiograph evidencing a separated file in the MB root of the upper left first molar referred for retreatment; (**b**) intraopera-tive radiograph with file by-passed; (**c**) clinical view showing the removed fragment; (**d**) final radiograph after retreatment; (**e**) 15-month follow-up showing healed periapical tissues

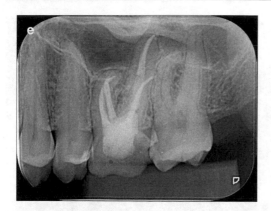

Fig. 7.12 (continued)

During all these procedures, a clinician may take the advantage of making a clear diagnosis through the use of a three-dimensional CBCT scan of the involved tooth, of working under the microscope magnification and illumination of the field to be more conservative on the residual tooth structure, of using ultrasonic inserts that are much more conservative than rotating burs, and of manipulating special modern materials and instruments that may guarantee a higher success and transform difficult procedures in more predictable treatments.

7.4 Predictability of Nonsurgical Retreatments

Nonsurgical endodontic retreatment, when properly indicated, is a treatment modality with a success rate above 85% and should be the treatment of choice in cases of failure of initial endodontic treatment [25, 26] (Fig. 7.15). Given this treatment outcome, there are not endodontic limitations to nonsurgical retreatment. Limiting factors are mainly due to excessive loss of tooth structure leading to unrestorability of the tooth and vertical root fracture. As a consequence, minimally invasive procedures are mandatory in all steps of endodon-

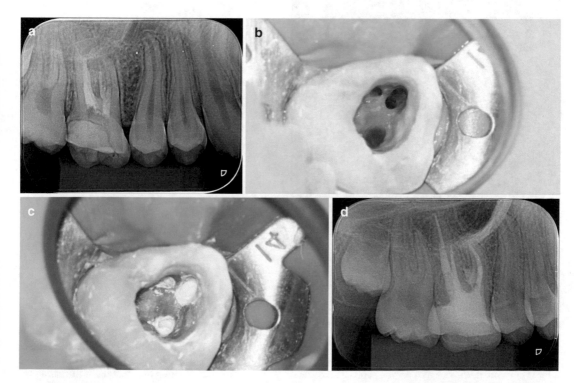

Fig. 7.13 Upper right first molar with a furcal perforation. (**a**) Initial radiograph; (**b**) clinical view after canal preparation and cleaning of the defect; (**c**) perforation treated with a hydraulic endodontic cement; (**d**) 9-month follow-up with evidence of bone repair in the furcation and periapical areas

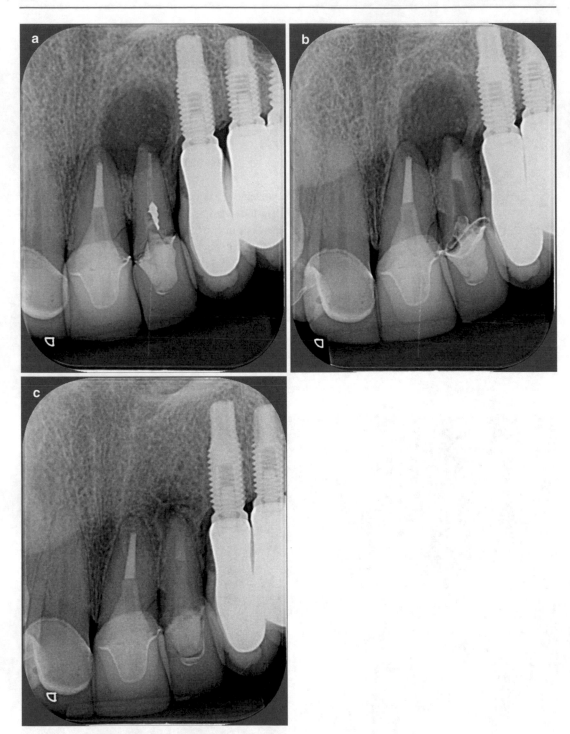

Fig. 7.14 (**a**) Initial radiograph of the upper left lateral maxillary incisor showing an open apex associated with a large periapical lesion, a broken post, and canal deviation; (**b**) radiograph after retreatment procedures and obturation with a plug of hydraulic endodontic cement for root repair; (**c**) 12-month follow-up with the new post and crown in position and healing of the periapical lesion

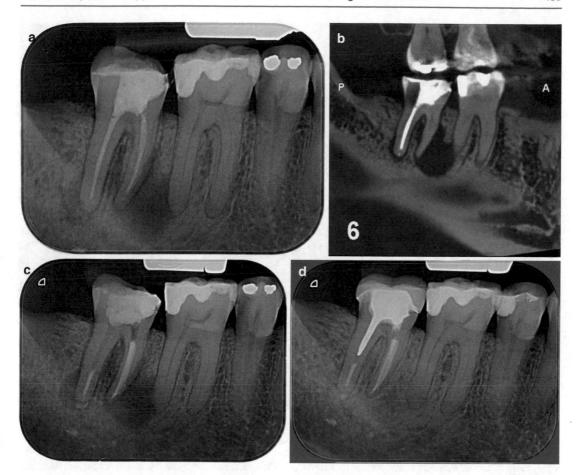

Fig. 7.15 Mandibular right second molar referred for retreatment. (**a**) Initial radiograph; (**b**) parasagittal CBCT showing a large bone loss; (**c**) radiograph immediately after retreatment and post space preparation; (**d**) 12-month follow-up with complete healing of the periapical lesion

tic treatment/retreatment to prevent unnecessary loss of sound tooth structure that may favor the conditions for a tooth to be lost for fracture.

In addition, procedural errors that may prevent the original canal from returning to its full extent have also been considered as risk factors that may negatively influence prognosis in cases of reintervention [26]. These may be the cases in which a microsurgical approach can be performed.

7.5 Endodontic Microsurgery

As seen earlier, endodontic retreatment has significant success rates. However, it cannot solve all endodontic failures. This means that even after a well-conducted endodontic retreatment, there will be cases of persistent periapical endodontic pathology.

The etiology of failure after endodontic retreatment is mainly related to the limitations of intracanal disinfection. These technical limitations are imposed by the complexities of internal root canal microanatomy.

Other etiological factors are extra-root infections, true cyst, and foreign body reactions by endogenous products, such as cholesterol crystals or exogenous dental materials extruded beyond the periapex [27]. In these clinical situations of persistent apical periodontitis, endodontic microsurgery is a conservative and highly successful clinical alternative (Fig. 7.16).

Since the introduction of new technical concepts such as the use of magnification-associated

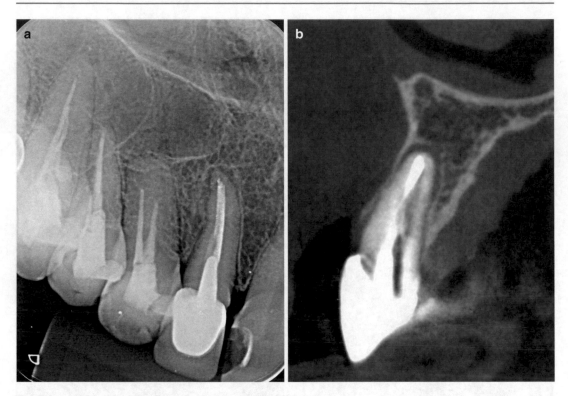

Fig. 7.16 (**a**) Preoperative radiograph; (**b**) preoperative CBCT

ultrasound and new calcium silicate-based hydraulic materials in apical surgery in the 1990s, the success rate of the now-called "Apical MICROsurgery" has increased significantly [28, 29]. A meta-analysis study showed that prior to this evolution (MACROsurgery), success rates were below 60%. However, with the application of these new technical concepts, MICROsurgery start to present a success rate of around 90% representing a significant evolution in this type of endodontic treatment [30].

Magnification contributed to microsurgical evolution mainly by allowing the visualization of details of anatomical structures not visible to the naked eye, as well as increasing the motor precision of the surgeon [31]. However, in order to be able to see, it is necessary to obtain an adequate visual access of the surgical field. In order to be able to manipulate structures, a cavity with a size compatible with the insertion and movement of the micro instruments is necessary since two objects cannot occupy the same place at the same time.

For this reason, the term MICROsurgery should never be related to the concept of minimally invasive surgical access that does not allow adequate access, visualization, and control of the ideal technical and environmental conditions of the operation field. By limiting the operator's vision and clinical performance, minimally invasive surgical accesses regarding the minimum cavity size are in the opposite direction to the evolution achieved in the last 20 years with the use of magnification in conventional endodontics and endodontic microsurgery.

Currently, the use of minimal surgical accesses is empirically based on better surgical precision and time, less postoperative inflammation and lower risks of gingival recessions while maintaining the same clinical efficiency. However, other areas of dentistry, such as the extraction of impacted third molars, have already shown that minimal surgical access does not allow adequate access, making surgical manipulation and the identification of anatomical structures difficult, leading to increased operating time [32]. As a consequence, it promotes worse postoperative conditions for patients [32–34].

In addition, the use of minimally invasive flaps and bone cavities may negatively interfere with the operative approach and postoperative recovery of endodontic MICROsurgery for several reasons such as:

- Promote insufficient mobility of the gingival flap leading to tension at the edges of the flap and consequent reduction of blood flow to the margins of the flap resulting in delayed repair or even gingival necrosis.
- Limit the visualization of the surgical field making the procedure more difficult and less accurate.
- Harm the illumination of the operating field by hindering the penetration of the powerful coaxial illumination provided by dental operating microscopes.
- Hinder the location of the ostcotomy starting point and the location of the periapical region in cases where the periapical lesion did not rupture the buccal cortical bone.
- Make curettage and removal of all periapical lesion difficult.
- Do not allow the visualization of the entire root extent not allowing the identification and access to lateral canals or cracks visualization on the coronal and middle third of the root.
- Prevent an accurate assessment of the anatomical microstructures and the identification of the possible cause that led the case to endodontic failure prior to microsurgery.
- Limit or prevent visualization of the main foramina and extra foramina located especially in the palatal or lingual area.
- Disrupt or prevent the correct positioning and working kinematics of the retropreparation ultrasonic tips.
- Impair or limit proper moisture control in retrograde preparations before retrofilling.
- Make delivery, placement, and compaction of retrograde filling material difficult in its cavity.
- Do not allow a tension-free flap for passive repositioning prior to suturing. This condition, besides interfering at the moment of suturing, may predispose to suture dehiscence during the initial healing period [35].
- Increase the surgical time causing more aggression to the body, producing greater inflammation and consequently worse postoperative recovery.

Therefore, the definition of MICROsurgery is not related to small cavities but to the possibility of detailed visualization and less traumatic manipulation of macro and microstructures involved in the surgery. Less operative trauma due to delicate and precise manipulation is the main factor that will provide less inflammation and better and faster postoperative for the patient and for tissue repair. Following this philosophy, the use of systems that allow the execution of a Full-Piezoelectric Endodontic Microsurgery should be strongly considered and its advantages will be addressed throughout this chapter.

Conventional endodontic surgery (Macro) differs from microsurgery not only using magnification. The main differences between traditional surgery and microsurgery are listed in Table 7.1.

Table 7.1 Technical differences between MACRO and MICROsurgery

Surgical steps	MACROsurgery	MICROsurgery
Magnification use	NO	YES
Bone crypt size	Large	Small (sometimes less than 3 mm)
Apicectomy angle	45°	90° (perpendicular to the long axis of the root)
Retropreparation	Drills	Ultrasonic tips
Retropreparation angle	30°/45° to the long axis of the root	In the long axis following the canal
Retrograde filling material	IRM/super EBA	Hydraulic calcium-silicate-based cements
Soft tissue management	Aggressive	Precise and delicate

7.6 Access to the Periapical Region

Access to the apical region involves three main steps: soft tissue management (incisions and flap design), hard tissue management (osteotomy), and apical curettage.

7.6.1 Flap Design

The use of semilunar and Lüebke-Ochsenbein submarginal "high flaps" was and is still very popular in endodontic surgery and microsurgery [28]. However, these types of flaps should have already been abolished from these procedures for several reasons:

- They do not allow visual access to the entire root extent. Thus, lateral canals, root fractures, and endodontic and periodontal lesions present in the cervical third and in the beginning of the middle third of the root would go unnoticed during the surgical procedure, compromising the effective control of the infection leading to a surgical failure.
- Unable to extend the flap, if needed.
- They are the flaps that most predispose the formation of gingival scars [36, 37].
- Incisions should not be made on bone defects as they facilitate the formation of gingival dehiscence. Horizontal incisions of these types of flaps can overlap areas of bone defects leading to unnecessary risks and also hinder proper repair of pink aesthetics [37].
- Predispose the suture to rupture in the initial postoperative period [32].
- Predispose necrosis of the edge of the wounds [36, 37].
- An adequate band of inserted gum is required which is not present in most cases [38].

As endodontic microsurgery always has an exploratory character to define the reason of the endodontic failure, the flaps should expose the entire root extension, starting from the cervical region with intrasulcular incisions and usually, with a releasing vertical incision. This way, the entire extent of the tooth will be exposed for transoperative evaluation.

With the most delicate and precise handling of microsurgery, the use of papilla-based flaps with one vertical incision release is favored [35, 37] (Fig. 7.17).

Obtaining a good hemostasis is of fundamental importance [39]. Hemostatic control favors the differentiation of anatomical structures such as root edges, bone, foramens, and cracks and provides a favorable environmental condition for the introduction of back-filling material in the retrocavity without the presence of blood. It is preferable to perform physical maneuvers to obtain hemostasis than chemical agents. The use of chemical agents can lead to postoperative damage as chemical irritation and the residues of these chemical agents in tissues lead to more inflammation and delayed repair [40], or even to a foreign body reaction [41].

Hemostatic control begins with the planning of the anesthetic technique and solution. The anesthetic solutions of choice are those containing the epinephrine vasoconstrictor in a concentration of 1:100,000. This way the practitioner can choose either 2% Lidocaine solution with Epinephrine 1:100,000 or 4% Articaine with Epinephrine 1:100,000 or 3% Mepivacaine with Epinephrine 1:100,000. The use of anesthetic solutions containing epinephrine in higher concentrations as 1:50,000 is unnecessary. The use of higher epinephrine concentrations increases the risk of tissue hypoxia, acidosis, and necrosis and may lead to the so-called reactive hyperemia rebound effect [42]. This physiological event leads to marked vasodilation in response to previous excessive vasoconstriction. This increases the risk of trans or postoperative bleeding [42].

Hemostatic control is favored by the use of a surgical piezoelectric ultrasonic system for the most diverse microsurgical steps. Its use reduces by 25–35% the intraoperative bleeding. Thus, it does not require the use of chemical hemostatic agents. The piezoelectric system acts on hemostasis because cavitation and the acoustic microstreaming flow formed in the fluid in the surgical cavity tamponade the vessels [43, 44] (Fig. 7.18).

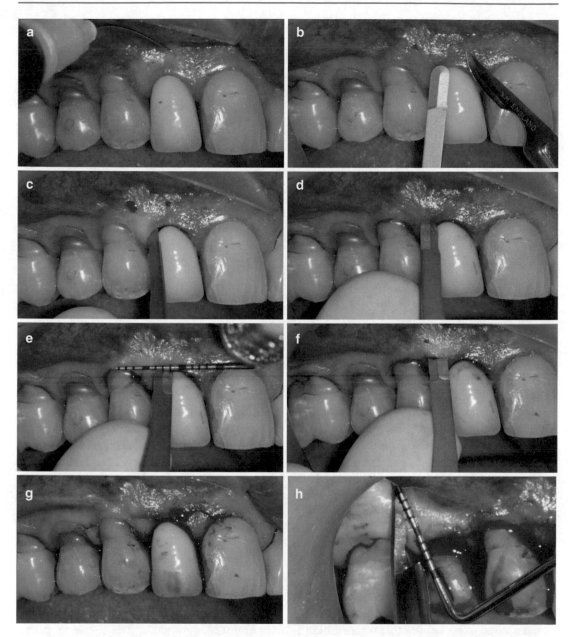

Fig. 7.17 (**a**) Complementary anesthesia at the mucogengival line for a better hemostatic control; (**b**) surgical Miniblades 6900 made by electropolishing provides thinner and precise incisions. Surgical Blades 15C are made by machining parts; (**c**) intrasulcular incision; (**d**) starting point to a papilla base incision. It must be perpendicular to the margin; (**e**) periodontal probe must be used as a guide for all incisions; (**f**) second papilla base incision with 45°; (**g**) papilla base incisions; (**h**) periodontal probe used as a guide for the vertical incision

7.6.2 Osteotomy

With the use of piezosurgical ultrasonic associated to magnification, osteotomy has become more conservative. In cases of small apical lesions, the osteotomy does not need to be larger than 3 mm. This size is sufficient to expose the apical third, allows the apicectomy to be performed, and provides space for the proper kinematics of the use of 3 mm long ultrasound tips for

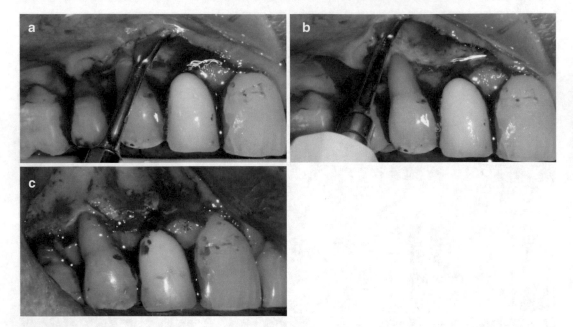

Fig. 7.18 (a) Piezo flap retraction using a ultrasonic tip with power adjustment in special mode; (b) exceptional bleeding control achieved by piezo flap retraction; (c) flap retracted

retrograde preparation and also for the retrograde filling procedure. The smaller the osteotomy, the faster the healing and the better the postoperative recovery [45].

Determining the starting point of osteotomy is a clinical step that causes insecurity in less experienced surgeons. However, its determination can be easily established using a North Carolina periodontal probe positioned on the long axis of the root to be operated (Fig. 7.19a). In addition, its execution is one of the simplest technical steps in all endodontic microsurgery.

It is facilitated in cases where there is already buccal bone wall fenestration allowing direct visual access. However, in cases where the cortical bone is intact it is up to the microsurgeon to determine the initial point of wear.

Considering that the roots of the permanent teeth have an average length of 10–12 mm, the point of choice for osteotomy can be easily determined by placing a North Carolina periodontal probe measuring 15 mm at the cement-enamel junction of the tooth to be operated (Fig. 7.19a). Osteotomy should begin at the same level as the tip of the probe where the periapical lesion will be present (Fig. 7.19b, c).

Recent static or dynamic guided surgery systems may be used for this purpose due to their accuracy and may be especially helpful in the most difficult anatomical situations to conservatively and safely solve them. The static system (3D physical printed guide) requires more preoperative clinical steps (digital workflow) such as CBCT, intraoral digital scanning, image matching, and 3D reconstruction in specific software, digital planning, and surgical guide design for later milling or 3D printing. These steps require the practitioner to master these technologies and add additional costs and time just to solve and performing one of the simplest steps of the microsurgical procedure. The dynamic guided surgery system unlike the static system does not require prior intraoral scanning. It also needs a prior CBCT scan and requires additional investment for the purchase of equipment and specific training. The learning curve is longer because the procedure is performed with the practitioner looking at the computer screen rather than the operation field. Like the static guided surgery system, the dynamic navigation is used only for the simplest steps of the microsurgical procedure.

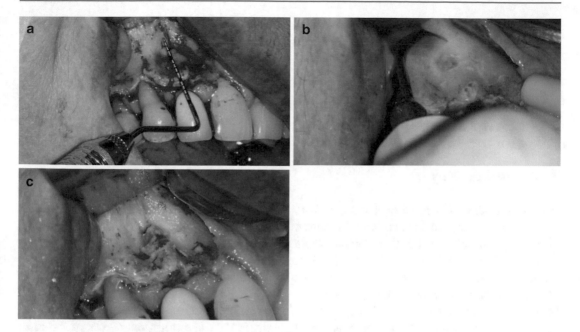

Fig. 7.19 (**a**) Determining the osteotomy site guided by a periodontal probe positioned in the long axis of the tooth; (**b**) piezo-osteotomy using an ultrasonic tip; (**c**) apical third exposed

Piezo-osteotomy increases cutting accuracy and provides more conservative bone cavity designs than circular osteotomies performed with drills. In addition, they allow the creation of bone cavities with non-standard circular design traditionally made with drills. Precise groove-shaped osteotomies, removing only enough bone quantity for penetration and movement of the retropreparation tips can be also carried out.

In addition, use of piezoelectric osteotomy system brings technical, biological, and clinical advantages when compared to the use of drills:

- The ultrasound tips have a long neck and do not interfere with the visualization of the surgical field as with the head of the high-speed handpieces when using drills.
- Ultrasound allows greater surgical precision with micrometer cuts by linear movements of amplitude between 50 and 200 μm only.
- Osteotomies performed with piezoelectric systems lead to the formation of less inflammatory cells. Consequently, there will be less postoperative discomfort [46].
- The use of piezo-osteotomy promotes a significant increase in the number of osteoblasts in the postoperative 45 days. The larger number of these cells leads to a faster initial repair [46].
- Piezosurgical systems generate less heating during bone cutting preserving cell viability and facilitating repair [46].
- Cutting selectivity is another advantage when compared to the use of drills. Piezoelectric systems cut only hard (mineralized) tissues such as bone and teeth, preserving soft tissues. This makes its use safer near nerves and membrane of the maxillary sinus.
- Cavitation formation, acoustic microstreaming, and intense irrigation promote optimal hemostatic control [43, 44].

7.6.3 Apical Curettage

Apical curettage can be performed before or after apicectomy. Due to the smaller size of bone areas in microsurgeries, apical curettage is usually performed after or with apicectomy. It can be performed with Lucas surgical curettes. In cases of larger apical lesions its curettage can be performed piezoelectrically with ultrasonic tips.

Removal of all soft tissue is of utmost importance to reduce the possibility of recurrence of periapical cysts and also to promote better hemostasis.

7.7 Surgical Management of the Apical Root Region

7.7.1 Apicectomy

Apicectomy should be performed at 3 mm from the root vertex. Root cutting at this level removes 98% of apical deltas and 97% of lateral canals [28]. In addition, the elimination of the final 3 mm of the root does not change the functional stability of the tooth after complete bone repair [47]. Apicectomies larger than 3 mm are not effective in removing 100% of the anatomical complexities and may even lead to tooth instability because of inadequate crown/root ratio [47].

Not only the amount of root to be removed in apicectomy is important, the cutting angle is also of fundamental importance in this process. As the lateral and delta canals are located on all root surfaces, the removal of 3 mm is fundamental by both buccal and palatal (or lingual) sides. Therefore, any type of bevel cutting should be avoided. Beveling does not allow for equal removal of 3 mm on all root faces. Therefore, apicectomy should always be performed perpendicularly along the root axis. This is the main difference between the apicectomy of the macrosurgery that was done at angles from 30 to 45° and the microsurgery that is done at 0°.

However, the use of high-speed drills does not always allow proper positioning for perpendicular cutting along the root axis in all cases. The use of piezoelectric ultrasonic inserts has become an effective alternative, giving rise to the so-called piezo-apicectomy [48]. Piezosurgical inserts are extremely efficient for performing apicectomies in 0° with the long axis of the roots (Fig. 7.20).

With the movement of the apical cutting instrument during apicectomy, the gutta-percha present in the remaining part of the root undergoes marginal misadaptation [48, 49]. This gap

formed between the canal wall and the filling material needs to be filled to prevent new bacterial growth.

7.7.2 Retropreparation

Retropreparation should be performed with a depth of 3 mm in the long axis of the root canal to ensure a good apical sealing [50]. To achieve this depth and pattern, the use of ultrasonic tips is critical during this microsurgery procedure step. Use of drills for this purpose is contraindicated because proper positioning and angles as described above are not possible.

In a study with bilaterally matched pairs of teeth in human cadavers, 100% of retropreparations with round bur showed deviation from long axis. In the same study, only 2.6% of the cases retro-prepared with ultrasonic tips showed deviation [51]. Wuchecich et al. [52] showed that retrograde preparations with burs produced cavities with 45° to 60° to the long axis of the root and achieved only an average depth of 1 mm. Moreover, ultrasonic root-end preparations produced cavities with less smear layer. This is clinically important since its presence may prevent intimate contact of the retrofilling material with the cavity

In order to prevent root cracks and chipping during the surgery or in the long term, a minimal invasive retrograde root canal preparation must be considered. Retrograde preparations with drills produced a root canal enlargement of 616% with a remaining thickness of 0.17 mm [53]. However, retropreparations with thin ultrasonic tips are less invasive than drills. They produced a root canal enlargement of 326% and remaining thickness wall of 0.43 mm [53]. A more conservative retrograde preparation is also important to prevent apical perforations. Therefore, the use of ultrasonic tips is less invasive than drills.

Another surgical drawback is the difficulty in removing gutta-percha. Diamond-coated retrotips are more abrasive than ultrasonic tips with a smooth surface. The abrasive properties might be advantageous in removing the gutta-percha. At the same time, these tips have more aggressive

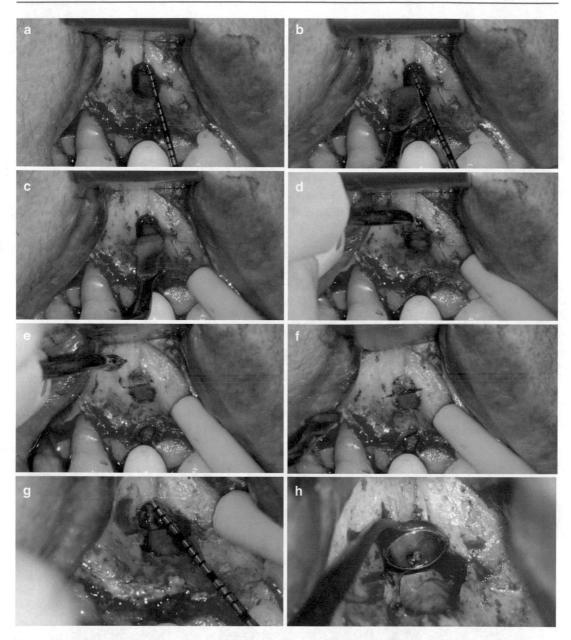

Fig. 7.20 (**a**) Determining the size of the apicectomy guided by the periodontal probe; (**b**) positioning the ultrasonic tip; (**c**) the power adjustment in the piezosurgery machine must be adjusted in cortical mode; (**d**) position- ing the tip perpendicular to the long axis of the root; (**e**) checking the angulation; (**f**) apicectomy precisely per- formed; (**g**) measurement of the bone crypt size; (**h**) rho- dium micromirror to analyze the root surface

cutting ability and must be gently used in order to not remove an excessive amount of sound dentin. Due to that, the ultrasonic power setting has to be adjusted to a maximum of 20%, with a continu- ous irrigation.

In cases with apical bone cavity smaller than 3 mm, it is not possible to insert and work with the ultrasonic tip into the long axis of the root (Fig. 7.21). The use of piezosurgery, a less inva- sive groove-shaped osteotomy, can be created allowing the proper use of the ultrasonic retro-preparation tips (Figs. 7.22, 7.23, and 7.24).

7.7.3 Retrofilling

In order to maintaining the disinfection achieved by the former surgical steps, the retrocavity must be filled.

Historically, several materials such as amalgam, endodontic sealers, temporary cements, hydroxyapatite, zinc-oxide eugenol (ZOE)-based

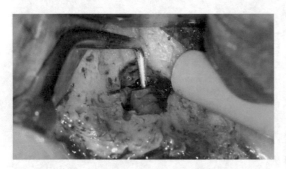

Fig. 7.21 The very conservative osteotomy did not allow a proper positioning of retrograde ultrasonic tip

cements, IRM, Super EBA, composite, and glass-ionomer have been used to fill the retrograde cavity. However, none of them have met all requirements to be considered an ideal retrofilling material.

The ideal material should be able to fill and seal the retrocavity, needs to be biocompatible, needs to have antibacterial properties, and should stimulate the cementogenesis. Moreover, these surgical sites are in contact with periodontal and bone tissues. These tissues have fluids and the environment around them is moist. Therefore, the retrofilling material should be able to work in a moist environment. Among all materials, the only types of material able to work in a moist environment are the hydraulic calcium-silicate-based materials.

Because they are bioactive and provide good filling, sealing, marginal adaptation, and biocompatibility, promote cementogenesis and biomineralization, are bacteriostatic, and perform well in wet environments, hydraulic cements are chosen for retrograde filling purposes [54–59]. This group of materials ranges from traditional MTA to new premixed or mixable materials (Fig. 7.25).

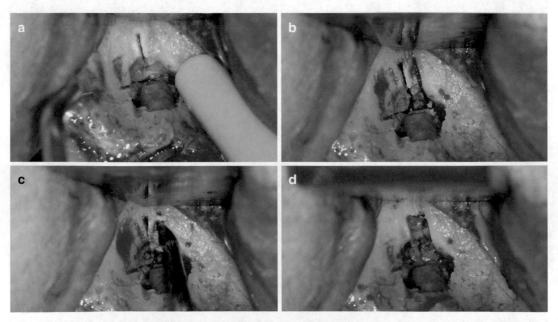

Fig. 7.22 (**a**) A precise grove can be create using piezo-osteotomy; (**b**) a second groove was created using a ultrasonic tip; (**c**) the bone between grooves was gently removed using a curette; (**d**) a very conservative bone resection was performed right over the dental root foramen

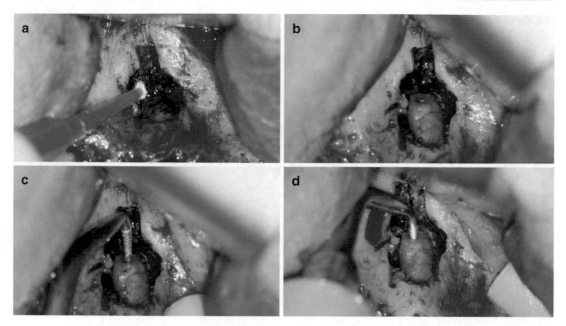

Fig. 7.23 (**a**) 2% Methylene blue was used to evidence small structures, accessory foramens, or root fractures; (**b**) direct view under 12.5× magnification provided by advanced three axis microscope; (**c**) the precise groove allowed the ultrasonic tip penetration; (**d**) piezo-osteotomy precision allows bone preservation and hemostatic control

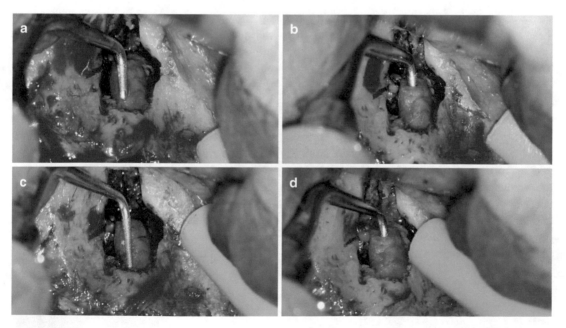

Fig. 7.24 (**a**) US Tip with 3 mm length; (**b**) retropreparation—3 mm in depth; (**c**) US Tip with 6 mm length; (**d**) retro-preparation—6 mm in depth

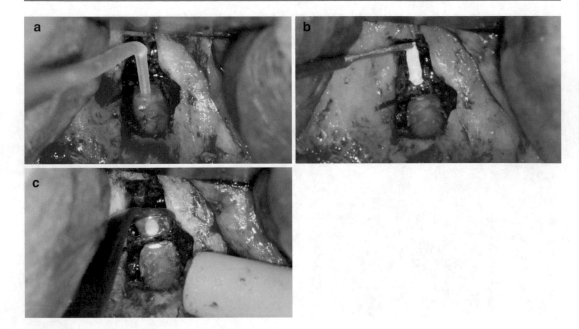

Fig. 7.25 (**a**) Drying the retrocavity using aspiration. Paper points should not be used because they can induce a postop foreign body reaction by leaving cellulose inside the bone crypt. Moreover, the hydraulic calcium-silicate-based materials need a moist environment to set; (**b**) retrograde filling with a hydraulic calcium-silicate-based cement; (**c**) checking the retrograde filling quality

7.8 Suture

The surgical closure is of utmost importance for the good and rapid recovery of the patient. The choice of microsurgery suture thread is subjected to non-resorbable monofilament threads (Nylon, Polypropylene or Polyamide). These threads cause less inflammation because they are smooth and make it difficult to accumulate biofilm over the sutures. Polypropylene threads are the first choice because they have good tension resistance and better shape memory control.

The use of small threads with atraumatic needles also aims to reduce surgical trauma and favor rapid repair. The 6-0, 7-0, 8-0, and 10-0 threads are used in microsurgeries. The 6-0 threads stabilize the flap while the 7-0, 8-0, or 10-0 threads are used for coaptation of the surgical wound edges (Fig. 7.26).

Microsutures should be carefully performed to avoid overlapping connective tissue in epithelial tissue and vice versa. This is the key to rapid soft tissue repair allowing suture removal between 48 and 72 h postoperatively (Fig. 7.27). Fast suture removal is another factor that aims to facilitate repair by decreasing postoperative inflammation caused by the presence of the suture and the biofilm formation on it.

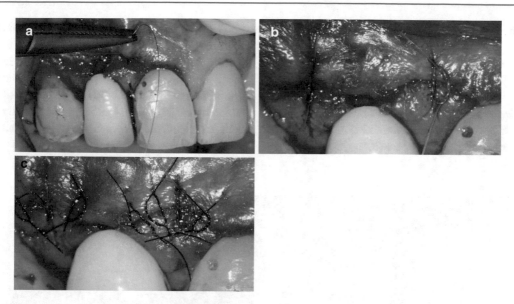

Fig. 7.26 (**a**) Special and precise forceps are necessary to handle 6-0 to 10-0 sutures; (**b**) stabilization suture with polypropylene 6-0; (**c**) geometry of papilla suture: coaptation sutures with polypropylene 7-0

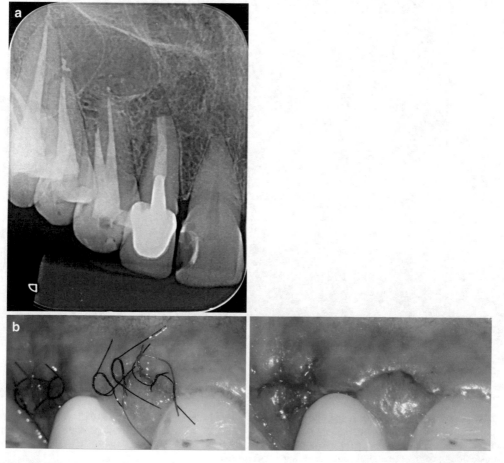

Fig. 7.27 (**a**) Follow-up 48 h after microsurgery; (**b**) initial fast healing and suture removal 48 h later

7.9   Conclusions

Technical development and greater microsurgical predictability have increased clinical indications, placing microsurgery as a direct alternative in some cases of primary endodontic failures because they show greater success than endodontic orthograde retreatment in some selected cases [60] (Fig. 7.28).

As a final remark, it is important to point out that nonsurgical endodontic retreatment or endodontic microsurgery, when adequately indicated, are a type of treatment associated with a high success rate and should be the treatment of choice for cases of failed initial endodontic treatment in patients motivated to maintain their natural teeth in the oral cavity.

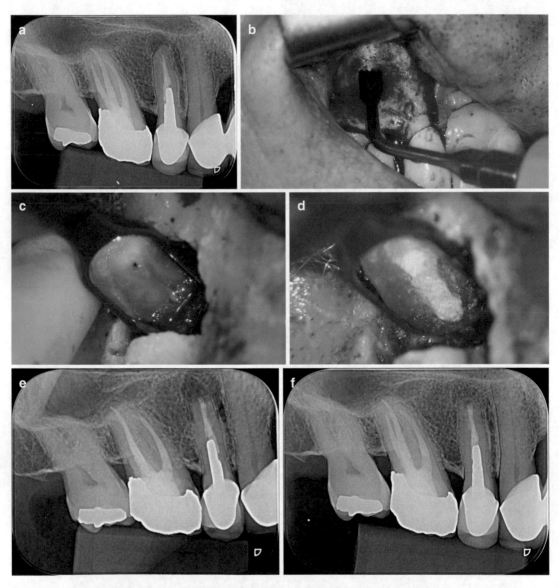

Fig. 7.28 Surgical retreatment in a maxillary right second premolar with a big metal post. (**a**) Initial radiograph showing a large periapical lesion; (**b**) piezosurgical ultrasonic osteotomy; (**c**) root resection showing an untreated canal in the buccal side. (**d**) retrofill with a hydraulic endodontic cement; (**e**) postoperative radiograph; (**f**) 12-month follow-up showing bone healing in the apical area

References

1. Zuolo ML, Kherlakian D, Mello JE Jr, Carvalho MC, Fagundes MI. Reintervention in endodontics. 1st ed. São Paulo: Quintessence; 2017.
2. Sung HK, Bom SK, Yemi K. Cracked teeth: distribution, characteristics, and survival after root canal treatment. J Endod. 2016;42:557–62.
3. Zuolo AS, Mello JE Jr, Cunha RS, Zuolo ML, Bueno CE. Efficacy of reciprocating and rotary techniques for removing filling material during root canal retreatment. Int Endod J. 2013;46:947–53.
4. Rios Mde A, Villela AM, Cunha RS, Velasco RC, De Martin AS, Kato AS, Bueno CE. Efficacy of 2 reciprocating systems compared with a rotary retreatment system for gutta-percha removal. J Endod. 2014;40:543–6.
5. Fruchi Lde C, Ordinola-Zapata R, Cavenago BC, Duarte MAH, Bueno CES, De Martin AS. Efficacy of reciprocating instruments for removing filling material in curved canals obturated with a single-cone technique: a micro-computed tomographic analysis. J Endod. 2014;40:1000–4.
6. Crozeta BM, Silva-Sousa YT, Leoni GB, Mazzi-Chaves JF, Fantinato T, Baratto-Filho F, Sousa-Neto MD. Micro-computed tomography study of filling material removal from oval-shaped canals by using rotary, reciprocating, and adaptive motion systems. J Endod. 2016;42:793–7.
7. Özyürek T, Demiryürek EÖ. Efficacy of different nickel-titanium instruments in removing Gutta-percha during root canal retreatment. J Endod. 2016;42:646–9.
8. Zuolo AS, Zuolo ML, Bueno CES, Chu R, Cunha RS. Evaluation of the efficacy of TRUShape and RECIPROC file systems in the removal of root filling material: an ex vivo micro-computed tomographic study. J Endod. 2016;2:315–9.
9. Ricucci D, Siqueira JF Jr. Biofilms and apical periodontitis: study of prevalence and association with clinical and histopathologic findings. J Endod. 2010;36:1277–88.
10. Wu MK, Wesselink PR, Walton RE. Apical terminus location of root canal treatment procedures. Oral Surg Oral Med Oral Pathol. 2000;89:99–103.
11. Leal Silva CJN, Menajed K, Ajuz N, Monteiro MRFP, Coutinho-Filho TS. Postoperative pain after foraminal enlargement in anterior teeth with necrosis and apical periodontitis: a prospective and randomized clinical trial. J Endod. 2013;39:173–6.
12. ElAyouti A, Dima E, Ohmer J, Sperl K, Von Ohle C, Löst C. Consistency of apex locator function: a clinical study. J Endod. 2009;35:179–81.
13. Wilcox LR, Van Surkum R. Endodontic retreatment in large and small straight canals. J Endod. 1991;17:119–21.
14. Wilcox LR, Swift ML. Endodontic retreatment in small and large curved canals. J Endod. 1991;17:313–5.
15. Nevares G, de Albuquerque DS, Freire LG, Romeiro K, Fogel HM, Dos Santos M, Cunha RS. Efficacy of ProTaper NEXT compared with Reciproc in removing obturation material from severely curved root canals: a micro-computed tomography study. J Endod. 2016;42:803–8.
16. Rödig T, Reicherts P, Konietschke F, Dullin C, Hahn W, Hülsmann M. Eficacy of reciprocating and rotary NiTi instruments for retreatment of curved root canals assessed by micro-CT. Int Endod J. 2014;47:942–8.
17. Baugh D, Wallace J. The role of apical instrumentation in root canal treatment: a review of the literature. J Endod. 2005;31:333–40.
18. Souza-Filho FJ, Benatti O, Almeida OP. Influence of the enlargement of the apical foramen in periapical repair of contaminated teeth of dog. Oral Surg Oral Med Oral Pathol. 1987;64:480–4.
19. Fornari VJ, Silva-Sousa YTC, Vanni JR, Pécora JD, Versiani MA, Sousa-Neto MD. Histological evaluation of the effectiveness of increased apical enlargement for cleaning the apical third of curved canals. Int Endod J. 2010;43:988–94.
20. Card SJ, Sigurdsson A, Ørstavik D, Trope M. The effectiveness of increased apical enlargement in reducing intracanal bactéria. J Endod. 2002;28:779–83.
21. Aminoshariae A, Kulild JC. Master apical file size—smaller or larger: a systematic review of healing outcomes. Int Endod J. 2015;48:639–47.
22. Alves FR, Roças IN, Almeida BM, Neves MAS, Zoffoli J, Siqueira JF Jr. Quantitative molecular and culture analyses of bacterial elimination in oval-shaped root canals by a single-file instrumentation technique. Int Endod J. 2012;45:871–7.
23. Somma F, Cammarota G, Plotino G, Grande NM, Pameijer CH. The effectiveness of manual and mechanical instrumentation for the retreatment of three different root canal filling materials. J Endod. 2008;34:466–9.
24. Nudera WJ. Selective root retreatment: a novel approach. J Endod. 2015;41:1382–8.
25. Friedman S, Mor C. The success of endodontic therapy. Healing and functionality. J Calif Dent Assoc. 2004;32:493–503.
26. Gorni FG, Gagliani MM. The outcome of endodontic retreatment: a 2-yr follow-up. J Endod. 2004;30:1–4.
27. Nair PN. On the causes of persistent apical periodontitis: a review. Int Endod J. 2006;39:249–81.
28. Kim S, Kratchman S. Modern endodontic surgery concepts and practice: a review. J Endod. 2006;32:601–23.
29. Tsesis I, Rosen E, Schwartz-Arad D, Fuss Z. Retrospective evaluation of surgical endodontic treatment: traditional versus modern technique. J Endod. 2006;32:412–6.
30. Setzer FC, Shah SB, Kohli MR, Karabucak B, Kim S. Outcome of endodontic surgery: a meta-analysis of the literature-part 1: comparison of traditional root-end surgery and endodontic microsurgery. J Endod. 2010;36:1757–65.

31. Bowers DJ, Glickman GN, Solomon ES, He J. Magnification's effect on endodontic fine motor skills. J Endod. 2010;36:1135–8.
32. Mobilio N, Vecchiatini R, Vasquez M, Calura G, Catapano S. Effect of flap design and duration of surgery on acute postoperative symptoms and signs after extraction of lower third molars: a randomized prospective study. J Dent Res Dent Clin Dent Prospects. 2017;11:156–60.
33. Chen YW, Lee CT, Hum L, Chuang SK. Effect of flap design on periodontal healing after impacted third molar extraction: a systematic review and meta-analysis. Int J Oral Maxillofac Surg. 2017;46:363–72.
34. Şimşek Kaya G, Yapıcı Yavuz G, Saruhan N. The influence of flap design on sequelae and quality of life following surgical removal of impacted mandibular third molars: a split-mouth randomised clinical trial. J Oral Rehabil. 2019;46:828–35.
35. Pini Prato G, Pagliaro U, Baldi C. Coronally advanced procedure for root coverage. Flap with tension versus flap without tension: a randomized controlled clinical study. J Periodontol. 2000;71:188–201.
36. Kramper BJ, Kaminski EJ, Osetek EM, Heuer MA. A comparative study of wound healing of three types of flap design used in periapical surgery. J Endod. 1984;10:17–25.
37. Velvart P. Papilla base incision: a new approach to recession-free healing of the interdental papilla after endodontic surgery. Int Endod J. 2002;35:453–60.
38. Lang NP, Löe H. The relationship between the width of keratinized gingiva and gingival health. J Periodontol. 1972;43:623–7.
39. Peñarrocha-Oltra D, Menéndez-Nieto I, Cervera-Ballester J, Maestre-Ferrín L, Peñarrocha-Diago M, Peñarrocha-Diago M. Aluminum chloride versus electrocauterization in periapical surgery: a randomized controlled trial. J Endod. 2019;45:89–93.
40. Clé-Ovejero A, Valmaseda-Castellón E. Haemostatic agents in apical surgery. A systematic review. Med Oral Patol Oral Cir Bucal. 2016;21:652–7.
41. Torabinejad M, Kang HJS, Maskiewicz R, Grandhi A. The haemostatic efficacy and foreign body reaction of epinephrine-impregnated polyurethane from in osseous defects. Aust Endod J. 2018;44:204–7.
42. Gutmann JL. Parameters of achieving quality anesthesia and hemostasis in surgical endodontics. Anesth Pain Control Dent. 1993;2:223–6.
43. Landes CA, Stübinger S, Rieger J, Williger B, Ha TK, Sader R. Critical evaluation of piezoelectric osteotomy in orthognathic surgery: operative technique, blood loss, time requirement, nerve and vessel integrity. J Oral Maxillofac Surg. 2008;66:657–74.
44. Spinelli G, Lazzeri D, Conti M, Agostini T, Mannelli G. Comparison of piezosurgery and traditional saw in bimaxillary orthognathic surgery. J Craniomaxillofac Surg. 2014;42:1211–20.
45. Rubinstein R, Kim S. Short-term observation of the results of endodontic surgery with the use of a surgical operation microscope and Super-EBA as root-end filling material. J Endod. 1999;25:43–8.
46. Preti G, Martinasso G, Peirone B, Peirone B, Navone R, Manzella C, Muzio G, Russo C, Canuto RA, Schierano G. Cytokines and growth factors involved in the osseointegration of oral titanium implants positioned using piezoelectric bone surgery versus a drill technique: a pilot study in minipigs. J Periodontol. 2007;78:716–22.
47. Jang Y, Hong HT, Roh BD, Chun HJ. Influence of apical root resection on the biomechanical response of a single-rooted tooth: a 3-dimensional finite element analysis. J Endod. 2014;40:1489–93.
48. Bernardes RA, de Souza Junior JV, Duarte MA, de Moraes IG, Bramante CM. Ultrasonic chemical vapor deposition-coated tip versus high and low-speed carbide burs for apicoectomy: time required for resection and scanning electron microscopy analysis of the root-end surfaces. J Endod. 2009;35:265–8.
49. Zerbinati LP, Tonietto L, de Moraes JF, de Oliveira MG. Assessment of marginal adaptation after apicoectomy and apical sealing with Nd:YAG laser. Photomed Laser Surg. 2012;30:444–50.
50. Gilheany PA, Figdor D, Tyas MJ. Apical dentin permeability and microleakage associated with root end resection and retrograde filling. J Endod. 1994;20:22–6.
51. Mehlhaff DS, Marshall JG, Baumgartner JC. Comparison of ultrasonic and high-speed-bur root-end preparations using bi-laterally matched teeth. J Endod. 1997;23:448–52.
52. Wuchenich G, Meadows D, Torabinejad M. A comparison between two root-end preparation techniques in human cadavers. J Endod. 1994;20:279–82.
53. Lin CP, Chou HG, Kuo JC, Lan WH. The quality of ultra-sonic root-end preparation: a qualitative study. J Endod. 1998;24:666–70.
54. Parirokh M, Torabinejad M. Mineral trioxide aggregate: a comprehensive literature review—Part I: chemical, physical, and antibacterial properties. J Endod. 2010;36:16–27.
55. Torabinejad M, Parirokh M. Mineral trioxide aggregate: a comprehensive literature review—Part II: leakage and biocompatibility investigations. J Endod. 2010;36:190–202.
56. Parirokh M, Torabinejad M. Mineral trioxide aggregate: a comprehensive literature review—Part III: clinical applications, drawbacks, and mechanism of action. J Endod. 2010;36:400–13.
57. Biočanin V, Antonijević Đ, Poštić S, Ilić D, Vuković Z, Milić M, Fan Y, Li Z, Brković B, Đurić M. Marginal gaps between 2 calcium silicate and glass ionomer cements and apical root dentin. J Endod. 2018;44:816–21.

58. Ferreira CMA, Sassone LM, Gonçalves AS, de Carvalho JJ, Tomás-Catalá CJ, García-Bernal D, Oñate-Sánchez RE, Rodríguez-Lozano FJ, Silva EJNL. Physicochemical, cytotoxicity and in vivo biocompatibility of a high-plasticity calcium-silicate based material. Sci Rep. 2019;9:3933.
59. López-García S, Lozano A, García-Bernal D, Forner L, Llena C, Guerrero-Gironés J, Moraleda JM, Murcia L, Rodríguez-Lozano FJ. Biological effects of new hydraulic materials on human periodontal ligament stem cells. J Clin Med. 2019;14:8.
60. Curtis DM, VanderWeele RA, Ray JJ, Wealleans JA. Clinician-centered outcomes assessment of retreatment and endodontic microsurgery using cone-beam computed tomographic volumetric analysis. J Endod. 2018;44:1251–6.

Strategies for the Restoration of Minimally Invasive Endodontically Treated Teeth

8

Gianluca Plotino and Matteo Turchi

Contents

8.1 Introduction

Numerous articles have been published about endodontically treated teeth over the past decades. Among all the articles on this topic the conclusion of a Cochrane review [1] is particularly interesting: until more evidence becomes available, clinicians should continue to choose how to restore root-filled teeth based on their own clinical experience. In fact, a lot of variables may play a great role in the restoration of endodontically treated teeth and, lacking a strong evidence, individual circumstances and patients' preferences may determine the rehabilitation strategy.

Endodontically treated teeth have a minimum loss of water content [2] and the proprioceptive perception of these teeth may change [3, 4], but the variations in their structure summarized by

G. Plotino
Private Practice, Grande, Plotino & Torsello – Studio di Odontoiatria, Rome, Italy

M. Turchi (✉)
General Dentistry and Orthodontics, Catholic University of the Sacred Heart, Rome, Italy

© Springer Nature Switzerland AG 2021
G. Plotino (ed.), *Minimally Invasive Approaches in Endodontic Practice*,
https://doi.org/10.1007/978-3-030-45866-9_8

Gutmann [5] do not affect the mechanical properties of dentin, as demonstrated by several tests (punch shear strength, toughness test, load to flexural fracture) performed on both vital and contralateral teeth endodontically treated at least 10 years before and then extracted for orthodontic reasons [6].

Researches on this topic mainly focused on the amount of the residual tooth structure as the most important issue influencing endodontically treated teeth resistance [7, 8]. Panitvisai and Messer [9] showed that the deflection of the cusps increases with increasing cavity size from an occlusal cavity to a mesio-occlusal (MO) or disto-occlusal (DO) cavity to a mesio-occluso-distal (MOD) cavity. Nevertheless, only performing the endodontic procedures showed a small effect on tooth stiffness. In this case, the 5% reduction in relative stiffness from endodontic treatment is contributed entirely by the access opening [7]. An occlusal cavity preparation due to an occlusal caries can show a fourfold greater decrease in tooth stiffness (20%) than the only endodontic access cavity preparation [7]. Both procedures involve the same tooth occlusal area, but a greater extension of the caries and consequently of the occlusal cavity on the marginal ridge area may explain this difference. Therefore, the relevance of the marginal ridge integrity comes out and its violation can be considered as the greatest contribution to loss of tooth strength. A two-surface cavity preparation requires the removal of only one marginal ridge, like in a MO or DO cavity. It results in a 46% loss in tooth stiffness, while extending the cavity preparation to a MOD cavity results in an average of 63% loss of cuspal relative stiffness [7].

Clearly, even if endodontic access cavity preparation itself was thought to make teeth more susceptible to fracture as a result of the loss of tooth vitality, restorative procedures due to the loss of tooth structures are the major factor in weakening the tooth [10]. Thus, the decision on the type of restoration for an endodontically treated tooth should take in greater account the loss of tooth structure, in particular of the marginal ridges rather than the endodontic procedure itself.

The golden rule in common with access cavity and root canal preparation is to preserve as much sound dentin as possible, following a minimally invasive approach. The prognosis of an endodontically treated tooth improves proportionally to the amount of sound tooth structure, regardless of the type of restoration that is subsequently provided [11, 12]. Factors that can impair resistance of the tooth removing enamel and dentin structure during the access approach and the root canal preparation have been clearly reported in the Chapters 3 and 4 of this book.

8.2 Minimally Invasive Approach to Restorative Procedures

Minimally invasive approaches in endodontic procedures may guarantee less sacrifice of sound tooth structure, especially at the level of the cervical area of the tooth, that is where coronal fractures mostly happen, thus influencing also the restorative algorithm [13]. In fact, clinicians should always start their endodontic procedures keeping in mind that endodontics does not represent only "white lines" on a radiograph, but should be part of a more complex treatment plan that aims to restore the tooth to its original function in the mouth system. Following this principle, endodontists should always perform their procedures having the vision on the final aim of their work: to put the tooth in function again. The great indiscriminate removal of dentin given by a traditional endodontic access cavity, which recommends in all cases a predefined shape of the occlusal cavity and a straight-line access for the stainless-steel files to the apical curvatures removing the coronal interferences [14–16], may reduce the resistance of the tooth [17] and impair the long-term prognosis [18]. A more conservative approach that takes in higher consideration the peri-cervical dentin, the axial wall dentin, and the soffit, representing the most relevant tooth structure to be maintained and preserved, may increase the resistance to fracture of an endodontically treated tooth and its long-term retention, following the simple principle that the greater amount of dentin is kept, the longer the tooth may be maintained [18] (Fig. 8.1). The possibility to

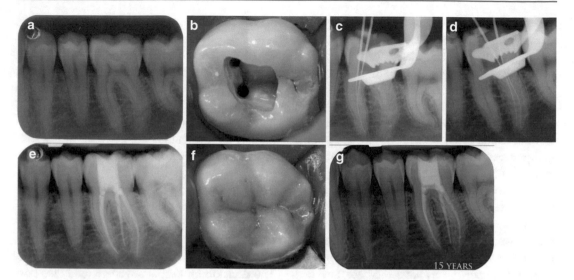

Fig. 8.1 Conservative approach in endodontics in a 15-year-old case demonstrating the way of thinking even when the actual technologies were not present. Preoperative view of the first lower left molar tooth with a deep occlusal caries (**a**). Conservative access cavity (**b**).

Scouting of the root canals (**c, d**). The final root canal therapy with the preservation of sound dentine permits a direct restoration without post placement (**e, f**). A 15-year control radiograph (**g**)

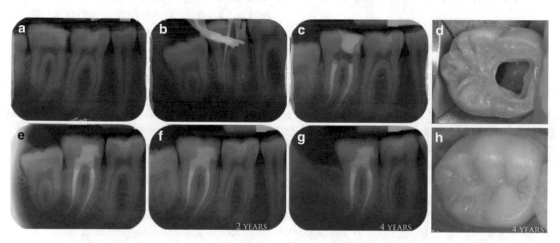

Fig. 8.2 Conservative approach in endodontics. Preoperative view of the second lower right molar with an old mesial restoration (**a**). Thanks to their higher flexibility, heat-treated NiTi alloys permits to shape successfully even severely curved canals, like the distal (**b**), with the

preservation of the original anatomy (**c**) and to be conservative even in the access cavity (**d**). Restoration with an indirect composite onlay (**e**) and 2- and 4-years follow-up radiographs (**f, g**) and image (**h**)

perform more conservative treatments with a dynamic approach given by the technological advancement of instruments, materials, and techniques [19], as demonstrated throughout all this book, permits the clinician to save tooth structure and influence the treatment plan from a restorative point of view (Fig. 8.2).

Technological advancements on the restorative field also permit today more conservative tooth preparations: the most modern restorative materials may be highly performant in much less thickness than before [20, 21], and the advancements in bonding technology [22] permit to create adhesive restorations in most of the cases of endodontically treated teeth except when a full crown is already present. Both these important technological advancements reduce the sacrifice of sound tooth structure required during restorative procedures and cavity preparation, as partial adhesive restorations with complete or partial cuspal coverage may be performed in most of the teeth endodontically treated following the minimally invasive procedures described in this book and given the fact that less extensive tooth preparation is today required for a full-crown restoration, when necessary [23, 24]. In any case, the dogmatic correlation between endodontics and full-crown restoration given by classic studies [25–27], in which a complete cuspal coverage with a full crown was advocated for any endodontically treated tooth, independently of the amount of residual tooth structure, to reduce the risk for fracture and improve the prognosis of these teeth, may be no more actual, given the present advancements described above.

8.3 Post-endodontic Restoration: How and Why

The type of restoration on an endodontically treated tooth may be strongly influenced by the amount of residual tooth structure and the need or not for a partial or complete cuspal coverage [28]. In case that a cuspal coverage may be not needed, an inlay restoration (direct or indirect) may be performed, while when a partial or complete cuspal coverage will be required it may be usually performed with an indirect restoration. The onlay restoration is represented by a partial cuspal coverage, usually involving the cusps and tooth structure near a marginal ridge missing, while an overlay restoration is a complete cuspal coverage with a partial tooth preparation that differs from a 360° full crown preparation because of coronal exposed margins saving more cervical toot structure [29]. Usually the cuspal coverage with onlays/overlays is performed with an indirect restoration, even if in some cases it can be accomplished even with a direct restoration [30].

A direct restoration involving partial or complete cuspal coverage should be considered as a compromise respect to an indirect one, not because it may reduce the fracture strength of the tooth, as it has demonstrated no difference between the two different types of restoration [31], but because it may be more related to the operator skills, given the higher difficulties to perform the correct occlusal and interproximal shape directly in the mouth.

An analysis of the variables that may influence the type of restoration required for an endodontically treated tooth is mainly needed in order to reduce the risk for tooth fracture, which is the most common reason for their failure [32]. The decision on cuspal coverage (and also post placement, as reported later on this chapter) is mainly based on the following parameters: the quantity and quality of residual tooth structure, mainly given by the number and thickness of the remaining cavity walls and the height and thickness of the prepared dentin to be covered (ferrule effect), in case of full-crown restorations.

Generally speaking, in the presence of only an occlusal endodontic cavity, cuspal coverage and post are not necessary and the clinician should only perform a simple direct filling of this space. If only one marginal ridge is lost, usually a post is not needed [33, 34], while the cuspal coverage may be suggested in posterior teeth depending on the quantity and quality of residual tooth structure [35]. Despite the rule should be to cover the cusps near the marginal ridge lost, in these cases the thickness of residual walls near the marginal ridge lost is a determining factor to decide when the cuspal coverage of the adjacent cusps is required: when this thickness is less than 2 mm, cuspal coverage may be suggested [36–38]. However, in these cases, a modern most conservative access cavity design and root canal preparation may preserve critical tooth structure [17], thus permitting in some selected situations a direct (or indirect) restoration without any cuspal coverage even when a marginal ridge is missing.

When both marginal ridges are lost, the result is a strong reduction in tooth stiffness [7] and complete cuspal coverage and post are usually required in almost all these cases. Given the most modern and conservative endodontic approaches described above and throughout all this book, most of these cases may be solved performing a complete cuspal coverage with a partial restoration adhesively cemented, while in case of further tooth structure loss, post and cuspal coverage with a full crown are more indicated. A direct restoration without cuspal coverage and post placement in these cases should be considered an extreme compromise for patients requiring it for a particular socio-economical situation [39].

The height and thickness of the prepared dentin to be covered by a full crown is related to the ferrule effect. A ferrule effect is defined as a "360° collar of the crown surrounding the parallel walls of the dentin extending coronal to the most cervical point of the preparation. The result is an elevation in resistance form of the crown from the extension of dentinal tooth structure" [40]. Therefore, the presence of circumferential 2 mm high parallel walls of dentin extending coronally from the crown margin provide a "ferrule": after being encircled by a crown, it provides a protective effect by reducing stresses within a tooth, called the "ferrule effect" [41]. Maintaining sound coronal and radicular tooth structure and cervical tissue to create a ferrule effect is crucial to optimize the biomechanical behavior of the restored tooth and to guarantee a better prognosis [12]. In fact, in addition to the relative consistency in literature supporting the 2 mm height rule, some authors have implicated even the thickness of residual axial tooth structure after coronal preparation to be significant for fracture resistance [42]. The thickness of the residual dentin after the preparation for the crown should be at least 1 mm [43]. Jotkowitz and Samet [42] also stressed the number of walls as another aspect that should be re-thought. Usually caries brings down some walls, and more frequently the proximal ones, while erosion and abrasion more commonly affect only the buccal walls. If the clinical situation does not provide a circumfer-

ential ferrule, an incomplete ferrule is always preferable than a complete lack of ferrule [44]. Furthermore, when an incomplete ferrule is present in anterior teeth, the presence of the palatal wall becomes more important than the other walls in terms of fracture resistance [44].

The clinician should also take a decision when to insert a root canal post or not, and this procedure is determined by more factors than just the number and thickness of the residual cavity walls and the height and quality of the ferrule present, as it will be reported in the last part of this chapter.

Additional parameters to be taken into consideration for the restoration of endodontically treated teeth that may influence the type of restoration required are: the position of the tooth in the arch (anteriors, premolars, molars), the role of the tooth in the rehabilitation (single-tooth, part of a bridge or of a full mouth restoration), and the strength of occlusal and shear stress (parafunctions, antagonist teeth, orthodontic class). In particular, if a tooth is part of a most complex restoration, it must be considered in a different way rather than if it is a single tooth restoration, as the loss of a tooth with a poor prognosis, but included in a full-arch restoration may impair the prognosis of the entire rehabilitation.

8.4 Parameters Influencing Restoration of Endodontically Treated Anterior Teeth

In anterior teeth, in cases of an intact crown where only the access cavity has been opened, a simple direct composite restoration may be performed to fill the palatal access [45] (Fig. 8.3). When a more incisal conservative access with a direction parallel to the long axis of the root following the principles given in Chap. 3 is performed (Fig. 8.4), a greater attention should be given to clean the mesial and distal pulp horns to prevent future crown discoloration and voids in the restoration in these points [46]. As a general

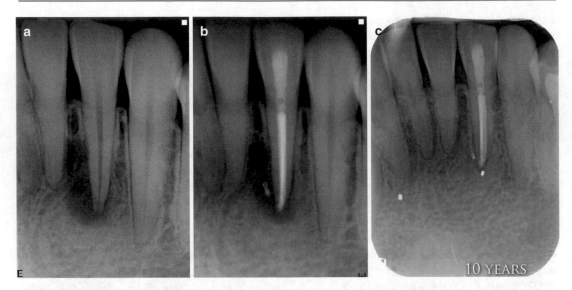

Fig. 8.3 Lower left lateral incisor with periapical lesion (**a**). Even after the endodontic treatment (**b**) the crown is intact overall. A direct restoration is satisfactory (**c**)

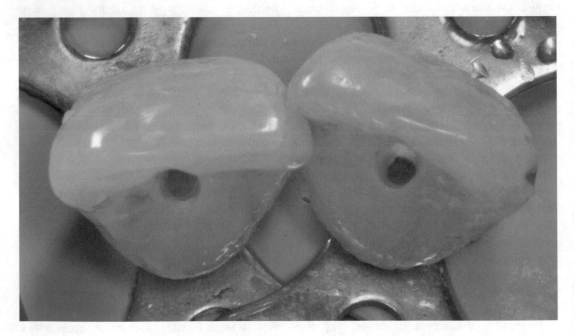

Fig. 8.4 Examples of more incisal access cavities

rule, gutta-percha filling should be limited 2 mm below the root canal orifices that should be adhesively sealed and filled with resin composite during the restorative process or by the endodontist specialist before to send back the case to the referral dentist (in cases in which a post will be not needed). This is of particular importance in the anterior teeth to prevent crown discoloration by the root canal filling materials in the cervical area, through the dentinal tubules that in this region of the tooth proceed in an apico-coronal direction from the canal to the enamel [47]. Thus, the dentinal tubules starting from the buccal part of the canal 2 mm below the CEJ will finish in the CEJ area, which in case of cemental defects may be stained by endodontic materials. In retreatment cases in which this discoloration is already present, an internal bleaching may be needed to solve it before completing the restoration [48, 49]. A flowable resin composite may be the material of choice to seal the root canal up to the orifices, moved by a thin sharp probe to reduce the inclusion of air bubbles between the gutta-percha and composite layers. In fact, inclusion of air bubbles in between the different layers of restorative materials may be difficult to be prevented when restoring a conservative access cavity with four walls, especially between the different layers of standard packable resin composite that should then be used in 2 mm thickness to complete the filling of the coronal access up to the occlusal surface [50]. In these cases, especially in posterior teeth with less esthetic requirements, clinicians may take the advantage of using bulk-fill flowable injectable resin composites with layer thickness of 4 mm to better fill undercuts and reduce air bubble inclusion [51]. The occlusal 1.5–2 mm layer should then always be filled with a packable standard composite with better mechanical properties than a flowable material.

In endodontically treated anterior teeth with a moderate loss of tooth structure, the clinician can decide case by case according to the different tooth characteristics to put a post or not and to perform a full crown or a veneer or a direct composite restoration. Usually, a fiber post or a full crown is not required in these cases [45] (Fig. 8.5), but some clinical exceptions to this rule should be considered. In case of the reattachment of a fragment, when a coronal fracture occurred in an anterior tooth, a strategical short post may be used to connect the fragment to the residual tooth structure, thus contrasting the harmful effects of lateral forces (Fig. 8.6). A strategical post may be also suggested in endodontically treated anterior teeth with incomplete root formation in young patients in which usually an apical plug with MTA has been performed to seal the open apex. Afterwards, a restoration using a fiber post may be performed to improve the resistance of the low thickness residual dentinal walls (Fig. 8.7). Similar indications to the use of a strategical post may exist when an unexpected big loss of coronal tooth structure may be a consequence of a complex endodontic clinical situation, such as to remove coronal calcifications to find a calcified root canal deep inside the root of a traumatized anterior tooth or in the presence of massive internal root resorptions (Fig. 8.8). Even the change of teeth axis during a prosthetic preparation in complex prosthetic rehabilitations may require the use of a strategical post to better maintain the core that will be extensively reduced by the circumferential tooth preparation.

An anterior tooth with a severe loss of tooth structure usually needs a fiber post placement and a full-crown restoration (Fig. 8.9). In these cases, a post is mainly needed to maintain the core and to better dissipate the functional stresses, especially to withstand the lateral forces, thus reducing the risks for a possible dramatic failure, and a full crown on a 2 mm circumferential ferrule is mandatory for a better long-term prognosis. In fact, it has been demonstrated that in these cases of big amount of loss of coronal tooth structure the presence of a post may reduce the number of catastrophic failures (mainly given by vertical unrestorable root fractures leading to the extraction of the tooth), increasing the possibility that the eventual failure may be more favorable and thus restorable,

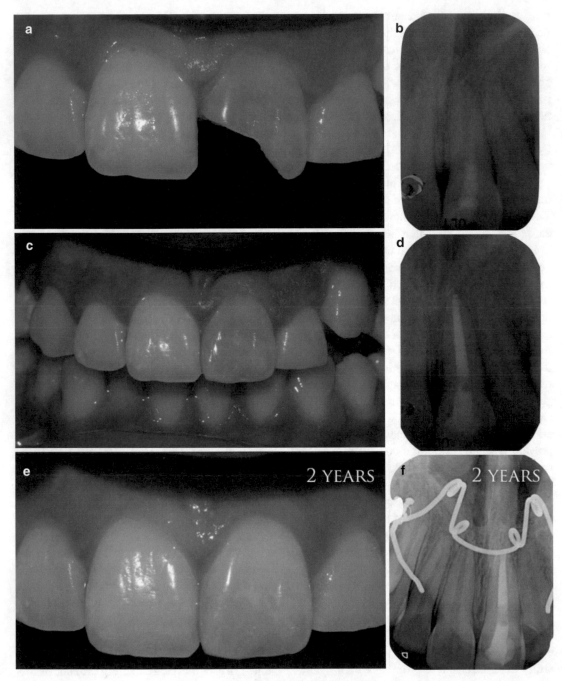

Fig. 8.5 Crown fracture of the maxillary left central incisor (**a**). The preoperative radiograph shows an incorrect endodontic treatment (**b**). The restoration was performed before the endodontic retreatment for esthetic request of the patient (**c**). Postoperative radiograph of the endodontic retreatment (**d**). Then a 2-week internal bleaching and a final direct restoration of the palatal access were performed because of tooth discoloration. 2-year follow-up of the endodontic treatment and the direct restoration (**e**, **f**)

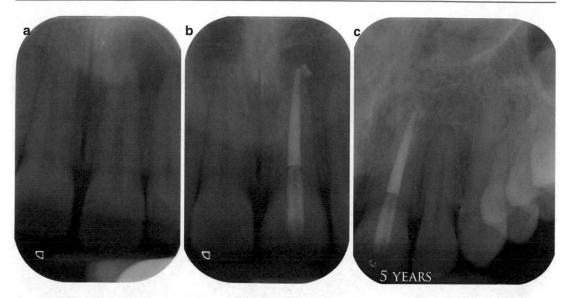

Fig. 8.6 Coronal fracture of a left maxillary central incisor (**a**). A short strategical fiber post was placed to connect the fragment to the remaining sound tooth structure (**b**). 5-year follow-up (**c**)

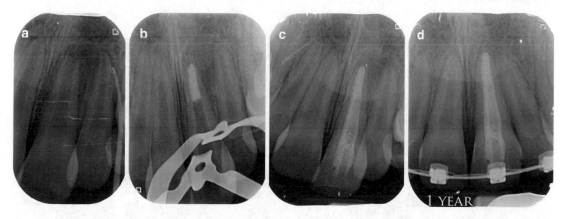

Fig. 8.7 Necrotic left central incisor with an incompletely formed root and low thickness of the residual dentinal root walls (**a**). A 4-mm apical plug of MTA was performed (**b**) and a strategical post was placed in order to reinforce the tooth structure (**c**). 1-year follow-up (**d**)

postponing the extraction of the tooth [52, 53]. When an old full crown should be substituted in the anterior teeth, different strategies may be followed and depending on the quantity and quality of the residual tooth structure a post may be inserted or not before performing a new restoration (Fig. 8.10).

Given the less occlusal stress and masticatory forces acting on the anterior teeth [54], in some situation when the loss of tooth structure involves the incisal tooth part up to the middle third of the crown and there are ideal conditions in terms of occlusion, a direct esthetic composite restoration may also be performed by a skilled clinician to restore the entire missing tooth structure. In these cases, the use of a post may be useful to better maintain the restoration and, above all, to withstand the lateral forces that may act to the restoration and promote its mechanical failure and detachment (Fig. 8.11).

On the contrary, when a complete loss of coronal tooth structure leaves the root without any ferrule, conservative treatments alternative to dental extraction and implant placement, such as

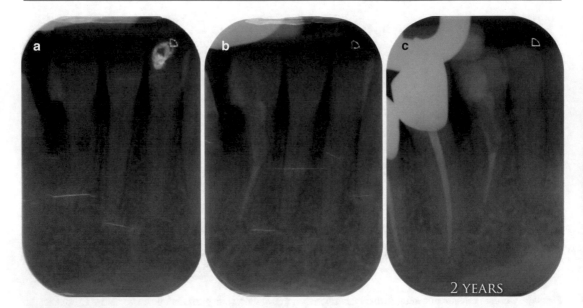

Fig. 8.8 Internal root resorption in a mandibular right lateral incisor (**a**). Endodontic therapy completed and strategical fiber-post placement (**b**). 2-year follow-up (**c**)

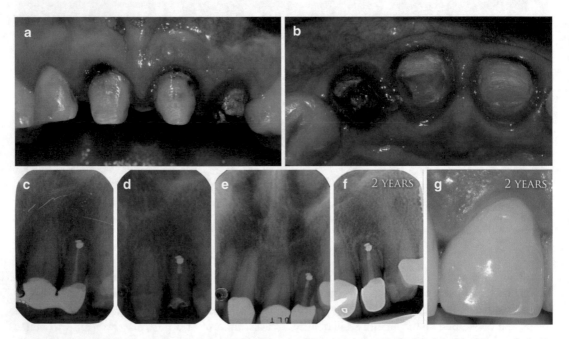

Fig. 8.9 Post and full crown need in a maxillary right lateral incisor with severe loss of tooth structure. Preoperative frontal (**a**) and occlusal (**b**) views. The preoperative radiograph shows an old retrograde filling with amalgam and a periapical lesion (**c**). After endodontic retreatment (**d**), post placement and full-crown restoration (Lab Loreti, Rome—Italy) (**e**). 2-year follow-up radiographical (**f**) and intraoral (**g**) views

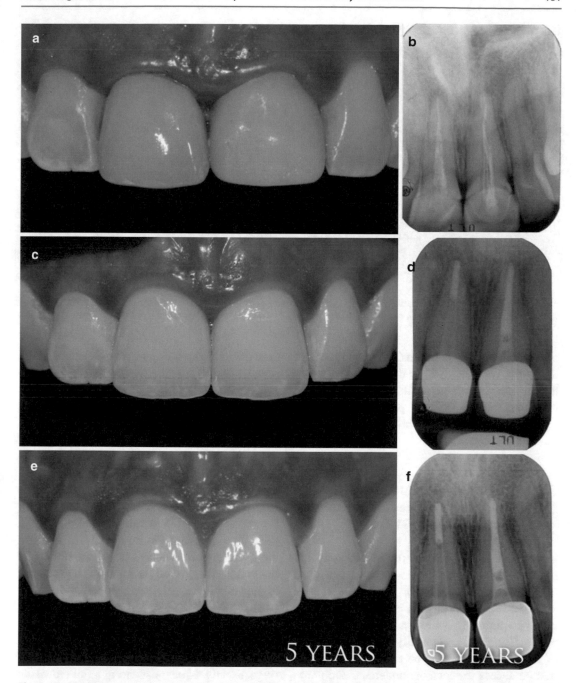

Fig. 8.10 Maxillary central incisors with bad conditions of the old full crowns and the surrounding soft tissues (**a**). Unacceptable root canal treatment for both quality and extent of the filling, with radiographic signs of periapical lesions (**b**). Full-crown restoration (Lab Loreti, Rome— Italy) (**c**) and post placement was performed in the right central incisor for the poor amount of residual tooth structure, while a post was not necessary in the other tooth (**d**). 5-year follow-up intraoral (**e**) and radiographical (**f**) views

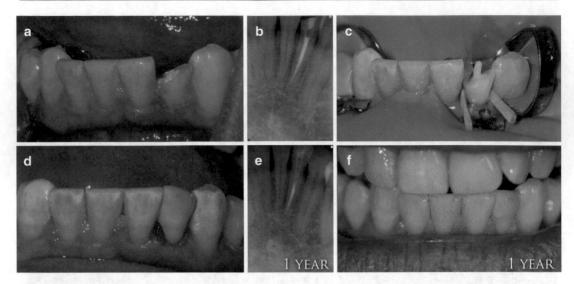

Fig. 8.11 Crown fracture of the mandibular left lateral incisor (**a**). After the endodontic treatment (**b**), a strategical post was used (**c**) to better retain the direct incisal restoration (**d**). 1-year follow-up radiographical (**e**) and intraoral (**f**) views

orthodontic or surgical extrusion, should be taken into great consideration, as described in the following chapter of this book. A surgical crown lengthening may be also performed in these cases, but with more contraindications being an esthetic anterior zone.

8.5 Parameters Influencing Restoration of Endodontically Treated Premolar Teeth

In premolars with intact crowns and only the presence of an endodontic access cavity, no fiber post nor full-crown or partial coverage is required, and the clinician can only perform a direct composite restoration to fill the occlusal cavity (Fig. 8.12). Generally speaking, the use of a liquid etchant may be suggested in a contracted access to reach the undercuts and penetrate such small spaces, given its decreased viscosity rather than acid gels. For the same reason, liquid acid can guarantee better etching in the apical region during post cementation [55]. Liquid etchants have better wettability and lower surface energy than acid gels, improving the capability of reaching the most difficult regions [55]. The use of small endodontic brushes to apply the adhesive system may be also suggested to better reach the less accessible

areas [56]. Light curing of the adhesive and the deepest layers of the restoration should be extended to 40 s in cases of areas with limited direct access [57]. Furthermore, the use of a flowable resin composite to build-up the deepest layer of the restoration may be helpful to permit the clinician to move this material inside the cavity [58], thus reaching more easily the undercuts and permitting to reduce the possible inclusion of air bubbles in the material layer [59]. Flowable bulk-fill materials may be used in these cases, having the possibility to increase the thickness of each layer to 4 mm instead of the standard 2 mm [60]. A standard light-curing highly filled packable resin composite is then used for the reconstruction of the last occlusal 1.5–2 mm layer, being more easily sculptable and more resistant to wear [50].

In premolar teeth with a loss of one marginal ridge, usually a fiber post and/or a full crown are not required and an adhesively cemented indirect restoration that will partially cover the cusps near the marginal ridge lost represents the solution of choice in these cases (Fig. 8.13). The decision generally is determined case by case depending on the amount of sound tooth structure, the thickness of the cusps near the marginal ridge lost, and the presence of further restorations (i.e., buccal restorations). In fact, in cases of interproximal caries-driven opportunistic

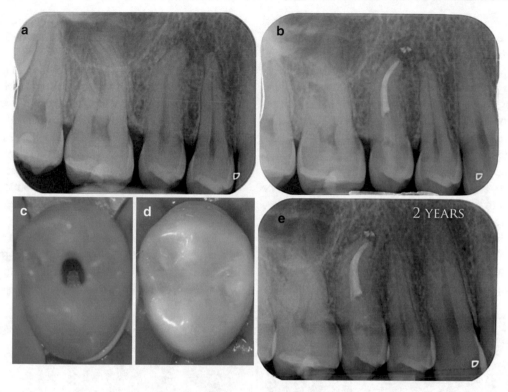

Fig. 8.12 Conservative approach in premolars. The second maxillary premolar tooth with a periapical lesion became necrotic probably for trauma (**a**). The absence of caries permitted a conservative access cavity and root canal treatment (**b**, **c**) and the restoration with a direct composite (**d**). Radiograph of the 2-year follow-up (**e**)

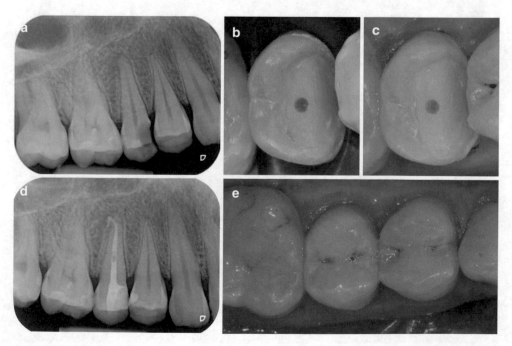

Fig. 8.13 Indirect restoration in a premolar with loss of one marginal ridge. The second maxillary premolar tooth shows a big mesial caries penetrating the pulp chamber (**a**). Preparation for the impression after the restoration with a fiber post (**b**, **c**). Radiographical (**d**) and intraoral (**e**) views after onlay cementation (Lab Loreti, Rome—Italy)

access cavity with the loss of only one marginal ridge with a well-represented thickness of the dentin at the bases of the buccal and lingual cusps, normally a direct resin composite restoration without any post can be also considered (Fig. 8.14). Conversely, when an indirect restoration with a partial cuspal coverage should be more indicated for the higher loss of sound tooth structure near the marginal ridge lost and a reduced cusp thickness, but the patient cannot afford it economically, a strategical post may be used to dissipate the stresses in a better way and a direct restoration removing all the undermined tooth structure may be performed with or without the direct cuspal coverage, as a compromise from an esthetic and functional point of view, given the difficulties in modelling the occlusal

surface in such big restorations. This choice may also allow the clinician to perform an indirect restoration even later.

When a full crown is indicated in cases of only one marginal ridge lost in premolars, because of the extension of the tooth structure lost, the presence of already existing restorations in other parts of the tooth, and/or the reduced thickness of both cusps, the use of a post may be recommended to better retain the core and dissipate the stress in a more favorable way, because of the further amount of tooth structure that will be lost after circumferential tooth preparation for the full crown (Fig. 8.15).

Clinicians may proceed similarly when in premolars the loss of both mesial and distal marginal ridges occurs: in these cases, a fiber post may be suggestable and a complete cuspal coverage is

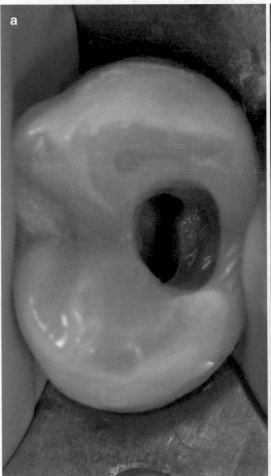
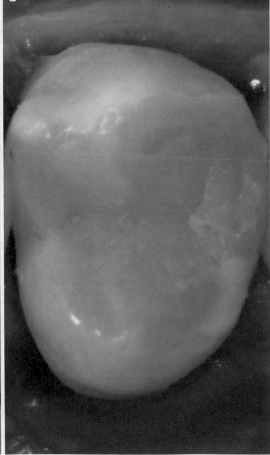

Fig. 8.14 Direct restoration in a premolar after the endodontic treatment performed with a conservative interproximal caries-driven access opened through the old interproximal restoration preserving all the residual coronal tooth structure (a, b)

always needed. A full crown or an overlay adhesive restoration may be performed depending on the quantity, quality, and thickness of the residual amount of tooth structure (Fig. 8.16).

In premolars with the loss of both marginal ridges together with a severe or complete loss of tooth structure, after the insertion of a post, a cus-

pal coverage with a full-crown restoration is the only possible choice. A surgical tooth crown lengthening (Fig. 8.17) or an orthodontic extrusion (Fig. 8.18) must be considered in these cases if there is not enough residual ferrule [61]. Crown lengthening has a significant biological cost that must be considered into the treatment decision-

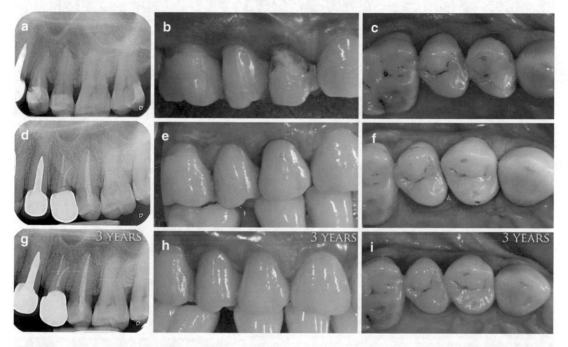

Fig. 8.15 Post and full-crown restoration in a first maxillary premolar tooth showing a significant loss of tooth structure in occlusal, mesial, and buccal area with a big old MO restoration and an extended cervical caries and an incomplete root canal treatment (**a–c**). After the endodontic retreatment, it was restored with a post and a full crown (Lab Loreti, Rome—Italy) (**d–f**). 3-year follow-up radiographical (**g**) and intraoral (**h, i**) views

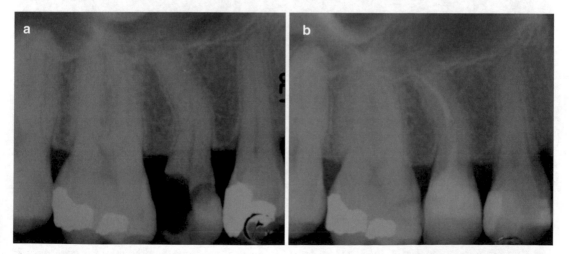

Fig. 8.16 Post and full-crown restoration in a second maxillary premolar tooth showing a significant loss of tooth structure with both mesial and distal marginal ridges missing (**a**). The decision was to restore it with a fiber post and a full crown (Lab Loreti, Rome–Italy) (**b, c**). 1-year follow-up (**d**)

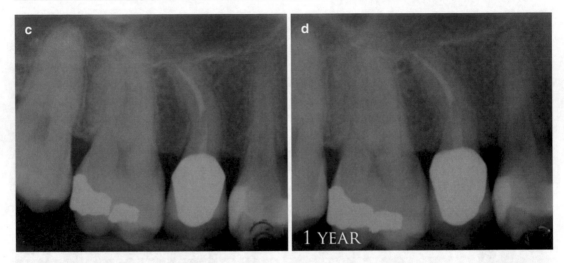

Fig. 8.16 (continued)

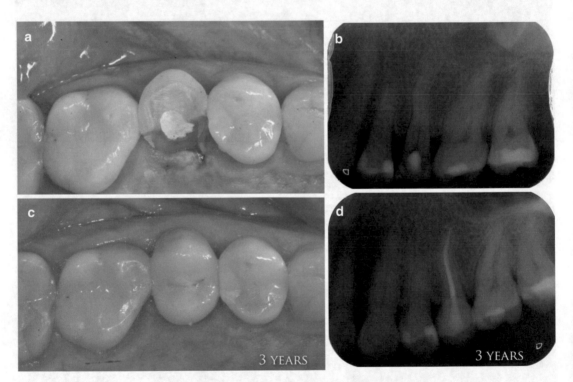

Fig. 8.17 Surgical crown lengthening. The second maxillary premolar tooth reported a fracture of the palatal cusp that invades the periodontal support (**a**), requiring endodontic treatment and crown lengthening (**b**). 3-year follow-up radiographical (**c**) and intraoral (**d**) views. (Surgical crown lengthening Dr. Guerino Paolantoni, prosthetic rehabilitation Dr. Fabio Teodori)

making process; in fact Gegauff [61] demonstrated a more favorable crown-root ratio with orthodontic extrusion than with crown lengthening that impairs tooth static load failure to a greater extent.

Patients may not accept the orthodontic extrusion because of longer treatment time and also because sometimes after the orthodontic extrusion a crown lengthening may be necessary if the clinician does not perform the fibrotomy weekly or if the bone follows the root [62–64]. Even if crown lengthening is performed after orthodontic extrusion, the same crown-root ratio is maintained in a more favorable way than with crown lengthening only, but in these cases an alternative treatment such as the surgical extrusion may be also taken into consideration as reported in Chap. 9. Extraction and implant placement remain the last option, having in any case a high success rate [65].

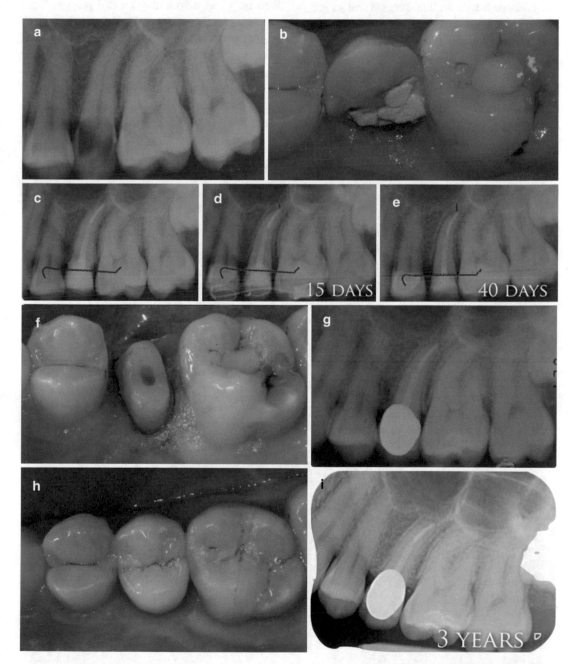

Fig. 8.18 Orthodontic extrusion. The second maxillary premolar tooth reported a fracture of the palatal cusp that invades the periodontal support caused by and extensive caries lesion (a, b). After endodontic treatment and post placement, orthodontic extrusion was performed in 40 days (c–e) and a full crown was chosen as final restoration (Lab Loreti, Rome—Italy) (f–h). 3-year follow-up radiograph (i). (Orthodontic extrusion Dr. Ferruccio Torsello)

8.6 Parameters Influencing Restoration of Endodontically Treated Molar Teeth

In molar teeth with an intact crown and an occlusal endodontic access cavity only, no fiber post nor full-crown or partial coverage restorations are needed, and the clinician can perform a direct composite restoration or eventually an indirect inlay without any cuspal coverage to fill the occlusal cavity, as already reported for premolar teeth (Fig. 8.19). The step-by-step restoration in these cases is similar to what has been already described for similar situations in anterior and premolar teeth with only an occlusal endodontic cavity.

In some cases, after the endodontic treatment both marginal ridges may be still present, but a greater extension of the caries (i.e., on the buccal-lingual surfaces) may cause a significant loss of tooth structure: a post is not needed to retain the material, but the clinician may perform an indirect onlay, with a partial cuspal coverage to better reconstruct the occlusal anatomy. Sometimes, when a big primary occlusal caries or a big old

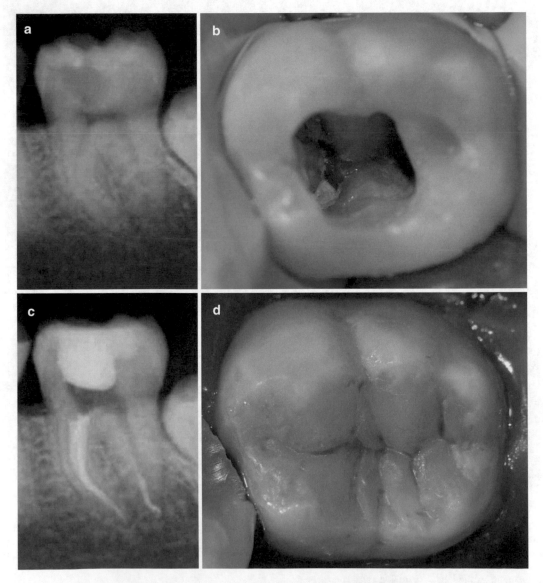

Fig. 8.19 Direct restoration in molars. The limited extension of the occlusal caries (**a**) allowed a conservative cavity access (**b**). The endodontically treated tooth (**c**) was restored with a direct composite (**d**)

occlusal restoration with recurrent caries are present, their removal can still lead to a class I cavity, but undermining the tooth structure with a poor amount of thickness of the residual walls circumferentially. In these cases, apparently intact teeth may also present mesial and/or distal vertical cracks, especially in amalgam-filled teeth [66, 67]. Sometimes cracks penetrate inside the pulp chamber, thus requiring an endodontic treatment [68] and an overlay adhesively cemented indirect restoration with a complete cuspal coverage to prevent cracks extension (Fig. 8.20). In these cases, usually clinicians should also perform a preventive cuspidectomy at the beginning of the endodontic treatment to reduce the risk for fracture of the thin residual walls under masticatory load between the appointments. When an indirect restoration is needed, a flowable bulk-fill resin composite may be used for the core build-up and the preparation for the cuspal coverage may be performed in tooth areas that are no more sustained by dentin. The cementation of a strategical fiber post may also be taken into consideration in these cases.

In molars with the loss of only one marginal ridge, a fiber post and a full crown are not usually needed because of the big amount of tooth structure maintained in the part of the tooth not involved in the pathology. A partial coverage of both the two cusps near the marginal ridge lost would be the ideal solution in these cases, even if a simple direct composite restoration may be performed without any cuspal coverage, depending on the amount of residual tooth structure and the thickness of the cusps near the marginal ridge lost. In fact, no post and a direct restoration can be a good solution for cases with a caries lesion penetrating the pulp, thus requiring endodontic treatment but involving only one marginal ridge, when a caries-driven conservative dynamic enlargement of the access is performed (Fig. 8.21). The stiffness of the cusps in this situation is similar to a class II cavity for the restoration of an interproximal caries, regardless that endodontic treatment is performed or not [69]. Treatment planning should be very important in these cases when the patient cannot afford a more expensive indirect restoration: performing a con-

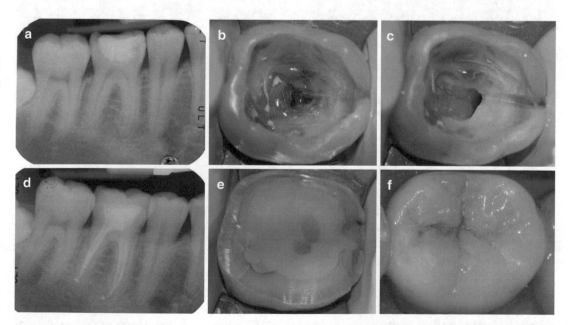

Fig. 8.20 Post and overlay restoration in molars. Old restoration with a big decay in the right mandibular first molar tooth (**a**). After the removal of the old restoration, a crack was appreciated in the cavity floor (**b**), that continued inside the pulp chamber and on the distal aspect (**c**). The tooth was endodontically treated, restored with fiber posts and an adhesively cemented lithium-disilicate ceramic overlay restoration (Lab Loreti, Rome—Italy) (**d–f**)

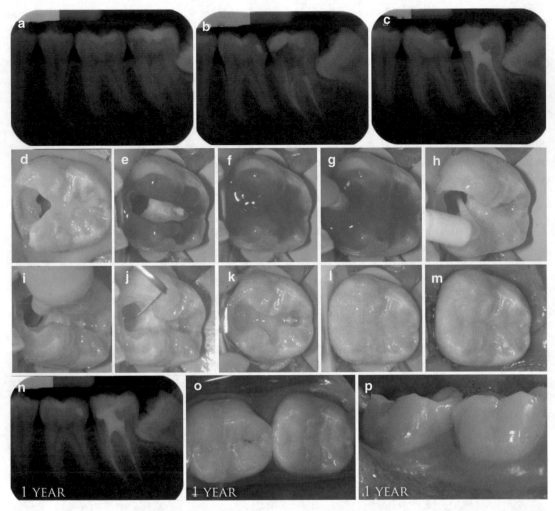

Fig. 8.21 Caries-driven interproximal conservative dynamic access and direct restoration. The mesial deep extension of the caries in the lower left second molar (**a**) required the root canal treatment (**b**), but a direct restora-tion without post was performed because of the only one marginal ridge lost and the conservative access opening (**c–m**). 1-year follow-up radiographical (**n**) and intraoral (**o, p**) views

servative endodontic treatment as described throughout all this book may help the clinician to perform a simple and less expensive direct resin composite class II restoration without cuspal cov-erage, without impairing too much the long-term outcome of these teeth. In similar cases but with a bigger loss of tooth structure, when the access is not much conservative and the thickness at the base of a cusp is less than 2 mm, a restoration can be performed also with the cementation of a strategical post and a direct partial coverage of the involved cusps (Fig. 8.22). In these cases, it may be advantageous to reduce these cusps 1.5–2 mm occlusally and restore the occlusal anatomy even with a direct restoration, thus not impairing the fracture resistance of these teeth with respect to an indirect restoration with cuspal coverage [31]. Direct restorations in these cases should be considered as an interim restoration waiting to perform a more performant indirect restoration: this is the reason of the insertion of the post. Strategical posts can be also used for prosthetic reasons after the endodontic treatment to better retain the core and avoid exposure of

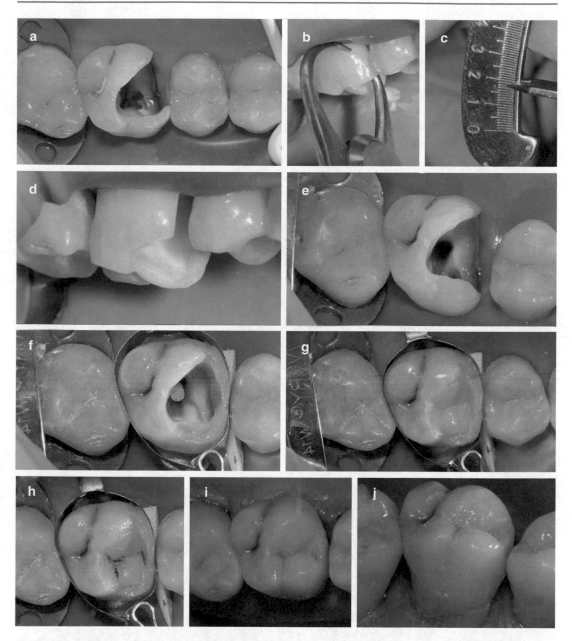

Fig. 8.22 An upper first molar with loss of one marginal ridge (**a**) and with a residual cusp thickness lower than 2 mm (**b**, **c**). Cusps were reduced (**d**, **e**) and tooth restored with a direct composite restoration using a strategical fiber post placement to dissipate the stress (**f**–**j**)

gutta-percha when root hemisection should be performed for periodontal reasons.

In molar teeth with the loss of both two marginal ridges, the use of a fiber post is suggestable and a complete cuspal coverage is always needed to protect the tooth from the high risk for fracture given by the reduced stiffness of the residual cusps and their higher deflection rate. As soon as both buccal and lingual walls are adequately maintained in these cases, a partial indirect adhesively cemented restoration with complete cuspal coverage (overlay) with or without the cementation of a fiber post may be the solution of choice to be conservative maintaining as much tooth structure as possible, while reducing the risk for cusp fracture (Fig. 8.23). Both a fiber post and a full-crown restoration are usually required in less conservative cases, with a massive loss of tooth structure because of big old restorations, caries, or fracture (Fig. 8.24). Surgical tooth crown lengthening should be also taken into consideration in cases of partial or complete lack of fer-

rule or loss of the biologic as width, but, if no ferrule is present at all, the clinician should also consider the extraction and implant placement as a predictable therapy or the surgical extrusion when ideal conditions are present for atraumatic extraction or tooth autotransplantation when an adequate donor tooth is available as described in Chap. 9.

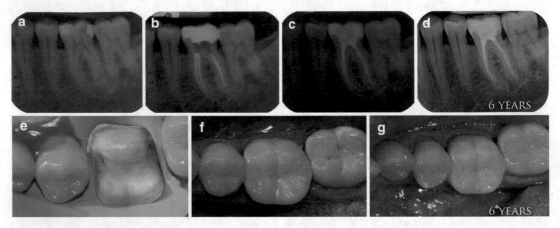

Fig. 8.23 Post and overlay restoration in molars. Mesial old restoration and distal caries under an old restoration in a mandibular first molar (**a**). After the endodontic therapy (**b**), the tooth was restored with a post (**c**) and prepared with cusp reduction and a build-up (**e**) for the cementation of a composite overlay (Lab Loreti, Rome—Italy) (**f**). 6-year follow-up radiographical (**d**) and intraoral (**g**) views

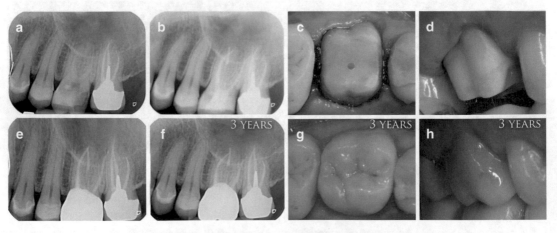

Fig. 8.24 Post and full-crown restoration in molars. Big amount of loss of tooth structure distally and big restoration mesially in an upper left first molar (**a**). After a pre-endodontic build-up with a bulk-fill material, the root canal treatment and the cementation of a fiber post were performed (**b**) and the tooth was prepared for a full crown (**c**, **d**). A monolithic full zirconia crown (Lab Loreti, Rome—Italy) was cemented (**e**). 3-year follow-up radiographical (**f**) and intraoral (**g**, **h**) views

8.7 Restoration of Endodontically Treated Teeth with Fiber Posts

8.7.1 Basic Concepts

Restoration of root-filled teeth may be carried out with or without a post [70]. The main reason to use a post is to retain a core when there is not enough residual coronal tooth structure [5, 71]. Different types of post have been available on the market. To achieve optimum results in post restoration, the materials that should be used to restore root-filled teeth should have physical and mechanical properties similar to that of dentin; they should be able to bond to the tooth structure and should be biocompatible in the oral environment [70]. Thus, it was suggested that the modulus of elasticity of a post should be as much as similar to that of dentin for a more uniform distribution of the stress along the post length [72–74].

Both cast gold post-and-cores and metal preformed posts distribute the stress along the post, concentrating it at the root area around the tip of the post, with a higher risk of root fracture [75]. On the other hand, the biomechanical properties of preformed fiber-reinforced posts have been reported to be close to that of dentin in terms of elastic modulus [76, 77], so that today they may be considered the gold standard for the restoration of endodontically treated teeth. In fact, the mean value of elastic modulus of dentin (Young's modulus) is around 15–20 GPa [77, 78], while fiber posts have registered the most similar modulus of elasticity to that of dentin, having the "white" glass fiber posts values nearer to that of dentin (24–28 GPa) [77] than "black" carbon fiber posts, that registered a little bit higher values (around 34 GPa) [77]. White fiber posts are recommended especially in esthetic areas, but today they are the most commonly used fiber posts in general [79], while in posterior teeth carbon fiber posts may be used to better withstand to the occlusal forces because they have a little bit

higher modulus of elasticity. Metal posts registered much higher values of elastic modulus than fiber posts (110 GPa for stainless-steel and 65 GPa for titanium), with gold posts having the lowest value (53 GPa) among different metals, more similar to that of fiber posts [77]. For this reason, when no more ferrule is present, the only alternative to fiber posts may be the use of a gold cast post-and-core [80], but in these cases clinicians should evaluate the long-term prognosis of no-ferrule teeth and also consider the possible implant alternative [81–84].

Teeth restored using fiber posts have demonstrated a good survival rate in clinical studies, with similar performance to cast post-and-cores [85]. Even metallic posts had a good clinical survival, but the associated failures were mostly irreversible, differently from what happened with fiber posts that reported with more restorable failures [85]. This is the most important reason today for using a fiber post instead of a metallic post. Several in vitro studies also confirmed that teeth restored with non-rigid (low modulus) posts (fiber posts) showed fewer catastrophic irreversible root fractures rather than teeth restored with rigid (high modulus) posts (metal posts) [84–87]. Endodontically treated teeth restored with glass fiber posts showed an increased fracture strength and a more favorable mode of fracture and therefore the use of fiber posts was highly recommended to achieve better clinical outcomes [88, 89], with also a higher survival rate of this type of restoration and of the tooth itself [90].

Furthermore, both in vivo and in vitro studies reported that teeth restored with fiber posts showed mostly restorable fractures, while the ones restored without posts displayed unrestorable failures, both when full coverage restorations were used or not [91–93]. Based on this statement, the use of strategical fiber posts to dissipate the stresses and protect against failure even when they are not strictly required only to retain the core have been mentioned several times previously in the present chapter.

8.7.2 Strategical Fiber Posts

Strategical fiber posts can be thus used in several clinical situations to enhance the biomechanical behavior to better dissipate the occlusal stresses on the tooth and to reduce the risks of a possible catastrophic non-restorable mechanical failure, even when it is not mandatory for their function to retain the core. This is the case, for example, of interproximal cavities with a marginal ridge lost in which an indirect adhesive restoration should be indicated in order to partially cover the undermined cusps near the marginal ridge lost, but the patient cannot afford an indirect restoration after the endodontic treatment [94]. In this border-line situation it is important to plan the treatment since the beginning, thus aiming to be as much conservative as possible, as indicated throughout all this book, to maintain as much tooth structure that may increase the prognosis of these teeth in which a compromise will be taken in the restorative phases. Thus, the clinician may perform in these cases a direct restoration with or without the partial reduction of the two cusps near the marginal ridge lost and a fiber post may be used to improve the mechanical behavior of the tooth (Fig. 8.22). Ideally, this restorative choice should be considered as a temporary compromise restoration and should be substituted by a more effective cuspal coverage as soon as possible.

A strategical post to better dissipate the forces can be also used when indirect adhesive restorations with partial/complete cuspal coverage (onlays/overlays) are performed and its use is not mandatory to retain the core (Fig. 8.13). As the absence of a post may impair fracture resistance and increase cusp strain, depending on the remaining tooth structure [95], the strategic purpose of inserting a post is to make an eventual mechanical failure more favorable and restorable, even if it will occur after several years [92, 96]. Being a circumferential tooth preparation for a full crown, the further step of the treatment, this strategy will make the reintervention easier, because a post placement is suggestable to retain the core in most of the cases when a full crown is required, as today this type of restoration is mainly performed in teeth with a severe loss of tooth structure.

8.7.3 Minimally Invasive Procedures for the Cementation of Fiber Posts

Fiber post placement, and a strategical post in particular, may also be suggested because of the possibility to perform these procedures with the maximum conservation of tooth structure, following the minimally invasive concepts described below.

In particular, the clinician must approach the phase of post-space preparation with the maximum conservative attitude, preserving as much sound dentin as possible, through the removal of the root canal filling material only and cleaning the root canal walls without an additional enlargement of the root canal after the endodontic treatment [11]. Removing a bigger amount of the remaining radicular and coronal tooth structure after the endodontic root canal preparation to insert a post does not lead to a concrete benefit and, on the contrary, it is detrimental for the long-term prognosis [97]. Thus, the most important message is that to insert a post the clinician should not enlarge the coronal part of the root canal more than what was required to perform the endodontic treatment. For this reason, the post-space tapered drills normally suggested to be used by post manufacturer are not compatible with a conservative preparation, because they are too big and rigid and always remove more dentin than needed and over-enlarge the canal. Gates-Glidden are the most preferable and conservative burs to be used in all cases: the rule to follow is to use a bur that is smaller than the root canal diameter, just to remove the filling material and respect the apical seal, maintaining at least 4–5 mm of gutta-percha apically [98, 99]. Largo burs may be also used but they are bigger and more rigid for their longer active part. If a vertical compaction of the gutta-percha technique is used to fill the root canals and a post is needed, it may be useful not to fill back the canal or to fill it back just as much as needed to leave the correct post-space length and just chemically clean the root canal walls before cementation.

Another important topic about the conservative approach in post-space preparation is the length of the post-space in relationship with the post length. In the metal post era, the length of a post was considered important since it was directly proportional to the amount of support offered to its retention and the resistance to root fracture [100]. From this retentive standpoint, not adhesively cemented metal posts were performed as long as possible, to increase the retaining and resistance properties [11, 101, 102]. These classic concepts are not valid anymore with fiber posts thanks to the adhesive procedures and because the insertion length does not influence the biomechanical performance and the fracture resistance of endodontically treated teeth restored with fiber posts [53, 79]. Therefore, the insertion of short posts became a valid alternative in the restoration of root-filled teeth [103], as adequate retentive values are achieved even with shorter posts [104]. The advantage of shortening the length of a post with the use of fiber posts is represented by the possibility to reduce the risks connected to a post-space preparation deep inside the root and the inevitable removal of more sound tooth structure. There are several factors that may influence the post length: when a strategical post is used post length may be reduced, as the main aim is not to retain the core (Fig. 8.13); the less is the residual tooth structure present, the longer should the post be to increase the retention and the fracture resistance (Fig. 8.24); the presence of a severe canal curvature in the middle third of the root canal may result in a reduction of the ideal post length up to the beginning of the curvature, regardless of the residual coronal tooth structure, as the clinician cannot straighten the curvature and reduce tooth resistance just to increase the length of the post [70, 105] (Fig. 8.16); usually the insertion of one fiber post is enough for the restoration of endodontically treated, but in multirooted teeth with severe loss of tooth structure the use of more than one post may be suggested: the length of the additional posts may be reduced in these cases as they only have an antirotational effect to act against lateral forces and/or act as support near the most damaged tooth areas; even in cases with a great amount of coronal tooth structure, a reduced periodontal support requires a longer post, as the crown-to-root ratio in these cases may be unfavorable because of the alveolar bone loss and the center of rotation moves apically reducing the tooth resistance to lateral forces [106]. To act against lateral forces in cases of alveolar bone loss, the clinician should insert the post below the bone level near the fulcrum, despite the amount of residual tooth structure.

While the post-space preparation is the most important step to increase the resistance of the tooth, being as much minimally invasive as possible [107], the post-space cleaning and disinfection is the crucial step to increase the retention of fiber posts. In fact, the most common type of failure with fiber-reinforced composite posts is not root fracture, but debonding [108, 109]. The post-space should be chemically cleaned using 17% EDTA or 2% CHX for 1–2 min after post-space preparation to remove debris and smear layer [110]. EDTA could also enhance the performance of self-etching primers [111, 112] and CHX may increase the retention of fiber post and the long-term stability of the adhesive system [113, 114]. A mechanical cleaning is also needed while using chemicals, performing a passive or active ultrasonic activation [115, 116] and/or using manual or mechanical brushes. Hydrogen peroxide and sodium hypochlorite liquids must be avoided in this cleaning step because they may interfere with the adhesive procedures [117, 118]. Even other materials can impair adhesives polymerization, for example, if the endodontic treatment and post placement are scheduled in the same visit, eugenol-based root canal sealers should be avoided [119], while bioceramic and resin-based root canal sealers are suggested. When bleaching is performed, adhesively cemented fiber post should also be performed at least 7–14 days after bleaching to reduce influence of peroxides generated by the bleaching agent on the adhesive procedures [48]. To increase retention of the fiber posts, posts with surface treatments made by the manufacturer should be selected to increase surface roughness and improve the surface area available for adhesion [120] and create a surface layer that may increase the bond strength of the composite resin to the fiber post [121, 122].

The shape of the post is also important in a minimally invasive restorative concept, as cylindrical fiber posts with parallel walls requests a less conservative preparation in the apical portion of the post-space removing sound dentin [123]. For this reason, a conical post with the same coronal taper of the last endodontic mechanical file used for the preparation of the root canal is the best choice possible to respect the original canal anatomy and do not further remove sound tooth structure important for its resistance. Furthermore, there was no statistical difference in the retention between tapered and parallel-sided posts when they were cemented with the same resin cement [104].

Following the concept that the post should be as similar as the residual canal after the endodontic treatment without further removal of tooth structure and that it must be the post to be adapted to the existing canal anatomy and not the canal to be adapted to the post, the golden rule to be followed in the choice of the correct tapered fiber post size should be that the biggest possible post that passively adapt to the root canal at the correct chosen length, without any friction on the walls and without any additional root canal enlargement is the correct post for that root canal. Usually, if the minimally invasive concepts described in this book will be followed, a very small post will be needed, but this will not affect the biomechanical performance of teeth restored with glass fiber posts to a significant degree [79].

It may be difficult to follow these concepts when the coronal portion of the canal is oval and a single circular preformed post should be inserted in a noncircular root canal. More than one post may be used in the same canal to fill the remaining space, reduce the amount of cement and contrast the C-factor during the polymerization, and increase the resistance of the tooth-restoration complex [124]. When using more posts, the amount of sealer is reduced, but a one-piece oval post would be even better to also increase its mechanical properties. For this reason, a minimally invasive technique to create anatomical fiber posts have been introduced [125] to reduce the amount of surrounding cement, thus reducing air bubble inclusion during cementation, distribute it in a regular thickness that may increase the retention of the post, while having a single piece of fiber-reinforced composite post that may increase the mechanical proprieties of the post and the tooth-post complex [77, 126, 127].

Once cemented, the fiber post should not be exposed to the oral environment for long time because humidity can alter the mechanical properties of fiber posts [128], so it is suggestable to always completely cover the post by the build-up material.

8.8   Conclusive Remarks

The survival of an endodontically treated tooth is dependent primarily on the amount of residual tooth structure. For this reason, over the last years all the efforts in endodontics and restorative dentistry have been directed toward a paradigm shift from the traditional rules to a more conservative and minimally invasive approach. The "golden rule" is now to preserve as much tooth structure as possible in all the procedures: from the access cavity preparation to the choice of the type of coronal restoration. The technical evolution has led to important changes in the clinical management of endodontically treated teeth, because new instruments, materials, and techniques have been introduced. In this perspective, the introduction of heat-treated NiTi alloys and new trends in access cavity opening has represented a conservative revolution in endodontics, such as the introduction of fiber-reinforcement for post fabrication has guaranteed a safer stress distribution and a higher preservation of sound intracanal dentin in post-space preparation than with the stiffer and wider metallic posts [129].

Despite all the innovations, a deep knowledge of occlusion still remains crucial to guide the clinician in a correct management of coronal restoration: direct composite, cusp reduction with an indirect restoration (onlay or overlay) and full crown are the treating options that the clinician can perform always taking into account both the amount and quality of the residual coronal tooth structure. In most destructive decays, even periodontal health must be considered, because usually a biological width violation may occur in these cases [130]. A particular concern should be reserved for crown-root ratio, and orthodontic extrusion and surgical crown lengthening can be performed to provide a favorable ferrule effect and improve biomechanical behavior of the restored tooth [131].

On the basis of these concepts it can be concluded that, before starting an endodontic treatment, the clinician should always keep in mind the final result of this procedure that must involve its restoration and the need to put the tooth in function again.

References

1. Fedorowicz Z, Carter B, de Souza RF, de Andrade Lima Chaves C, Nasser M, Sequeira-Byron P. Single crowns versus conventional fillings for the restoration of root filled teeth. Cochrane Database Syst Rev. 2012;5:CD009109.
2. Helfer AR, Melnick S, Schilder H. Determination of the moisture content of vital and pulpless teeth. Oral Surg Oral Med Oral Pathol. 1972;34:661–70.
3. Loewenstein WR, Rathkarnp R. A study on the pressoreceptive sensibility of the tooth. J Dent Res. 1955;34:287–94.
4. Randow K, Glantz PO. On cantilever loading of vital and non-vital teeth: an experimental clinical study. Acta Odontol Scand. 1986;44:271.
5. Gutmann JL. The dentin-root complex: anatomic and biologic considerations in restoring endodontically treated teeth. J Prosthet Dent. 1992;67:458–67.
6. Sedgley CM, Messer HH. Are endodontically treated teeth more brittle? J Endod. 1992;18:332–5.
7. Reeh ES, Messer HH, Douglas WH. Reduction in tooth stiffness as a result of endodontic and restorative procedures. J Endod. 1989;15:512–6.
8. Reeh ES, Douglas WH, Messer HH. Stiffness of endodontically-treated teeth related to restoration technique. J Dent Res. 1989;68:1540–4.
9. Panitvisai P, Messer HH. Cuspal deflection in molars in relation to endodontic and restorative procedures. J Endod. 1995;21:57–61.
10. Taha NA, Palamara JE, Messer HH. Cuspal deflection, strain and microleakage of endodontically treated premolar teeth restored with direct resin composites. J Dent. 2009;37:724–30.
11. Stankiewicz NR, Wilson PR. The ferrule effect: a literature review. Int Endod J. 2002;35:575–81.
12. Juloski J, Radovic I, Goracci C, Vulicevic ZR, Ferrari M. Ferrule effect: a literature review. J Endod. 2012;38:11–9.
13. Gutmann JL. Minimally invasive dentistry (Endodontics). J Conserv Dent. 2013;16:282–3.
14. Riitano F. La Tecnica Tre Tempi. Dental Cadmos. 1976;4:10–7.
15. Ruddle CJ. Current concepts for preparing the root canal system. Dent Today. 2001;20:76–83.
16. Ruddle CJ. Cleaning and shaping root canal systems. In: Cohen S, Burns RC, editors. Pathways of the pulp. 8th ed. St. Louis, MO: Mosby; 2002. p. 231–91.
17. Plotino G, Grande NM, Isufi A, Ioppolo P, Pedullà E, Bedini R, Gambarini G, Testarelli L. Fracture strength of endodontically treated teeth with different access cavity designs. J Endod. 2017;43:995–1000.
18. Clark D, Kadhemi J. Modern molar endodontic access and directed dentin conservation. Dent Clin N Am. 2010;54:249–73.
19. Shen Y, Zhou HM, Zheng YF, Peng B, Haapasalo M. Current challenges and concepts of the thermomechanical treatment of nickel-titanium instruments. J Endod. 2013;39:163–72.
20. Wilson NHF. Minimally invasive dentistry—the management of caries. London: Quintessence Publishing Co.; 2007.
21. Kidd E. Clinical threshold for caries removal. Dent Clin N Am. 2010;54:541–9.
22. Sabbagh J, McConnell RJ, McConnell MC. Posterior composites: update on cavities and filling techniques. J Dent. 2017;57:86–90.
23. Mannocci F, Bertelli E, Sherriff M, Watson TF, Ford TR. Three-year clinical comparison of survival of endodontically treated teeth restored with either full cast coverage or with direct composite restoration. J Prosthet Dent. 2002;88:297–301.
24. Nagasiri R, Chitmongkolsuk S. Long-term survival of endodontically treated molars without crown coverage: a retrospective cohort study. J Prosthet Dent. 2005;93:164–70.
25. Sorensen JA, Martinoff JT. Intracoronal reinforcement and coronal coverage: a study of endodontically treated teeth. J Prosthet Dent. 1984;51:780–4.
26. Sorensen JA, Martinoff JT. Clinically significant factors in dowel design. J Prosthet Dent. 1984;52:28–35.
27. Goodacre CJ, Spolnik KJ. The prosthodontic management of endodontically treated teeth: a literature review. Part I. Success and failure data, treatment concepts. J Prosthodont. 1994;3:243–50.
28. Seow LL, Toh CG, Wilson NH. Remaining tooth structure associated with various preparation designs for the endodontically treated maxillary second premolar. Eur J Prosthodont Restor Dent. 2005;13:57–64.
29. Veneziani M. Posterior indirect adhesive restorations: updated indications and the Morphology Driven Preparation Technique. Int J Esthet Dent. 2017;12:204–30.
30. Jackson RD. Indirect resin inlay and onlay restorations: a comprehensive clinical overview. Pract Periodontics Aesthet Dent. 1999;11:891–900.
31. Plotino G, Buono L, Grande NM, Lamorgese V, Somma F. Fracture resistance of endodontically

treated molars restored with extensive composite resin restorations. J Prosthet Dent. 2008;99:225–32.

32. Kishen A. Mechanisms and risk factors for fracture predilection in endodontically treated teeth. Endod Top. 2006;13:57–83.

33. Sorrentino R, Monticelli F, Goracci C, Zarone F, Tay FR, García-Godoy F, Ferrari M. Effect of post-retained composite restorations and amount of coronal residual structure on the fracture resistance of endodontically-treated teeth. Am J Dent. 2007;20:269–74.

34. Zhu Z, Dong XY, He S, Pan X, Tang L. Effect of post placement on the restoration of endodontically treated teeth: a systematic review. Int J Prosthodont. 2015;28:475–83.

35. Salameh Z, Sorrentino R, Papacchini F, Ounsi HF, Tashkandi E, Goracci C, Ferrari M. Fracture resistance and failure patterns of endodontically treated mandibular molars restored using resin composite with or without translucent glass fiber posts. J Endod. 2006;32:752–5.

36. Magne P, Harrington D, Harrington S. Semi-direct techniques. Chapter III. In: Esthetic and biomimetic restorative dentistry. Manual for posterior esthetic restorations. St. Louis (MO): Elsevier Mosby; 2005. p. 44–59.

37. Deliperi S, Bardwell DN. Multiple cuspal-coverage direct composite restorations: functional and esthetic guidelines. J Esthet Restor Dent. 2008;20:300–12.

38. Scotti N, Rota R, Scansetti M, Paolino DS, Chiandussi G, Pasqualini D, Berutti E. Influence of adhesive techniques on fracture resistance of endodontically treated premolars with various residual wall thicknesses. J Prosthet Dent. 2013;110:376–82.

39. Leprince JG, Leloup G, Hardy CMF. Considerations for the restoration of endodontically treated molars. In: The guidebook to molar endodontics. Berlin Heidelberg: Springer-Verlag; 2017. p. 169–205.

40. Sorensen JA, Engelman MJ. Ferrule design and fracture resistance of endodontically treated teeth. J Prosthet Dent. 1990;63:529–36.

41. Stankiewicz N, Wilson P. The ferrule effect. Dent Update. 2008;35:222–4.

42. Jotkowitz A, Samet N. Rethinking ferrule— a new approach to an old dilemma. Br Dent J. 2010;209:25–33.

43. Tjan AH, Whang SB. Resistance to root fracture of dowel channels with various thicknesses of buccal dentin walls. J Prosthet Dent. 1985;53:496–500.

44. Ng CC, Dumbrigue HB, Al-Bayat MI, Griggs JA, Wakefield CW. Influence of remaining coronal tooth structure location on the fracture resistance of restored endodontically treated anterior teeth. J Prosthet Dent. 2006;95:290–6.

45. Morgano S. Restoration of pulpless teeth: application of traditional principles in present and future contexts. J Prosthet Dent. 1996;75:375–80.

46. Ahmed HMA, Abbott PV. Discolouration potential of endodontic procedures and materials: a review. Int Endod J. 2012;45:883–97.

47. Ioannidis K, Beltes P, Lambrianidis T, Kapagiannidis D, Karagiannis V. Crown discoloration induced by endodontic sealers: spectrophotometric measurement of Commission International de l'Eclairage's L∗, a∗, b∗ chromatic parameters. Oper Dent. 2013;38:E1–12.

48. Plotino G, Buono L, Grande NM, Pameijer CH, Somma F. Nonvital tooth bleaching: a review of the literature and clinical procedures. J Endod. 2008;34:394–407.

49. Del Curto F, Rocca GT, Krejci I. Restoration of discolored endodontically treated anterior teeth: a minimally invasive chemomechanical approach. Int J Esthet Dent. 2018;13:302–17.

50. Ferraris F, Diamantopoulou S, Acunzo R, Alcidi R. Influence of enamel composite thickness on value, chroma and translucency of a high and a nonhigh refractive index resin composite. Int J Esthet Dent. 2014;9:382–401.

51. Jang P, Hwang I, Hwang IN. Polymerization shrinkage and depth of cure of bulk-fill resin composites and highly filled flowable resin. Oper Dent. 2015;40:172–80.

52. Salameh Z, Ounsi HF, Aboushelib MN, Sadig W, Ferrari M. Fracture resistance and failure patterns of endodontically treated mandibular molars with and without glass fiber post in combination with a zirconia-ceramic crown. J Dent. 2008;36:513–9.

53. Borelli B, Sorrentino R, Zarone F, Ferrari M. Effect of the length of glass fiber posts on the fracture resistance of restored maxillary central incisors. Am J Dent. 2012;25:79–83.

54. Kumagai H, Suzuki T, Hamada T, Sondang P, Fujitani M, Nikawa H. Occlusal force distribution on the dental arch during various levels of clenching. J Oral Rehabil. 1999;26:932–5.

55. Salas MM, Bocangel JS, Henn S, Pereira-Cenci T, Cenci MS, Piva E, Demarco FF. Can viscosity of acid etchant influence the adhesion of fibre posts to root canal dentine? Int Endod J. 2011;44:1034–40.

56. Ferrari M, Vichi A, Grandini S, Geppi S. Influence of microbrush on efficacy of bonding into root canals. Am J Dent. 2002;15:227–31.

57. Akram S, Ali Abidi SY, Ahmed S, Meo AA, Qazi FU. Effect of different irradiation times on microhardness and depth of cure of a nanocomposite resin. J Coll Physicians Surg Pak. 2011;21:411–4.

58. Lokhande NA, Padmai AS, Rathore VP, Shingane S, Jayashankar DA, Sharma U. Effectiveness of flowable resin composite in reducing microleakage - an in vitro study. J Int Oral Health. 2014;6:111–4.

59. Baroudi K, Rodrigues JC. Flowable resin composites: a systematic review and clinical considerations. J Clin Diagn Res. 2015;9:ZE18–24.

60. Benetti AR, Havndrup-Pedersen C, Honoré D, Pedersen MK, Pallesen U. Bulk-fill resin composites: polymerization contraction, depth of cure, and gap formation. Oper Dent. 2015;40:190–200.

61. Gegauff AG. Effect of crown lengthening and ferrule placement on static load failure of cemented cast post-cores and crowns. J Prosthet Dent. 2000;84:169–79.
62. Potashnick SR, Rosenberg ES. Forced eruption: principles in periodontics and restorative dentistry. J Prosthet Dent. 1982;48:141–8.
63. Pontoriero R, Celenza F Jr, Ricci G, Carnevale G. Rapid extrusion with fiber resection: a combined orthodontic-periodontic treatment modality. Int J Periodontics Restorative Dent. 1987;7:30–43.
64. Kozlovsky A, Tal H, Lieberman M. Forced eruption combined with gingival fiberotomy. A technique for clinical crown lengthening. J Clin Periodontol. 1988;15:534–8.
65. Avila G, Galindo-Moreno P, Soehren S, Misch CE, Morelli T, Wang HL. A novel decision-making process for tooth retention or extraction. J Periodontol. 2009;80:476–91.
66. Seo D-G, Yi Y-A, Shin S-J, Park J-W. Analysis of factors associated with cracked teeth. J Endod. 2012;38:288–92.
67. Danley BT, Hamilton BN, Tantbirojn D, Goldstein RE, Versluis A. Cuspal flexure and stress in restored teeth caused by amalgam expansion. Oper Dent. 2018;43:300–7.
68. PradeepKumar AR, Arunajatesan S. Cracks and fractures in teeth. Restor Dent Endod. 2017;2:25–30.
69. Burke FJ. Tooth fracture in vivo and in vitro. J Dent. 1992;20:131–9.
70. Fernandes AS, Shetty S, Coutinho I. Factors determining post selection: a literature review. J Prosthet Dent. 2003;90:556–62.
71. Assif D, Gorfil C. Biomechanical considerations in restoring endodontically treated teeth. J Prosthet Dent. 1994;71:565–7.
72. Grandini S, Goracci C, Tay FR, Grandini R, Ferrari M. Clinical evaluation of the use of fiber posts and direct resin restorations for endodontically treated teeth. Int J Prosthodont. 2005;18:399–404.
73. Naumann M, Sterzenbac G, Alexandra F, Dietrich T. Randomized controlled clinical pilot trial of titanium vs. glass fiber prefabricated posts: preliminary results after up to 3 years. Int J Prosthodont. 2007;20:499–503.
74. Al-Omiri MK, Rayyan MR, Abu-Hammad O. Stress analysis of endodontically treated teeth restored with post-retained crowns: a finite element analysis study. J Am Dent Assoc. 2011;142:289–300.
75. Martínez-Insua A, da Silva L, Rilo B, Santana U. Comparison of the fracture resistances of pulpless teeth restored with a cast post and core or carbon-fiber post with a composite core. J Prosthet Dent. 1998;80:527–32.
76. Duret B, Reynaud M, Duret F. Un nouveau concept de reconstitution corono-radiculaire: le composi-post. Chir Dent France. 1990;60:131–41.
77. Plotino G, Grande NM, Bedini R, Pameijer CH, Somma F. Flexural properties of endodon-tic posts and human root dentin. Dent Mater. 2007;23:1129–35.
78. Kinney JH, Marshall SJ, Marshall GW. The mechanical properties of human dentin: a critical review and re-evaluation of the dental literature. Crit Rev Oral Biol Med. 2003;14:13–29.
79. Rodríguez-Cervantes PJ, Sancho-Bru JL, Barjau-Escribano A, Forner-Navarro L, Pérez-González A, Sánchez-Marín FT. Influence of prefabricated post dimensions on restored maxillary central incisors. J Oral Rehabil. 2007;34:141–52.
80. Fokkinga WA, Kreulen CM, Bronkhorst EM, Creugers NHJ. Up to 17-year controlled clinical study on post-and-cores and covering crowns. J Dent. 2007;35:778–86.
81. Iqbal MK, Kim S. A review of factors influencing treatment planning decisions of single-tooth implants versus preserving natural teeth with nonsurgical endodontic therapy. J Endod. 2008;34:519–29.
82. Zitzmann NU, Krastl G, Hecker H, Walter C, Weiger R. Endodontics or implants? A review of decisive criteria and guidelines for single tooth restorations and full arch reconstructions. Int Endod J. 2009;42:757–74.
83. Soares CJ, Valdivia AD, da Silva GR, Santana FR, Menezes Mde S. Longitudinal clinical evaluation of post systems: a literature review. Braz Dent J. 2012;23:135–40.
84. Asmussen E, Peutzfeldt A, Heitmann T. Stiffness, elastic limit, and strength of newer types of endodontic posts. J Dent. 1999;27:275–8.
85. Mannocci F, Sherriff M, Watson TF. Three-point bending test of fiber posts. J Endod. 2001;27:758–61.
86. Drummond JL, Bapna MS. Static and cyclic loading of fiber-reinforced dental resin. Dent Mater. 2003;19:226–31.
87. Lassila LV, Tanner J, Le Bell AM, Narva K, Vallittu PK. Flexural properties of fiber reinforced root canal posts. Dent Mater. 2004;20:29–36.
88. Ferrari M, Cadigiaco MC, Goracci C, Vichi A, Mason PN, Radovic I, Tay F. Long-term retrospective study of the clinical performance of fiber posts. Am J Dent. 2007;20:287–91.
89. Jindal S, Jindal R, Mahajan S, Dua R, Jain N, Sharma S. In vitro evaluation of the effect of post system and length on the fracture resistance of endodontically treated human anterior teeth. Clin Oral Investig. 2012;16:1627–33.
90. Signore A, Benedicenti S, Kaitsas V, Barone M, Angiero F, Ravera G. Long-term survival of endodontically treated, maxillary anterior teeth restored with either tapered or parallel-sided glass-fiber posts and full-ceramic crown coverage. J Dent. 2009;37:115–21.
91. Salameh Z, Sorrentino R, Ounsi HF, Goracci C, Tashkandi E, Tay FR, Ferrari M. Effect of different all-ceramic crown system on fracture resistance and failure pattern of endodontically treated maxillary premolars restored with and without glass fiber posts. J Endod. 2007;33:848–51.

92. Salameh Z, Sorrentino R, Ounsi HF, Sadig W, Atiyeh F, Ferrari M. The effect of different full-coverage crown systems on fracture resistance and failure pattern of endodontically treated maxillary incisors restored with and without glass fiber posts. J Endod. 2008;34:842–6.

93. Sherfudhin H, Hobeich J, Carvalho CA, Aboushelib MN, Sadig W, Salameh Z. Effect of different ferrule designs on the fracture resistance and failure pattern of endodontically treated teeth restored with fiber posts and all-ceramic crowns. J Appl Oral Sci. 2011;19:28–33.

94. Hurst D. Indirect or direct restorations for heavily restored posterior adult teeth? Evid Based Dent. 2010;11:116–7.

95. Santana FR, Castro CG, Simamoto-Jùnior PC, Soares PV, Quagliatto PS, Estrela C, Soares CJ. Influence of post system and remaining coronal tooth tissue on biomechanical behavior of root filled molar teeth. Int Endod J. 2011;44:386–94.

96. Hitz T, Ozcan M, Göhring TN. Marginal adaptation and fracture resistance of root-canal treated mandibular molars with intracoronal restorations: effect of thermocycling and mechanical loading. J Adhes Dent. 2010;12:279–86.

97. Pilo R, Tamse A. Residual dentin thickness in mandibular premolars prepared with gates glidden and ParaPost drills. J Prosthet Dent. 2000;83:617–23.

98. Mattison GD, Delivanis PD, Thacker RW Jr, Hassel KJ. Effect of post preparation on the apical seal. J Prothet Dent. 1984;51:785–9.

99. Kvist T, Rydin E, Reit C. The relative frequency of periapical lesions in teeth with root canal-retained posts. J Endod. 1989;15:578–80.

100. De Sort KD. The prosthodontic use of endodontically treated teeth: theory and biomechanics of post preparation. J Prosthet Dent. 1983;49:203–6.

101. Standlee JP, Caputo AA, Hanson EC. Retention of endodontic dowels: effects of cement, dowel length, diameter, and design. J Prosthet Dent. 1978;39:400–5.

102. Macedo VC, Faria e Silva AL, Martins LR. Effect of cement type, relining procedure, and length of cementation on pull-out bond strength of fiber posts. J Endod. 2010;36:1543–6.

103. Scotti N, Scansetti M, Rota R, Pera F, Pasqualini D, Berutti E. The effect of the post length and cusp coverage on the cycling and static load of endodontically treated maxillary premolars. Clin Oral Investig. 2011;15:923–9.

104. Borer RE, Britto LR, Haddix JE. Effect of dowel length on the retention of 2 different prefabricated posts. Quintessence Int. 2007;38:e164–8.

105. Nissan J, Dmitry Y, Assif D. The use of reinforced composite resin cementas compensation for reduced post length. J Prosthet Dent. 2001;86:304–8.

106. Grossmann Y, Sadan A. The prosthodontic concept of crown-to-root ratio: a review of the literature. J Prosthet Dent. 2005;93:559–62.

107. Büttel L, Krastl G, Lorch H, Naumann M, Zitzmann NU, Weiger R. Influence of post fit and post length on fracture resistance. Int Endod J. 2009;42:47–53.

108. Cagidiaco MC, Goracci C, Garcia-Godoy F, Ferrari M. Clinical studies of fiber posts: a literature review. Int J Prosthodont. 2008;21:328–36.

109. Ferrari M, Vichi A, Fadda GM, Cagidiaco MC, Tay FR, Breschi L, Polimeni A, Goracci C. A randomized controlled trial of endodontically treated and restored premolars. J Dent Res. 2012;91:72S–8S.

110. Zehnder M. Root canal irrigants. J Endod. 2006;32:389–98.

111. Guerisoli DM, Marchesan MA, Walmsley AD, Lumley PJ, Pecora JD. Evaluation of smear layer removal by EDTAC and sodium hypochlorite with ultrasonic agitation. Int Endod J. 2002;35:418–21.

112. Zhang L, Huang L, Xiong Y, Fang M, Chen JH, Ferrari M. Effect of post-space treatment on retention of fiber posts in different root regions using two self-etching systems. Eur J Oral Sci. 2008;116:280–6.

113. da Silva RS, de Almeida Antunes RP, Ferraz CC, Orsi IA. The effect of the use of 2% chlorhexidine gel in post-space preparation on carbon fiber post retention. Oral Surg Oral Med Oral Pathol Oral Radiol Endod. 2005;99:372–7.

114. Mohammadi Z, Abbott PV. The properties and applications of chlorhexidine in endodontics. Int Endod J. 2009;42:288–302.

115. Serafino C, Gallina G, Cumbo E, Monticelli F, Goracci C, Ferrari M. Ultrasound effects after post space preparation: an SEM study. J Endod. 2006;32:549–52.

116. Plotino G, Pameijer CH, Grande NM, Somma F. Ultrasonics in endodontics: a review of the literature. J Endod. 2007;33:81–95.

117. Morris MD, Lee KW, Agee KA, Bouillaguet S, Pashley DH. Effects of sodium hypochlorite and RC-prep on bond strengths of resin cement to endodontic surfaces. J Endod. 2001;27:753–7.

118. Erdemir A, Ari H, Güngüneş H, Belli S. Effect of medications for root canal treatment on bonding to root canal dentin. J Endod. 2004;30:113–6.

119. Linard GL, Davies EH, von Fraunhofer JA. The interaction between lining materials and composite resin restorative materials. J Oral Rehabil. 1981;8:121–9.

120. Monticelli F, Osorio R, Sadek FT, Radovic I, Toledano M, Ferrari M. Surface treatments for improving bond strength to prefabricated fiber posts: a literature review. Oper Dent. 2008;33:346–55.

121. Magni E, Mazzitelli C, Papacchini F, Radovic I, Goracci C, Coniglio I, Ferrari M. Adhesion between fiber posts and resin luting agents: a microtensile bond strength test and an SEM investigation following different treatments of the post surface. J Adhes Dent. 2007;9:195–202.

122. Rathke A, Haj-Omer D, Muche R, Haller B. Effectiveness of bonding fiber posts to root canals and composite core build-ups. Eur J Oral Sci. 2009;117:604–10.

123. Fernandes AS, Dessai GS. Factors affecting the fracture resistance of post-core reconstructed teeth: a review. Int J Prosthodont. 2001;14:355–63.

124. Haralur SB, Al Ahmari MA, AlQarni SA, Althobati MK. The effect of intraradicular multiple fiber and cast posts on the fracture resistance of endodontically treated teeth with wide root canals. Biomed Res Int. 2018;1:1–6.

125. Grande NM, Butti A, Plotino G, Somma F. Adapting fiber-reinforced composite root canal posts for use in noncircular-shaped canals. Pract Proced Aesthet Dent. 2006;18:593–9.

126. Plotino G, Grande NM, Pameijer CH, Somma F. Influence of surface remodelling using burs on the macro and micro surface morphology of anatomically formed fibre posts. Int Endod J. 2008;41:345–55.

127. Grande NM, Plotino G, Ioppolo P, Bedini R, Pameijer CH, Somma F. The effect of custom adaptation and span-diameter ratio on the flexural properties of fiber-reinforced composite posts. J Dent. 2009;37:383–9.

128. Vichi A, Vano M, Ferrari M. The effect of different storage conditions and duration on the fracture strength of three types of translucent fiber posts. Dent Mater. 2008;24:832–8.

129. Sterzenbach G, Franke A, Naumann M. Rigid versus flexible dentine-like endodontic posts—clinical testing of a biomechanical concept: seven-year results of a randomized controlled clinical pilot trial on endodontically treated abutment teeth with severe hard tissue loss. J Endod. 2012;38:1557–63.

130. Schmidt JC, Sahrmann P, Weiger R, Schmidlin PR, Walter C. Biologic width dimensions—a systematic review. J Clin Periodontol. 2013;40:493–504.

131. Mamoun JS. On the ferrule effect and the biomechanical stability of teeth restored with cores, posts, and crowns. Eur J Dent. 2014;8:281–6.

Minimally Invasive Alternatives to Dental Extraction and Implant Placement

9

Francesc Abella Sans

Contents

9.1 Introduction to Autotransplantation of Teeth

The classic autotransplantation technique involves transplantation of an erupted or even an unerupted tooth from one site of the mouth to an extraction site or surgically prepared socket in the same person [1]. As a successfully transplanted tooth can function like a normal tooth, autotransplantation has become a viable treatment option to replace either a missing tooth or one with a poor prognosis [2].

However, the autotransplantation technique includes two additional procedures:

1. Surgical extrusion: intra-alveolar transplantation using a simple extraction to extrude teeth in a more coronal position [3].
2. Intentional replantation: a recognized endodontic procedure, used to correct a

F. Abella Sans (✉)
Department of Odontology, Universitat Internacional de Catalunya, Barcelona, Spain
e-mail: franabella@uic.es

© Springer Nature Switzerland AG 2021
G. Plotino (ed.), *Minimally Invasive Approaches in Endodontic Practice*,
https://doi.org/10.1007/978-3-030-45866-9_9

radiographic or clinical endodontic failure, whereby a tooth is extracted, treated outside the oral cavity, and then reinserted into its socket. This procedure is sometimes preferred over conventional apical surgery [4].

9.1.1 Clinical Examination and Diagnosis

Candidates for autotransplantation are examined and diagnosed based on their clinical and radiographic information. At present, the three-dimensional (3D) cone beam computed tomography (CBCT) radiographic assessment of teeth and their surrounding structures is desirable for planning an autotransplantation procedure [5]. Key information required includes the anatomic shape and root development of the donor tooth, bone dimension of the recipient socket, as well as the compatibility of the size of donor tooth with the size of the recipient site.

While successful autotransplantation can yield long-term results, patients should be informed that the procedure might have to be interrupted in the event of complications both in the donor tooth extraction and in the recipient site (such as insufficient alveolar bone), as well as unforeseen difficulties [6]. It is essential that the patient will be self-motivated when faced with a complex and somewhat uncertain procedure.

9.1.2 Advantages and Disadvantages

The main advantages offered by the technique are:

1. Preservation of the periodontal ligament (PDL) and the alveolar bone.
2. Ability to be performed in a growing child/adolescents as well as in adult patients.
3. Preservation of the natural shape of the attached gingiva while achieving an esthetic and optimal function.
4. Possibility, if necessary, of performing orthodontic treatment to properly position the transplanted tooth.

5. A viable alternative to dental implants, fixed bridgework, resin-bonded restorations, and removable partial dentures.

The main disadvantages are summarized thus:

1. Somewhat more aggressive and complicated surgery than conventional extraction.
2. Treatment outcome may be difficult to predict in some cases, despite digital planning.
3. Possible complications such as inflammatory root resorption, replacement root resorption, or loss of clinical attachment level, which may result in loss of the tooth.

9.2 Biological Basis

In recent decades the understanding of the wound healing process following transplantation and replantation has markedly improved the success rate of these procedures [7]. However, autotransplantation is frequently overlooked in patients with missing teeth or it is ruled out because of possible transplant-related complications. This is unfortunate because autotransplantation could become a highly relevant treatment option for single-tooth replacement, particularly since the transplanted tooth can function as a normal tooth [8]. An update of the biological basis would provide a better understanding of the high success and tooth survival rates after autotransplantation, replantation, and surgical extrusion, which would help the clinician to have in mind this procedure in specific cases.

9.2.1 Periodontal Ligament (PDL) and Bone Healing

Regardless of the procedure to be performed (autotransplantation, replantation or surgical extrusion), favorable PDL healing is the key to success [9]. Ideal PDL healing occurs when the extracted tooth is replanted in the original extraction socket in a very short extraoral time, when most of their cells are still alive. This type of healing, described as a reattachment of the PDL, consists of connecting the connective tissue to the root surface [7]. However, PDL cells can be mechanically damaged during extraction or be affected by changes in pH values, osmotic pressure, dehydration, etc. Therefore, an atraumatic removal of the donor tooth is critical to successful PDL healing. Indeed, during the extraction process and extraoral storage, extreme care should be taken to protect Hertwig's epithelial root sheath (HERS) and maintain pulp vitality [10].

Since events occur quickly, by the third and fourth week post-replantation, fibroblasts and regularly aligned bundles of collagen fibers proliferate, indicating functional alignment of the PDL tissue, which, according to the literature, is the ideal healing process [11]. At 8 weeks, a near normal PDL and alignment of collagen fiber bundles are observed, meaning that if necessary, a definitive direct or indirect restoration could be performed, particularly in donor teeth with closed apex [12]. Although there is a logical variability in this time frame, the process appears to take more than 1 month. As the PDL is normally separated in the middle of the root, the reattachment of the PDL located in the gingival area occurs sooner and takes only 1–3 weeks. The PDL is severed at the center of the root during donor tooth extraction, leaving a layer of PDL containing cells (e.g., cementoblasts, fibroblasts, pericytes, epithelial cells of Malassez) on the root surface, which are essential to prevent root resorption. It is desirable to extract a tooth containing as much PDL as possible, even though the cementoblast layer by itself seems to be sufficient in preventing root resorption [13].

The most frequently performed autotransplant is done immediately after the extraction of the tooth in question. However, we sometimes encounter scenarios in which the patient presents with congenitally missing teeth or early tooth loss, implying that the recipient site destined for autotransplantation needs to be created surgically [14]. The main difference with respect to replantation and transplantation to existing sockets is the absence of PDL fibers on the walls of the surgically prepared sockets [15]. During the first weeks, the blood clot is gradually replaced by granulation tissue that supplies nutrients and sets the stage for connective tissue reattachment [16].

Over the next 2–6 months, mature bone and tooth-bone reattachment progressively replaces the granulation tissue and the immature bone [11].

One downside of autotransplantation in surgically prepared sockets is that it produces a slower revascularization and insufficient nutrition to the apical tissues. Thus, the vitality of HERS is affected by this delayed revascularization and inadequate nutrition [17, 18]. Postoperative root development dependent upon the preserved activity of HERS reduces root development after transplantation to surgically created sockets [19, 20]. The trauma triggered by preparation of a new socket induces delayed revascularization and increases the risk of thermal bone damage [15].

Clinically, however, satisfactory healing appears to take place in autotransplantation to surgically prepared alveolar sockets. In most cases no root resorption is observed, the PDL space is maintained, and physiological tooth mobility is achieved [14]. There may be situations where we encounter cases with marked buccolingual alveolar bone atrophy, where promising and optimal functional outcomes can be also achieved with guided bone regeneration [21]. Modified surgical techniques to ensure minimally traumatic removal of donor teeth help to increase the success rate of mature molar autotransplantation, especially embedded or impacted third molars. In this context, piezosurgery is beneficial in socket preparation and atraumatic extraction of third molars [22]. Nevertheless, the clinician must bear in mind that the PDL attached to the bony walls of recipient sockets plays an important healing role.

Replantation studies have demonstrated that PDL deficits on the root surface are repaired by new attachment, defined as joining connective tissue to a root surface derived from its PDL. The new attachment mechanism results from the formation of connective tissue between the exposed root surface and its surrounding tissue (bone or gingival connective tissue) by proliferating the PDL cells around the exposed root surface with the addition of cementum and Sharpey's fiber. Bone graft materials are unnecessary between bone walls and transplant roots even if the space is wide [23]; this is a significant advantage over the use of implants. Garcia and Saffar transplanted 20 roots into surgically prepared bone cavities in the edentulous areas of 5 dogs [24]. The PDL of the roots implanted in the lower and upper right cavities remained intact, while the grafted roots in the left cavities were planed and dried. The authors of this study found that the preservation of the PDL cells benefited bone growth around the transplanted root. PDL cells are a heterogeneous cell population that can be genetically divided into three types of cells: fibroblasts, cementoblasts, and osteoblasts [25]. PDL cells induce bone regeneration in the surroundings after transplantation thanks to their high proliferative capacity, multilineage differentiation potential, capability to form PDL-like tissue, and high level of alkaline phosphatase activity [26, 27].

When donor teeth are placed into recipient sites with an insufficiently wide buccolingual space, a protrusion of the roots through bone dehiscence and a subsequent resorption of the alveolar ridge may be observed [28]. For this reason, the clinician must be able to anticipate this situation through adequate 3D planning. In such a scenario, as recommended by Imazato and Fukunishi [29], autogenous materials can be grafted over the exposed root to make way for bone regeneration. If this regeneration procedure is performed adequately, the outcome should be almost similar to that of a conventional autotransplant technique without guided bone regeneration [14]. Briefly, the narrower the recipient site is, the higher the number of failures [30].

If the area of root damage of the transplanted tooth is small, progenitor cells usually cover the area and new PDL is formed, as described by Tsukiboshi et al. [7], which is termed surface resorption or cemental healing. This transient process gives way to resorption cavities that are shallow and will heal by placement of new cementum and PDL fibers. However, in larger areas of damage, replacement resorption occurs. The damaged root surface is resorbed, leading to bone deposition and finally ankylosis. This situa-

tion is believed to be irreversible and progressive until tooth loss. The speed of the root replacement depends on the patient's age, meaning the younger the patient, the more rapid the process.

Hence, it is crucial to maintain PDL cellular viability of the donor tooth outside the mouth to ensure a long-term retention. An appropriate storage medium will preserve or improve cell viability during the extra-alveolar period, avoiding their desiccation [31]. The key factors for suitable cell growth and survival are physiologic osmolality, pH, and temperature [32]. Cellular reactions are dependent upon the pH of the environment since alterations may affect biological processes. The optimal pH and osmolality for cell growth should be in the region of 6.6–7.8 and 230–400 mosmol/kg, respectively [33]. In 1981, Andreasen [10] studied the effect of extra-alveolar time and storage media on periodontal and pulpal healing following replantation in green vervet monkeys (*Cercopithecus aethiops*). The results showed a significant relationship between the frequency of root resorption, extra-alveolar time, and storage medium, which was especially evident after dry storage. A sharp decrease in PDL survival was clearly observed after 30 min of dry storage. In sum, Andreasen demonstrated that prolonged non-physiologic storage time of the teeth was more important to prognosis than the entire extra-alveolar time.

Various storage media such as Hank's balanced salt solution (HBSS), tap water, coconut water, milk, egg white, pooled saliva, propolis, and Gatorade have been studied for their ability to preserve cell viability [34]. Osmanovic et al. [34] observed that media showing poorly conserved PDL cells after 2 h were tap water (53.4%), saliva (28.6%), and Gatorade (5.4%). HBSS is a storage medium that, thanks to its ability to provide long-term PDL, is considered the gold standard in cases of avulsion, but it is routinely unavailable in dental offices. Accordingly, the most practical choice of medium in autotransplant cases would be physiologic saline or milk because these products have also shown excellent PDL cell survival [7].

9.2.2 Pulp Regeneration and Root Development

Tooth transplantation, replantation, and surgical extrusion interrupt vascular supply to HERS. Experimental investigations have shown that after transplantation of immature teeth only a small apical part of the pulp tissue turns necrotic [35]. Skoglund et al. [36] studied revascularization of pulp of replanted and autotransplanted teeth with open apex in dogs. The transplant revascularization commenced on the fourth postoperative day with an ingrowth of new vessels, which were visible in the whole pulp at approximately 1 month. Therefore, pulp regeneration can be expected in replantation and transplantation of immature teeth. Andreasen et al. [37] have proposed that the diameter of the apical foramen should be greater than 1 mm for an autotransplanted tooth for revascularization. Pulp canal obliteration, a defense response of revascularized pulp, is frequently observed after tooth transplantation procedures, dental trauma injury, and orthodontic movement [38]. Abd-Elmeguid et al. [39] found that pulp canal obliteration was the most common outcome of pulpal healing, with 96% of healed pulps. Their study detected the first obliterations at 3–14 months with a mean time of 9.5 months. In such an event, the clinician must carry out a clinical and radiographic follow-up to check for apical periodontitis. Partial pulp canal obliteration, therefore, is a sign that the pulp is still vital during healing.

However, since revascularization and pulpal healing are far less probable in teeth with closed apex, endodontic treatment is considered a routine procedure to avoid pulp necrosis with subsequent periapical inflammation and inflammatory root resorption [40–42]. Endodontic treatment can be applied either preoperatively, extraorally during autotransplantation surgery, or within 2 weeks post-surgery [43]. However, some authors, including Andreasen et al. [37], Marques-Ferreira et al. [44], and Gaviño et al. [45], have suggested that revascularization can be achieved when the root is shorter than 8.07 mm and the diameter of the apical foramen is larger than

1 mm. These results are controversial, since studies by Iohara et al. [46], Laureys et al. [47], and Fang et al. [48] achieved a revascularization and regeneration in foramina of less than 1 mm. Prospective controlled clinical studies on extraoral apicoectomy are required to validate these findings, and this clinical procedure is yet to be recommended.

Autotransplantation performed with donor teeth of an ideal root developmental stage and using a procedure that avoids damaging the PDL and HERS enables continuing root growth [49]. Nonetheless, the extent of root elongation does not always occur and is difficult to predict [37]. The most common classifications of root stage development, according to the literature, are those described by Moorrees et al. [50] and Demirjian et al. [51]. Moorrees et al. [50] categorized development in stages 1 (beginning of root formation), stage 2 (one-fourth root formation), stage 3 (half root formation), stage 4 (three-fourths root formation), stage 5 (complete root formation with wide-open apex), stage 6 (complete root formation with half closed apex), and stage 7 (complete root formation with a substantially closed apex). Since no additional root development is possible, some clinicians have recommended that donor teeth should be transplanted between stage 3 and 5.

Van Westerveld et al. [52] evaluated the preoperative root development stage and the radiographic width of the apex as root-elongation predictors post autotransplantation. From a total of 58 transplanted premolars, 53 (91.4%) presented root elongation and the remaining 5 (8.6%) had no root elongation after autotransplantation. The mean length of root elongation at the end of follow-up measured 1.9 mm (range, 0.0–4.3 mm; SD, 1.2 mm). A wider open apex (≥ 2 mm) was statistically associated with root elongation post autotransplantation. These findings suggest that an ideal tooth autotransplantation should be performed when the root length of the donor tooth is approximately 50–75% of the total estimated, leaving the apical foramen with the potential for pulp regeneration (apex opening at least >1 mm radiographically).

9.3 Mechanisms of Root Resorption

During any of these three surgical procedures (autotransplantation, replantation, and surgical extrusion), the clinician may find three resorption situations: replacement resorption, inflammatory resorption, and surface resorption or cemental healing. Depending on whether pulp infection is present and on the state of the PDL, one of these three may occur, although sometimes combined resorption may occur. The main characteristics of each of them are explained below.

9.3.1 Replacement Resorption or Ankylosis (Fig. 9.1)

If the transplanted or replanted tooth has been exposed to air or stored in an inadequate medium for long periods or has been traumatically extracted, the PDL will become necrotic, thus making healing with a normal PDL impossible [53]. In such condition, the necrotic PDL will promote bone ingrowth, gradually substituting

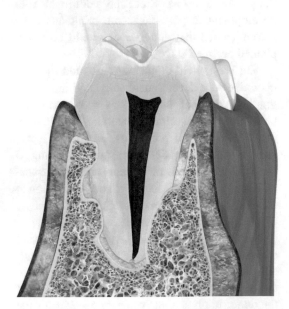

Fig. 9.1 Replacement resorption or ankylosis. Root dentin is replaced by bone, which results in a fusion of bone to tooth (ankylosis). This phenomenon occurs when there is an extensive loss of vital PDL

the tooth by bone [54]. The remodeling of the bone tissue is continuous as part of homeostasis [7]. When there is contact between the roots with necrotic or lost PDL and bone and its osteoclasts, cementum and dentin contribute to the bone remodeling process and root resorption and bone apposition occurs simultaneously on the root surface. This type of resorption is termed ankylosis, or replacement resorption. Ankylosis is nearly always progressive and will likely, over time, replace the tooth with bone, which may eventually result in tooth loss [55]. However, there is a very low risk of ankylosis occurring during any of these three surgical procedures because the clinician will have exhaustively planned the treatment in advance.

The rate of root resorption may progress depending on the rate of the patient's skeletal growth. Andersson et al. [55] found that root resorption progressed faster in younger (8–16 years) than in older patients (17–39 years). The mean resorption time for a replanted tooth ranges between 3 and 7 years in younger individuals, although in older patients such teeth may function for decades or for life.

The clinician detects the first sign of an ankylosed tooth through a metallic percussion, followed by reduced mobility, replacement resorption, and a gradual infra-position in growing individuals [56]. Infra-positioning is a condition that results from the local arrest of the surrounding alveolar bone growth simultaneously with the individual's continuous skeletal growth. This condition advances irreversibly and there is currently no means of arresting it. Consequently, infra-positioning leads to an unesthetic dento-gingival effect and aggravates future prosthetic rehabilitation.

However, in some instances a phenomenon known as partial ankylosis may occur. This is difficult to detect as some of these affected teeth present some mobility and respond normally to percussion test. For this reason, long-term radiographic evaluation is the only way to determine whether a partial ankylosis will evolve into a total replacement resorption or will heal by a new attachment.

9.3.2   External Inflammatory Resorption (Fig. 9.2)

In order for an inflammatory resorption to occur in a replanted or transplanted tooth, two conditions are required [57]:

1. The root canal system is, or has been, infected by bacteria.
2. There has been mechanical damage to the cementum during the extraction or the extra-oral manipulation, resulting in a loss of cementum, such that the dentinal tubules are exposed to the surrounding PDL and bone.

An inflammatory reaction in the host tissue takes place when bacteria and their by-products migrate through the tubules to the root surface [7]. This resorption is characterized by the radiographic appearance of loss of tooth substance (1–2 months after transplantation or replantation) as well as a radiolucency affecting the adjacent PDL and bone [11]. This is due to the presence of granulation tissue that contains capillary vessels

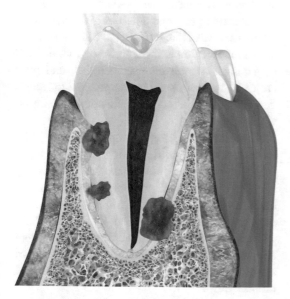

Fig. 9.2 External inflammatory resorption. The resorption of tooth structure is the result of adjacent inflammatory tissue, induced by infected pulp tissue. Resorption cavities can be observed in both the root and the adjacent bone, which are filled with granulation tissue. This is a reversible phenomenon, as if the infected pulp is removed, resorption will cease

in the resorption fossa, converting the area in radiolucency. Teeth with an inflammatory resorption will not respond to pulp sensibility testing and may be associated with other symptoms or clinical signs, according to general state of the tooth and surrounding tissues [19]. Most cases show no symptoms or signs, except when the infected root canal system is causing acute apical periodontitis or when an abscess develops. External inflammatory resorption may occur anywhere along the length of the root; characteristically it is observed laterally and apically post-trauma or autotransplantation surgery.

When faced with an established resorptive process, the clinician can interrupt this resorption and encourage hard tissue repair through root canal treatment. A corticosteroid-antibiotic intracanal medicament is recommended to prevent and manage external inflammatory resorption [57]. Calcium hydroxide is not recommended as an immediate medicament owing to its irritant properties, but it is useful as a subsequent medicament to promote hard tissue repair where required [7]. After root canal treatment, in normal conditions, the clinician will observe a healing by new attachment due to the fact that the granulation tissue will be replaced with PDL tissue. Therefore, the clinician should always monitor the pulp state, especially that of donor teeth with open apex. As mentioned above, autotransplanted immature teeth are able to revascularize, allowing tooth root development. However, upon detection of an inflammatory resorption, root canal treatment should be commenced at the earliest opportunity since it will provide a new attachment.

9.3.3   External Surface Resorption (Fig. 9.3)

External surface resorption is a type of healing response to limited partial damage of the PDL. In this type of resorption, macrophages and osteoclasts reabsorb the cementum adjacent to the damaged PDL, causing a saucer-shaped cavity on the root surface [58]. When the closest cementoblast layer is integral and the underlying dentinal

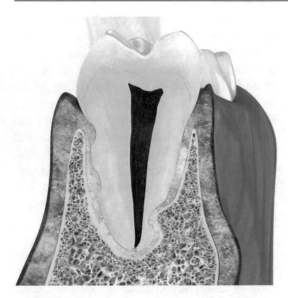

Fig. 9.3 External surface resorption. Surface resorption is the result of minor and partial damage to the PDL and is transient when repaired

tubules are uncovered, the cementoblasts will restore the damaged root surface and new cementum together with new Sharpey's fibers will repair the resorptive cavity. The surface resorption is self-limiting and repair-related, making it a non-progressive process. After the repair process, the clinician will observe a normal PDL width that follows the contours of the root defect. In both cases of minor trauma (concussion and subluxation) and replanted and transplanted teeth, surface root resorption is viewed as a favorable healing outcome [24].

9.4   Clinical Indications and Procedures

9.4.1   Classification

Knowing that surgical extrusion and intentional replantation follow an identical healing process to that of autotransplantation, these procedures fall within the same category. Autotransplantation can be classified into these three groups: (1) surgical extrusion, (2) intentional replantation, and (3) conventional autotransplantation. The main indications and step-by-step procedures are discussed below.

9.4.2   Surgical Extrusion: Indications and Technique

When restoring severely damaged teeth, an adequate biologic width and distance between the crown margin and alveolar crest should be ensured [59, 60]. In the case of insufficient tooth structure, the clinician may consider three options: surgical crown lengthening, orthodontic extrusion, or surgical extrusion [61]. Surgical extrusion, also referred to as intra-alveolar transplantation, entails the displacement of the remaining root to a more coronal position with a view to restorability based upon a sufficient ferrule [62]. The choice of one technique over another depends upon several patient-related factors: esthetics, clinical crown-to-root ratio, root proximity, root morphology, furcation location, individual tooth position, and strategic tooth position [63, 64].

The conditions of certain clinical situations are not conducive to surgical and restorative procedures. Extensive osseous surgery may produce increased pocket depth and mobility, furcation involvement, poor crown-to-root ratio, and loss of supporting periodontal tissues of the neighboring teeth or implants [65]. In the case of surgical crown lengthening in the anterior region, the loss of papillae, uneven gingival margins, and poor crown-to-root ratios might compromise the situation from the esthetic and functional point of view [66].

An alternative treatment approach would be an orthodontic forced extrusion [63]. This treatment is considered less invasive because it actually improves rather than compromises aesthetics, without interfering with the periodontal support of neighboring teeth [61]. Yet, these procedures have limitations, including patient acceptance, treatment duration, availability of appropriate orthodontic anchorage, and risk of relapse [66].

An alternative treatment is found in surgical extrusion, defined as a procedure in which the remaining tooth structure is repositioned more supra-gingivally in the same socket [67]. Tegsjö et al. [68] first developed the intra-alveolar transplantation or surgical extrusion of teeth fractured

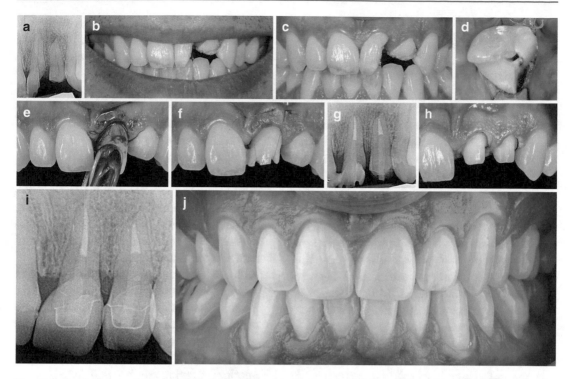

Fig. 9.4 Surgical extrusion after dental trauma. (**a**) Preoperative clinical examination of fractured maxillary left central and lateral incisors. (**b**) Image of preoperative periapical radiograph showing intact PDL space with no evidence of root fracture. (**c**) Oblique complicated crown-root fracture in tooth 21 revealing subgingival fracture margin, and middle-third fracture of crown in tooth 22. (**d**) Emergency endodontic treatment in tooth 21. (**e**) Surgical extrusion procedure using forceps. (**f**) Tooth 21 fixed with a suture and a fiber-reinforced composite bonded to tooth 11. (**g**) Radiographic detail of surgical extrusion and teeth restored with fiber post and composite build-up. (**h**) Teeth before final impression. (**i**) Radiographic examination at 7 years post-surgery showing no evidence of root resorption, crestal bone resorption, or endodontic problems. (**j**) Clinical aspect of crowns at 7 years post-surgical extrusion. (Courtesy of Dr. Ramón Gómez-Meda)

by trauma in youngsters. This procedure, based on the biological behavior of dental replantation following avulsion, allows the clinician a direct observation of the root, thereby favoring the treatment planning. Khanberg [62] advocates bypassing both the osteotomy and bone graft in the root apical area and instead performing just a careful and gentle root luxation until the desired extrusion of the tooth is achieved. It is important to note that, apical root resorption and marginal bone loss occasionally occur; these phenomena are believed to be the result of surgical trauma [69].

This treatment is perfectly viable when the affected teeth have complete root formation and the remaining root in the socket is long enough to support a new restoration, such as a core-retained crown [70] (Fig. 9.4). It is widely agreed that the key to a successful surgical extrusion mainly hinges on an atraumatic extraction with minimal damage to the cementoblast layer on the root surface [71].

Traditional extraction techniques involve the use of elevators and periotomes, which unavoidably traumatize the alveolar bone and the root surface to some extent [72]. It is for this reason that techniques involving only forceps or specially designed extrusion instruments for vertical tooth extraction are recommended [71]. Minimally invasive vertical tooth extraction was introduced mainly to enable extraction of severely damaged teeth, without the need for flap-raising, thus reducing the degree of alveolar bone resorption [72–74].

9.4.2.1 Diagnosis and Treatment Planning

- It is essential to take the patient's medical history and ascertain whether they have any contraindications. Abnormal metabolic conditions or immunosuppressive risk factors can delay healing and reduce the prognosis of the technique. It is also important to have in mind the patient's age, as the procedure in older patients is more challenging due to their higher alveolar bone density.
- The ideal candidate teeth for this technique are monoradicular, particularly the conical shaped ones. The standard procedure for multirooted teeth is not recommended, especially in teeth with short root trunks, since they tend to develop periodontal furcation defects. The root minimum length needed for proper function should leave a minimum coronoradicular ratio of 1:1.
- In posterior teeth it is essential to take a bitewing radiograph to correctly measure the distance from the healthy margin of the tooth to the alveolar ridge.
- With this information, the clinician can plan the type of final restoration. The root length to extrude will vary in accordance with the tooth preparation selected. It should be taken into account that a preparation for an adhesive partial restoration preserves a larger amount of healthy tissue than one for a metal-free full-crown.

9.4.2.2 Surgical Procedure

- Whenever possible it is recommended to initially restore the tooth with a post or composite build-up to minimize the risk of fracture during surgical extrusion or uprighting. If this procedure is performed in conditions of absolute isolation, endodontic treatment or nonsurgical retreatment is also advised. If this is not possible, the root canal treatment should be immediately planned after replantation.
- After local anesthesia, a small scalpel blade or a micro-periosteal elevator can be used to carefully separate the gingival fibrous attachment, taking extreme care not to induce mechanical damage on the root surface. Subsequently, the clinician can luxate the tooth with the aid of forceps. However, in extremely difficult cases, such as teeth with very long roots and a completely missing coronal tooth structure, a vertical extraction device can be used [75]. It should be noted that in most cases there is no need to raise a flap when performing surgical extrusion.
- It is crucial to work under magnification to rule out cracks or fractures on the root surface. Depending on the site of the marginal defect, the tooth may even be rotated by 180° before replantation, facilitating the restoration and reducing the amount of extrusion needed.
- With the tooth placed in the optimum coronal position, the clinician can splint the tooth for 2 weeks using one of several flexible splinting methods, such as suture, stainless-steel wire and acid etch-composite resin or resin activated glass-ionomer cement [76].
- Surgical dressing can be used for 3–5 days to improve soft tissue healing and prevent contamination. The mismatch between the socket and the extruded root means that the splinting period may require up to 6 weeks in cases of high mobility of the extruded root [74]. Regardless of the type of restoration, the clinician must leave the tooth margin at least 3 mm from the bone crest (Figs. 9.5 and 9.6).
- If endodontic treatment has not been performed previously, it should be commenced within the first 2 weeks to avoid inflammatory root resorption [77]. If needed, an antibiotic-corticosteroid paste as an intracanal dressing may be recommended instead of calcium hydroxide, which may have a possible negative impact on periodontal healing [78].
- Extraoral root canal treatment is usually not recommended, since extra-alveolar conditions are not conducive to PDL survival. The longer the extra oral time, the greater the risk of root resorption [10]. However, it is advantageous if the clinician can perform this procedure with a maximum extraoral time of 12 min, because the most complex part at the endodontic level

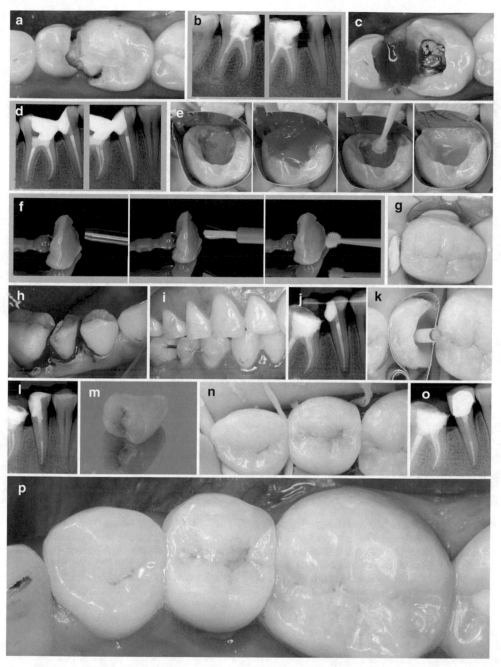

Fig. 9.5 Surgical extrusion to save a mandibular premolar. (**a**) Clinical examination showing extensive secondary decay in the mandibular right first molar and partial destruction of crown structure in the mandibular right second premolar. (**b**) No signs of apical lesions were observed in either tooth. (**c**) Image after removal of decay and composite from both teeth. (**d**) Endodontic treatment of tooth 45 and nonsurgical retreatment of tooth 46. (**e**) Deep margin elevation or coronal margin relocation in tooth 46. (**f**) Step-by-step adhesive preparation of the workpiece. (**g**) Occlusal view of restored molar 1 week after luting. (**h**) Atraumatic surgical extrusion locating the tooth margin at least 3 mm from the bone crest. (**i**) Splinting the tooth with a stainless-steel wire and acid etch-composite resin. (**j**) Periapical radiograph showing space gained. (**k**) Tooth restored with fiber post and composite build-up. (**l**) Radiographic aspect at 4 weeks post-surgery. (**m**) Monolithic zirconia crown. (**n**) Placement of the zirconia crown on the surgically extruded tooth. Follow-up at 36 months: (**o**) periapical radiograph; (**p**) clinical aspect

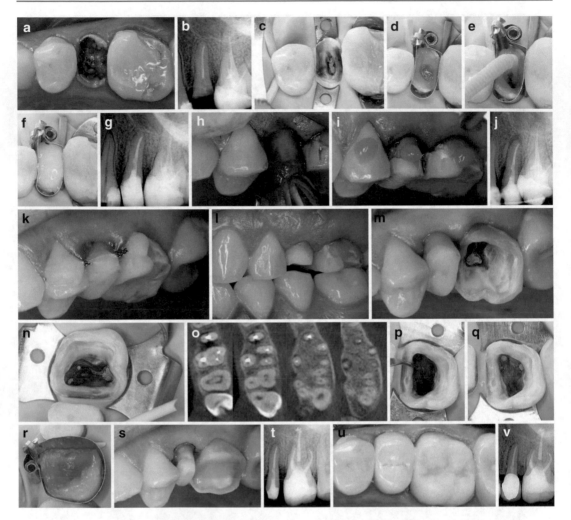

Fig. 9.6 Management of a severely damaged maxillary premolar. (**a**) Deep decay affecting the maxillary left second premolar. (**b**) Periapical radiograph showing a previous endodontic treatment and an extensive subgingival decay compromising the biologic width. (**c**) Initial view of the tooth under rubber dam isolation before the nonsurgical retreatment. (**d–f**) A fiber post was placed to maintain material for a coronal restoration through radicular anchoring. (**g**) Radiographic aspect just after the nonsurgical retreatment and the composite build-up. (**h**) Surgical extrusion procedure. (**i–k**) Semi-rigid splint of the tooth by a wire-fixed composite. (**l, m**) Clinical aspect at 4 weeks post-surgery. (**n**) Tooth 26 isolation before the nonsurgical retreatment. (**o**) A limited volume cone beam computed tomography (CBCT) scan taken of the maxillary left quadrant to manage the tooth 26. (**p**) Location of the secondary mesiobuccal canal (MB2). (**q**) Nonsurgical retreatment completed. (**r**) Orthophosphoric acid etching. (**s**) Details of the preparation of both teeth. (**t**) Radiographic control at 8 weeks. (**u, v**) At 24 months, clinical and radiographic examination showed a healthy gingival condition associated with a normal periodontal contour

(apical area) is removed at once. Obviously, a key factor such as root length can limit its use. For example, this technique cannot always be applied in surgical extrusion, since the root reduction would be excessive and would compromise the coronoradicular ratio.

- Restorative treatment, whether direct or indirect, is usually carried out from 6 to 8 weeks post-surgical extrusion. Although systemic antibiotics have been prescribed for surgical extrusion, there is insufficient evidence to support or reject their indication [79].

9.4.3   Intentional Replantation: Indications and Technique

Intentional replantation is a useful endodontic procedure for correcting an evident endodontic failure in which a tooth is intentionally extracted, manipulated extraorally, and then replanted in its original site [4, 80] (Fig. 9.7). It differs from surgical extrusion in that this procedure entails positioning the tooth at the same bone level without having to position it more coronally than when it was surgically extruded. However, in some cases the clinician can combine the two techniques and thus improve both the restorability and the periapical condition of the tooth that needs to be treated.

Intentional tooth replantation, described as a treatment option for different selected and challenging situations, is all the rage among clinicians, yet this procedure is nothing new. According to Dryden and Arens [81], Pierre Fauchard first described its use in the eighteenth century. Over time, thanks to greater in-depth knowledge of wound healing processes, the indications for this procedure have evolved and increased. Intentional tooth replantation can be applied in a broad range of situations [4, 82, 83], including root canal treatment failure, anatomic limitation, accessibility problems, persistent chronic pain, external root resorption, vertical root fracture, accidental exarticulation, involuntary rapid orthodontic extrusion, patients with objections to apical microsurgery or trismus, and cases in which patients meet the expense of longer and/or costly expensive treatments. Given the almost 90% success rates shown in recent studies [84, 85], intentional replantation with more modern techniques are considered an accepted treatment modality [86].

Single-rooted and conical teeth are more favorable for extraction without producing major damage to the root surface while reducing the risk of fracture. Furthermore, it is important to take into account that extraoral time should be kept as short as possible [83]. The literature on avulsed teeth has contributed to our understanding of the implication of extraoral time, particularly dry time [87]. An extraoral time lasting more than 30 min increases the likelihood of replacement resorption [88].

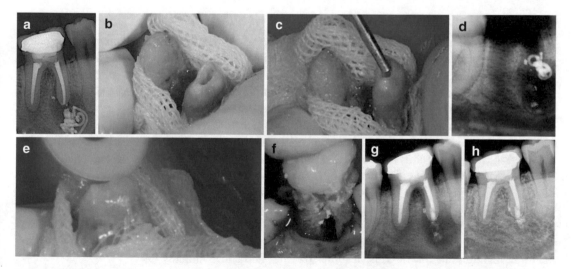

Fig. 9.7 Intentional replantation of a mandibular first molar. (**a**) Large amount of extruded material associated with a radiolucent lesion in the mesial root. (**b**) The coronal two-thirds of the root surface gently covered with gauze soaked with copious saline. Detail of the retrograde preparation. (**c**) Placement of a dual-cured resin-modified glass ionomer (Geristore; DenMat, Santa Maria, CA) as a retrograde filling. (**d**) Removal of the periapical granulation tissue and the extruded material while taking care to avoid damaging the socket wall. (**e**) Final polishing before tooth placement in the recipient site. (**f**) Digital pressure to place the tooth in its original position. (**g**) Immediate radiographic control after intentional replantation. (**h**) Periapical radiograph at 24 months post-replantation. (Courtesy of Dr. Miguel Roig and Dr. Fernando Durán-Sindreu)

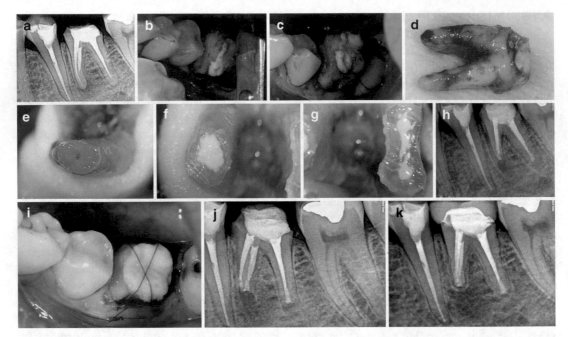

Fig. 9.8 Management of an endodontic failure. (**a**) Periapical radiolucency is visible in the area of the mandibular left first molar of a 34-year-old male. Fragments of broken instruments are observed in the apical part of both roots. Patient ruled out an apical microsurgery. (**b, c**) Extraction of the tooth using forceps. (**d**) The extracted tooth. Note that the tooth had an intact PDL covering the root. (**e**) Three millimeters of root resection were performed extraorally. Detail of one of the broken fragments under magnification. (**f, g**) Retrofilling with Biodentine (Septodont, Saint-Maur-des-fossés, France). (**h**) Postoperative periapical radiograph. (**i**) Fixation of the replanted tooth using sutures. (**j**) Three months after replantation. (**k**) Four years after replantation. Note an external surface resorption, a type of healing response to limited partial damage of the PDL

Recent advances in apical microsurgery have provided the clinician with solutions to some of the shortcomings for orthograde retreatment [89]. However, there are even cases that cannot be treated adequately with apical microsurgery, either due to anatomical factors (i.e., proximity to the mental nerve or maxillary sinus, buccal plate thickness or inoperable sites such as lingual surfaces of mandibular molars) or due to financial factors, which preclude conventional implant placement [90]. When both nonsurgical and surgical retreatments have a low prognosis or cannot be feasible, intentional replantation provides a solution resulting in fewer complications [82, 91]. In the event of a failed intentional replantation, we will have delayed time in placing an implant, as opposed to whether the implant was placed from the outset [85].

The principal advantage of intentional replantation is that tooth surfaces, including inaccessible areas, can be directly examined and repaired under magnification, reducing potential damage in the PDL (Fig. 9.8). This technique is potentially more cost-effective and less time consuming than the alternatives [90]. Originally, clinicians were recommended to carefully select each case and to inform the patient of a low probability of success. More recent studies have reported intentional replantation in previously insurmountable situations, such as teeth with vertical root fractures [92, 93], periodontally hopeless teeth [94, 95], or invasive cervical resorptions in which the clinician cannot access and seal the lesion conventionally [96].

Clearly, there are some contraindications that clinicians should know as: a more favorable prognosis with either conventional endodontic surgery or implant placement, an uncontrolled periodontal disease, a non-restorable tooth, an extraction requiring hemi-section or osseous recontouring, a tooth that is part of a multiple-tooth prosthesis or when roots are divergent [97]. In the cases involving individual teeth with divergent roots, one clinician should perform a small osteotomy in the alveolar socket with the help of a 3D-printed tooth, while a second clinician performs the extra-alveolar apical surgery. This protocol significantly reduces extra oral time while avoiding the excessive friction over the tooth surface.

9.4.3.1 Diagnosis and Treatment Planning

- On the first visit, the patient must be informed of the different treatment options available and each one of their benefits and risks explained. Once the patient has understood what intentional replantation consists of, they must sign an informed consent. Needless to say, the patient's medical and dental history must be taken and any contraindications ascertained.
- Clinical and radiographic examination. Different tests should be performed such as periodontal probing, mobility, percussion, bite tests, acquisition of periapical radiographs, and limited CBCT images, if indicated. These tests will allow the clinician to assess both the endodontic status of the tooth (i.e., anatomical difficulty of the root canal system, presence of a separated instrument or a perforation, size and length of a post) and its anatomic relationship with neighboring structures, such as the mental nerve, inferior alveolar nerve, and maxillary sinus. It is also important to have in mind the patient's age, as the procedure in older patients is more challenging due to their higher alveolar bone density.
- Contraindications for intentional replantation include teeth that are candidates for apical microsurgery and teeth diagnosed with a vertical root fracture. In contrast, among the indications are teeth that could not be properly treated with apical microsurgery due to anatomic limitations and thick buccal bone and teeth with low accessibility to manage a radicular groove, endodontic perforation, or invasive cervical resorption.

- A small field of view CBCT scan allows the clinician not only a 3D assessment of the area of interest, but also the possibility of segmenting the tooth to be treated and manufacturing a 3D-printed tooth replica. This step substantially reduces extraoral time, particularly in multirooted teeth where replantation into the socket is challenging.
- A preoperative orthodontic movement for 2–3 weeks to mobilize the tooth is recommended in the intentional replantation of teeth with a complicated root structure and high risk of fracture during extraction [91].

9.4.3.2 Surgical Procedure

- One hour before the procedure, the patient should rinse with chlorhexidine gluconate 0.12% and take 600 mg of ibuprofen. A systematic antibiotic prophylaxis (i.e., amoxicillin/clavulanic acid) can lower the failure rate after intentional replantation [42]. The presence of two clinicians throughout the procedure can expedite management and reduce chair time.
- After local anesthesia, the clinician should extract the tooth as carefully as possible to avoid damaging the root surface, as described for the surgical extrusion. A #15 blade or similar can be inserted in parallel to the PDL space and gently tapped with a mallet. Then, using forceps, the clinician luxates the tooth slowly but steadily in the buccolingual direction until it is vertically displaced. Placement of a rubber band around the handles of the forceps may be useful in securing this step. An elevator must not be used during extraction to avoid any unnecessary damage to the root surface and alveolar bone crest. In some situations, a mucoperiosteal flap is an option to access the tooth apical to the crown margin, avoiding damage to the crown. Finally, the patient is instructed to bite on wet sterilized gauze while the tooth is being managed extraorally to maintain the recipient site contamination free.
- Once the tooth is extracted, it is submitted to treatment procedures in accordance with current standards of apical microsurgery [98]. Any granulation tissue attached to the root is

carefully removed and the tooth is placed under an operating microscope to examine for abnormalities such as fractures, cracks, and accessory canals. The coronal two-thirds of the root surface should be gently covered with gauze soaked with copious saline or HBSS.

• While one clinician is performing the extra-oral apical microsurgery, a second clinician removes the periapical granulation tissue taking care to avoid damaging the socket wall. If there is 3D printed tooth replica available, it can be used to modify the socket until the fit of the replica fits smoothly and snugly in the recipient socket.

• Then the socket is rinsed with sterile saline solution and the tooth is replanted gently. If the tooth is stable, it is not strictly necessary to splint; the patient need only bite on gauze. However, an unstable tooth must be semi-rigidly splinted (i.e., resin wire splint or interrupted sutures) for 2 weeks. In addition, a surgical dressing can be applied to enhance healing and protect the area from infection and preserve the blood clot. Occlusal adjustment to minimize occlusal force for the first months may be indicated.

• In the event of an endodontic perforation or an invasive cervical resorption, the clinician should proceed in the same way, only by selecting one or another material according to each case.

9.4.4 Conventional Tooth Autotransplantation: Indications and Technique

Conventional autotransplantation is commonly indicated when a tooth is unrestorable and another tooth, such as a third molar or a malpositioned tooth, is not in function, or in cases of orthodontic problems [99]. However, the clinician should only propose this procedure when an appropriate donor tooth can be used without subsequent negative effects [7, 100] and when other treatment options (orthodontics, implants, fixed or removable partial dentures) are unfavorable in some aspects, such as function, time, cost, or

long-term prognosis. There has been a renewed interest in this procedure, especially in growing patients, since it promotes functional adaptation and alveolar bone induction, thus re-establishing of a normal alveolar process [7].

Tooth autotransplantation is widely used to replace a single tooth, both in patients who have not completed craniofacial development and in adult patients. Therefore, as explained in the introduction, this therapeutic option is valid in many circumstances, including deep caries, trauma, periodontitis and endodontic problems, as well as in cases with tooth impact or agenesis. However, from all these situations, the clinician must clearly detect two highly different situations: one in which there is an early loss of a permanent tooth in a growing patient and the other in a patient who has already finished growing and has the option under normal conditions to have an implant placement.

Today, dental implants are a very common and predictable procedure for the rehabilitation of partially and completely edentulous arches, even in the area of esthetics, providing better outcomes compared to conventional fixed bridgework, resin-bonded restorations and removable partial dentures [101, 102]. Nonetheless, this treatment approach can frequently present technical complications and biological ones, including peri-implant diseases [103, 104]. These complications may have substantial economic implications [105] for patients and for their perception of the treatment [91]. In addition, implant dentistry is categorically contraindicated in growing patients because the implant cannot follow the maxillofacial development and it would remain in malocclusion during growth [106, 107].

The volume of the alveolar bone decreases significantly following extraction, creating a challenge for the prosthetic rehabilitation, particularly in growing patients [8]. The clinical consequences of these physiological hard and soft tissue changes may affect the outcome of ensuing therapies aimed at restoring lost teeth [108]. When considering implants, the clinician must often first carry out a bone augmentation technique. Therefore, it would be preferable to offer the patient autotransplantation, which main-

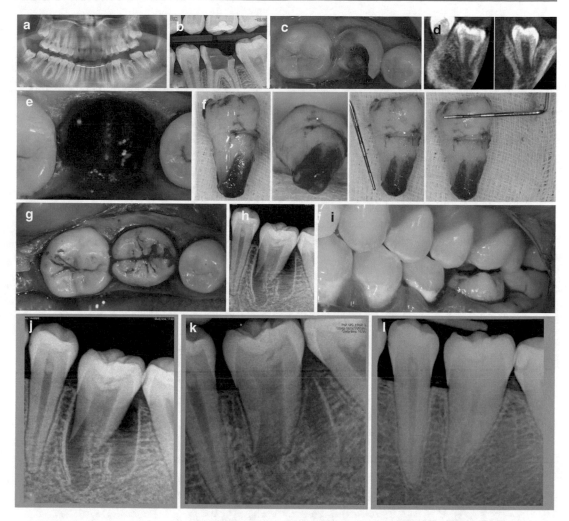

Fig. 9.9 Conventional autotransplantation of an immature tooth. (**a, b**) Preoperative radiographs of a severely damaged mandibular first molar in a 16-year-old female. (**c**) The first molar was non-restorable. The treatment plan was to transplant the patient's mandibular third molar. (**d**) Checking the suitability of the size and shape of the donor tooth through a limited CBCT. (**e**) The recipient site after the extraction of the first molar. The removal of alveolar septum was necessary. (**f**) The donor tooth (mandibular left third molar). Note that the tooth had an intact follicle. (**g**) After transplantation of the donor tooth. (**h**) Verification of donor tooth's position in the modified recipient site. (**i**) The transplanted tooth positioned 2 mm below the occlusal contact. (**j**) Radiographic aspect at 4 weeks post-surgery. (**k**) Follow-up at 3 months. (**l**) After healing (3 years after the procedure), root canal treatment was not necessary because the immature apex promoted revascularization, healing of the pulp, and continuation of root development. (Courtesy of Dr. Alejandro Núñez and Nacho Cañameras)

tains bone structure and adapts to both growth and developmental changes (Fig. 9.9). This treatment does entail potential complications, including pulp necrosis and infection, replacement resorption and stunted root development, among others. However, Rohof et al. [109] states that this type of complication has an incidence of <5%. It is important, therefore, to assess each patient to consider the immediate and short-term outcome, as well as the long-term outcome and alternative treatment options. A multidisciplinary approach is expected to enhance these outcomes for autotransplantation in children-adolescents and adults patients [110].

9.4.4.1 Diagnosis and Treatment Planning

- Before establishing candidates for a transplantation, a careful clinical (including photographs), radiographic, and periodontal examination should be performed. The clinician should take care to evaluate soft tissues and caries risk presented by the patient. As with any surgical procedure and the procedures mentioned above, medical and dental specialty consultations are required. To ensure a desirable antibiotic level in the patient's bloodstream, both during and after surgery, antibiotics should be prescribed a few hours prior to the procedure.

- Potential donor teeth for extraction must be analyzed to ascertain suitability of shape. At present, a limited CBCT scan of the area in question facilitates the evaluation and allows the clinician to select an ideal donor tooth. In addition, surgical planning software can be used to plan the tooth's ideal final position in the recipient site (Fig. 9.10). It is essential to measure the basic parameters, such as the mesiodistal and buccolingual widths of the alveolar ridge and the placement of the mandibular canal or maxillary sinus. The root development stage in growing patients should be 4 or 5.

- Oral hygiene phase. An oral hygiene, scaling, and root planing must be performed prior to,

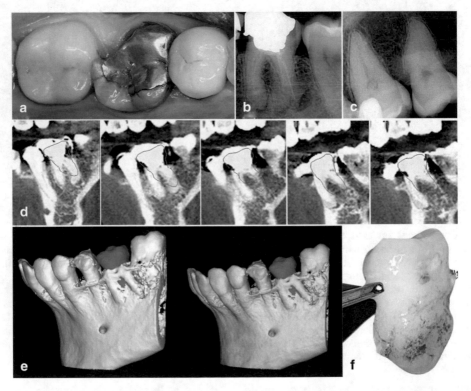

Fig. 9.10 Immediate autotransplantation in a fresh extraction socket. (**a**) Fracture of an amalgam restoration in the mandibular left first molar. (**b**) Preoperative periapical radiograph showing the presence of an accessory distolingual (DL) root (radix entomolaris). (**c**) Radiographic aspect of the donor tooth (maxillary left third molar). (**d**) Autotransplant digital planning. (**e**) Simulation of the 3D position of tooth 28 in the recipient site. (**f**) Tooth 28 after atraumatic extraction. (**g**) Post-extraction alveolar ridge.

(**h**) Position of the donor tooth in the recipient site as digitally planned. (**i**, **j**) Semi-rigid splinting with adjacent teeth for 4 weeks. (**k**) Note the minimally invasive access cavity. (**l**, **m**) Follow-up at 1 month post-surgery. (**n**) Preparation completed and ready for adhesive cementation. (**o**) Lithium disilicate overlay. (**p**) Three years and 4 months after the procedure. A normal lamina dura and PDL space can be observed

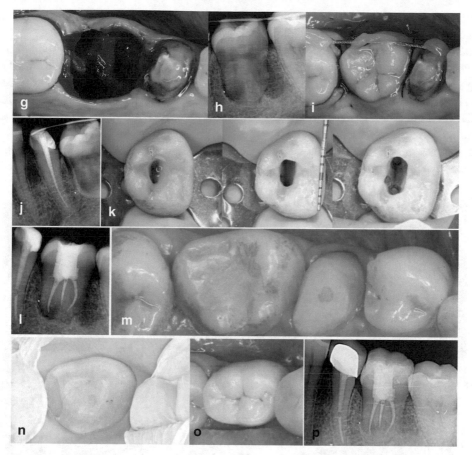

Fig. 9.10 (continued)

or at the same time as, the surgical procedure. Before considering surgery, the clinician must be sure the patient has good oral hygiene habits. If they are not willing to change their habits, autotransplantation must be ruled out.

- Timing of extraction. Determining the right moment to extract the damaged donor tooth is not always easy, and factors such as pain or the root development of the donor tooth may hasten or delay the transplantation date. If tooth extraction and transplantation can be performed simultaneously, the PDL present in the extraction socket promotes healing while saving the patient undergoing a second surgery. However, in some situations the clinician may prefer or be forced to postpone the transplant: These cases may include acute or chronic infection or sinus tract at the extrac-

tion site, pregnant women, patients not available for an earlier surgery, congenitally missing teeth or early tooth loss, or an insufficient mesiodistal space in the recipient site and need for prior orthodontic treatment. Transplantations should be performed within 2 months post extraction, since extensive bone resorption may occur after that period.

- Timing of root canal treatment. In cases of fully developed teeth, it is necessary in most cases to perform an endodontic treatment. This can be done before, during, or 2 weeks post-transplantation, according to the position of the donor tooth and its anatomical complexity. The treatment aim is to prevent inflammatory root resorption.

- Fabrication of surgical models: 3D tooth replicas and guiding templates. 3D radiologic data can be used to print tooth replicas that help clinicians prepare the recipient site, thus reducing possible injury to the donor tooth during the procedure and the extra oral time (Figs. 9.11 and 9.12).

9.4.4.2 Surgical Procedure (Fig. 9.13)

- Simultaneous anesthesia of the donor tooth and the recipient area. Anesthesia without vasoconstrictor is recommended if the donor

tooth has an immature root, which is likely revascularize.

- Extraction of the damaged tooth. An atraumatic extraction should be performed as soon as possible, since both the bone surrounding the tooth and the PDL maintained in the recipient socket are key factors in the case of prognosis.
- Tooth replica try-in. The recipient site should be modified according to the dimensions of

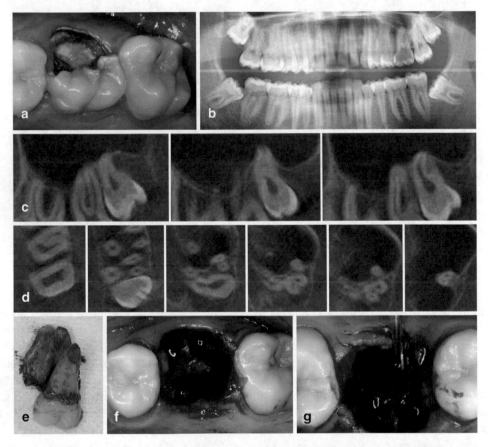

Fig. 9.11 Autotransplantation of a mature third molar. (**a**) An 18-year-old male with a chief complaint of pain around the maxillary left first molar. A deep caries was found and the tooth was planned to be replaced by the maxillary third molar. (**b**) The panoramic view at the first examination. (**c, d**) A limited CBCT showing the position of the maxillary left third molar. (**e**) The extracted maxillary first molar. (**f**) The recipient site post-extraction. (**g**) Preparation of the socket for the autotransplantation replacing the maxillary first molar. (**h**) 3D-printed tooth

replica and the donor tooth. (**i**) Clinical view immediately after transplantation. Note that the position of the tooth was reversed, leaving the palatal root in the buccal area. (**j**) After autotransplantation of the donor tooth and suturing of the flap. No accessory fixation to the suture was needed since the primary stability was excellent. (**k**) Periapical radiograph after the procedure, and at 3 weeks post-endodontic treatment. (**l**) Occlusal view of the restored molar immediately after luting. (**m**) Radiograph 4 years later showing a normal PDL space

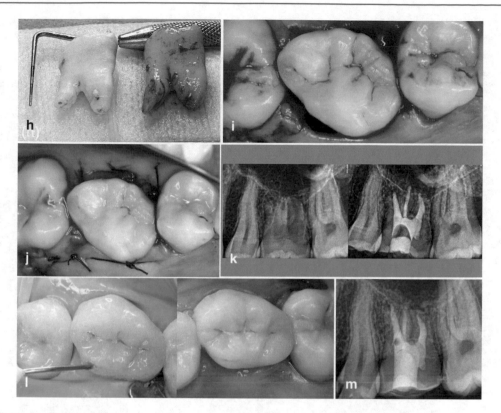

Fig. 9.11 (continued)

the tooth replica, with the aim of placing it in the same position previously digitally planned. Accordingly, the clinician can use 3D-printed guiding templates to ensure a faster and more accurate definitive placement of the tooth replica. Surgical round burs, at low speed but with water cooling, or piezoelectric inserts are recommended for this procedure. After removing any granulation tissue from the extraction socket, the alveolar septum should be removed in most cases of posterior teeth. Once the donor tooth replica fits passively and frictionlessly, the clinician may consider the modification of the alveolus finished.

- Extraction of the donor tooth. To perform this step, the clinician should use only forceps and avoid the use of luxators to preserve as much PDL as possible. Sometimes it is advisable to make a slight intra-crevicular incision before luxation. With a previous digital planning, the clinician will know whether it is necessary to reduce the length of the root or eliminate some of the root canal curvature to facilitate placement in the recipient socket or the future endodontic treatment. The donor tooth must be kept in appropriate storage conditions, such as commercial tooth storage media, Hank's balanced salt solution, or saline solution. The donor tooth is placed in the recipient site at the earliest opportunity, leaving it in a slight infraposition free from occlusal forces. In children, where the donor tooth is partially erupted with an immature root development, it should be placed at its original level of eruption to allow it to erupt, since the root formation continues after revascularization.

- Fresh extraction socket. In most cases of immediate autotransplant, it is not necessary to raise a flap. However, if tooth extraction at the recipient site has been performed within a

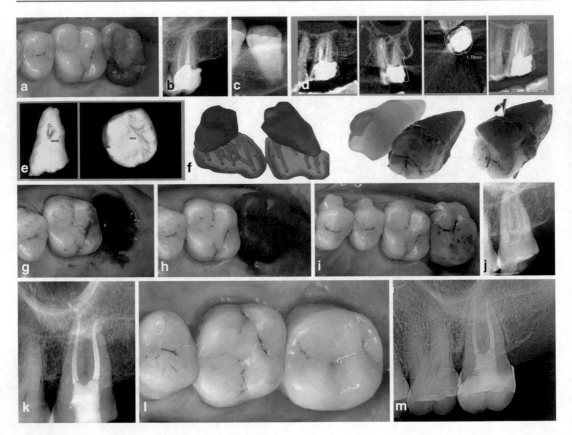

Fig. 9.12 Autotransplantation of a tooth with completed root formation. (**a**) A secondary decay of the maxillary left second molar in a 68-year-old male. The tooth could not be restored. (**b**) Radiograph of the affected tooth. (**c**) Radiograph of the donor tooth. The mandibular left third molar was considered to be the best candidate for transplantation. (**d**) Digital segmentation of the donor tooth. (**e**) Final segmentation of the tooth before printing the replica. (**f**) Comparison between the 3D-printed tooth replica and the donor tooth. (**g**) The recipient site post-extraction. (**h**) The replica tooth used to check the recipient socket. (**i**) The transplanted tooth with fixation in situ. (**j**) Radiograph immediately after transplantation. (**k**) Endodontic treatment performed 2 weeks post-surgery. (**l**) Occlusal view of the restored molar 1 month after luting. (**m**) Two-year radiographic follow-up

few weeks before the surgery, a full-thickness flap must be raised to expose the recipient site.

- Absence of recipient socket. When there is almost no extraction socket (i.e., temporary tooth) or none at all (i.e., teeth lost years ago or congenitally missing teeth), the recipient site must be surgically created or modified. This step can be taken more predictably if it is done using 3D technology. Otherwise, it is recommended to mark different reference points on the alveolar bone surface. Implant drills, surgical round burs, or even trephine burs, always irrigated with saline, can be used to perform the osteotomy in the recipient socket.

- Insufficient recipient socket. There are circumstances in which the clinician cannot ensure a sufficiently large recipient site [7, 8] for a predictable tooth autotransplantation. For buccal or lingual alveolar bone loss, the clinician should carry out guided tissue regeneration or an autogenous bone graft at the recipient site simultaneously with the transplant [29]. The mechanisms of action of these approaches are based primarily on separating the gingival connective tissue from the PDL, maintaining a space for the osteoblastic cells to proliferate.

- Primary stability and occlusal adjustment. The type of fixation and its duration depends on

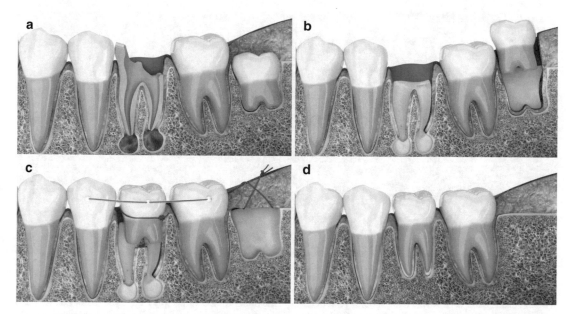

Fig. 9.13 Simulation of an immediate autotransplantation in a fresh extraction socket. (**a**) Situation before procedure. The mandibular first molar is non-restorable and the immature third molar is suitable in size and shape. (**b**) After the extraction of the unrestorable tooth, the recipient site is examined and the donor tooth is atraumatically extracted. (**c**) Transplantation of donor tooth with resin wire splint and interrupted sutures. (**d**) After healing, pulp vitality is maintained and root development is completed

several factors, the primary stability being one of the most important. In the event of a good initial primary stability, the postoperative fixation can be performed by suturing at the occlusal or buccal level. It is important to remember that the occlusal adjustment should be prior to fixation. The suture should be removed between 5 and 7 days. In the case of poor initial stability, a buccal/lingual acid-etch composite and flexible wire splint is indicated for a period of 4–8 weeks. In such case, the occlusal adjustment is advisable once the splint has been placed. During the first 2 or 3 days, a surgical dressing can be placed to protect the transplant against infection.

- Radiographic evaluation. The clinician should take a periapical radiograph before and after splinting to check the position of the donor tooth in the recipient socket. However, if the position of the donor tooth is the same as the tooth replica, this step can be omitted.
- Removal of the fixation. If the primary stability of the donor tooth has been adequate, the fixation can be removed at 4 weeks. However, if it has not been good, the fixation can be extended to 8 weeks. It is important to check that the transplanted tooth must stable before the splint is removed.
- Root canal treatment. Pulp healing is expected with transplanted immature teeth, making endodontic treatment unnecessary in most cases. Therefore, in normal conditions, root development will take place and the tooth will respond positive to electric pulp tests. If the roots do not continue developing and symptoms of pulp pathology (essentially, inflammatory root resorption) appear, the root canal treatment should be started immediately. If a mature donor tooth is accessible, the endodontic treatment can be completed before surgery. This approach can be highly advantageous, since in the hypothetical case of an intraoperative accident (i.e., separated instrument) during the endodontic treatment, the problem can be solved during autotransplant surgery. However, if the donor tooth is impacted or

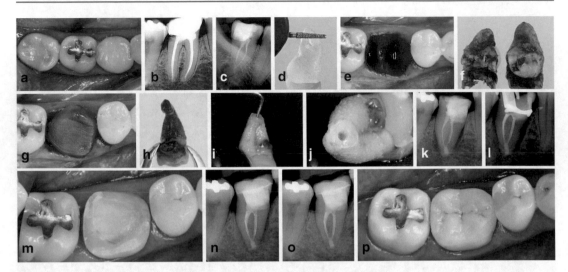

Fig. 9.14 Autotransplantation of a mature tooth combined with extraoral apicoectomy. (**a**) The patient was a 44-year-old female with a chief complaint of pain in teeth 46 and 48. Planning of the transplantation of the mandibular right third molar to the area of the non-restorable mandibular first molar. (**b**) Preoperative periapical radiograph. (**c**) Periapical radiograph of the donor tooth. (**d**) Simulation of the apical microsurgery in the printed replica. (**e**) The recipient site post-extraction. (**f**) Extraction of the non-restorable mandibular first molar. (**g**) Placement of the replica in the recipient site before extraction of the donor tooth. (**h**–**j**) The apicoectomy performed extraorally on the donor tooth, which was then replanted in the modified extraction socket. (**k**) Periapical radiograph immediately after transplantation. Note the apical retrofilling. (**l**) Nonsurgical retreatment performed 3 weeks post-surgery. (**m**) Cavity before impression. (**n**) Radiographic aspect of the restored molar 2 months after transplantation. (**o**) Three-year radiographic follow-up. (**p**) Three-year clinical follow-up showing excellent esthetic maintenance

erupted in a position that makes endodontic access difficult, root canal treatment should be started 2 weeks post surgery before removing the splint. The clinician may opt to complete the endodontic treatment in the same visit or place an interim dressing of calcium hydroxide in the root canal system. How long the intracanal medication is left inside the root canal depends on the clinician's criteria. Alternatively, root canal treatment can be performed extraorally during transplantation; however, this is not generally recommended, as there is a clear risk of damage to the PDL during the procedure (Fig. 9.14).

- Orthodontic and restorative treatment. After removal of the splint, the transplanted tooth normally sits naturally in its new position, especially when the donor tooth has an immature apex. It is vital to continuously check the position of the tooth to ensure there is no type of occlusal interference. In cases of autotransplantation to the anterior region, minor modifications of the morphology should be performed as soon as possible according to the esthetics and function of the tooth. One of the main advantages of the autotransplant technique is that it allows the clinician to work in a very conservative way and to finish the preparation on the enamel where the adhesion is superior to that of the dentin [111]. If necessary, an external bleaching can be performed when the tooth is still vital, or an internal bleaching in cases of an endodontically treated tooth. There are other scenarios where the clinician has no other choice than to perform an indirect restoration to place the tooth in an adequate occlusion and with the appropriate contact points with the neighboring teeth.

- A very frequent topic that clinicians ask themselves concerns the application of orthodontic forces to these transplanted teeth. In fact, there are no papers on the effectiveness or success of orthodontic forces of autotransplanted teeth [109]. Despite the lack of randomized controlled trials (RCTs), the influence of orthodontic movements on transplanted teeth seems to have minimal or little relevance [112–114]. However, as any traumatized tooth with a PDL injury, it is generally accepted that orthodontic forces should not be applied to a transplanted tooth for at least 6 months post-surgery [115, 116]. In cases of autotransplantation of immature teeth, orthodontic treatment should ideally be started after complete PDL healing, but preferably before the bone alveolar has fully formed. Therefore, the onset time can vary from 8 weeks to 3–9 months post-transplantation [117, 118].

- Periodical follow-up. Once transplanted teeth have healed, they are prone to the same risks as any natural tooth regarding caries and periodontal disease. Thus, these teeth require a periodic follow-up, just as the other teeth in the mouth. The patient's proactiveness is crucial to ensure positive long-term results.

9.5   Concluding Remarks

In the last 30 years, a better understanding of wound healing processes following transplantation, replantation, and surgical extrusion has significantly increased the success of these procedures. However, there is no general consensus as to the criteria used, making success rates vary within studies. It is evident that regardless of the study assessed, the clinician can expect the same level of success from these procedures as can be expected from dental implants. Thus, in specific and properly selected cases, autotransplantation and replantation are highly effective procedures. In this aspect, the clinician must know the fundamental healing mechanisms of the PDL, the alveolar bone, and the gingival tissue and the pulp.

With careful case selection based on indications, autotransplantation can prove to be a sufficiently predictable treatment, with success rates of 70–95% over 5 years. Naturally, the individual clinician's skill and ability in the final results is also a determining factor. An autotransplantation can be made even more predictable by combining digital planning, experience, skill, and good judgment in case selection.

However, surgical extrusion, intentional replantation, and autotransplantation have low level of scientifically based evidence due to a lack of randomized controlled trials (RCTs). Adequately designed prospective studies with an agreed definition of success are indispensable for a more comprehensive insight into the success rates of these treatments. Detection of root resorption following replantation may take up to 3 years, implying that more investigation is necessary with a sufficient sample size that includes long-term follow-ups. Multicenter collaborative efforts to study this could yield the sample size required to draw meaningful conclusions.

References

1. Natiella JR, Armitage JE, Greene GW. The replantation and transplantation of teeth. A review. Oral Surg Oral Med Oral Pathol. 1970;29:397–419.
2. Sugai T, et al. Clinical study on prognostic factors for autotransplantation of teeth with complete root formation. Int J Oral Maxillofac Surg. 2010;39:1193–203.
3. Krastl G, Filippi A, Zitzmann NU, Walter C, Weiger R. Current aspects of restoring traumatically fractured teeth. Eur J Esthet Dent. 2011;6:124–41.
4. Peer M. Intentional replantation—a "last resort" treatment or a conventional treatment procedure? Nine case reports. Dent Traumatol. 2004;20:48–55.
5. Anssari Moin D, Verweij JP, Waars H, van Merkesteyn R, Wismeijer D. Accuracy of computer-assisted template-guided autotransplantation of teeth with custom three-dimensional designed/printed surgical tooling: a cadaveric study. J Oral Maxillofac Surg. 2017;75:925.e1–7.
6. Almpani K, Papageorgiou SN, Papadopoulos MA. Autotransplantation of teeth in humans: a systematic review and meta-analysis. Clin Oral Investig. 2015;19:1157–79.
7. Tsukiboshi M. Autotransplantation of teeth: requirements for predictable success. Dent Traumatol. 2002;18:157–80.
8. Kafourou V, Tong HJ, Day P, Houghton N, Spencer RJ, Duggal M. Outcomes and prognostic factors that influence the success of tooth autotransplanta-

tion in children and adolescents. Dent Traumatol. 2017;33:393–9.

9. Andreasen JO, Paulsen HU, Yu Z, Ahlquist R, Bayer T, Schwartz O. A long-term study of 370 autotransplanted premolars. Part I. Surgical procedures and standardized techniques for monitoring healing. Eur J Orthod. 1990;12:3–13.

10. Andreasen JO. Effect of extra-alveolar period and storage media upon periodontal and pulpal healing after replantation of mature permanent incisors in monkeys. Int J Oral Surg. 1981;10:43–53.

11. Tsukiboshi M. Autotransplantation of teeth. Chicago, IL: Quintessence Pub Co; 2001.

12. Zufía J, Abella F, Trebol I, Gómez-Meda R. Autotransplantation of mandibular third molar with buccal cortical plate to replace vertically fractured mandibular second molar: a novel technique. J Endod. 2017;43:1574–8.

13. Proye MP, Polson AM. Repair in different zones of the periodontium after tooth reimplantation. J Periodontol. 1982;53:379–89.

14. Yu HJ, Jia P, Lv Z, Qiu LX. Autotransplantation of third molars with completely formed roots into surgically created sockets and fresh extraction sockets: a 10-year comparative study. Int J Oral Maxillofac Surg. 2017;46:531–8.

15. Bauss O, Zonios I, Rahman A. Root development of immature third molars transplanted to surgically created sockets. J Oral Maxillofac Surg. 2008;66:1200–11.

16. Skoglund A, Hasselgren G. Tissue changes in immature dog teeth autotransplanted to surgically prepared sockets. Oral Surg Oral Med Oral Pathol. 1992;74:789–95.

17. Andreasen JO, Kristerson L, Andreasen FM. Damage of the Hertwig's epithelial root sheath: effect upon root growth after autotransplantation of teeth in monkeys. Endod Dent Traumatol. 1988;4:145–51.

18. Kristerson L, Andreasen JO. Autotransplantation and replantation of tooth germs in monkeys. Effect of damage to the dental follicle and position of transplant in the alveolus. Int J Oral Surg. 1984;13:324–33.

19. Andreasen JO, Paulsen HU, Yu Z, Bayer T. A long-term study of 370 autotransplanted premolars. Part IV: root development subsequent to transplantation. Eur J Orthod. 1990;12:38–50.

20. Bauss O, Schwestka-Polly R, Schilke R, Kiliaridis S. Effect of different splinting methods and fixation periods on root development of autotransplanted immature third molars. J Oral Maxillofac Surg. 2005;63:304–10.

21. Bauss O, Engelke W, Fenske C, Schilke R, Schwestka-Polly R. Autotransplantation of immature third molars into edentulous and atrophied jaw sections. Int J Oral Maxillofac Surg. 2004;33:558–63.

22. Nagori SA, Jose A, Bhutia O, Roychoudhury A. Evaluating success of autotransplantation of embedded/impacted third molars harvested using

piezosurgery: a pilot study. Acta Odontol Scand. 2014;72:846–51.

23. Adreasen JO. Interrelation between alveolar bone and periodontal ligament repair after replantation of mature permanent incisors in monkeys. J Periodontal Res. 1981;16:228–35.

24. Garcia A, Saffar JL. Bone reactions around transplanted roots. A 5-month quantitative study in dogs. J Clin Periodontol. 1990;17:211–6.

25. Lekic P, Rojas J, Birek C, Tenenbaum H, McCulloch CA. Phenotypic comparison of periodontal ligament cells in vivo and in vitro. J Periodontol Res. 2001;36:71–9.

26. Seo BM, Miura M, Gronthos S, et al. Investigation of multipotent postnatal stem cells from human periodontal ligament. Lancet. 2004;364:149–55.

27. Ogata Y, Niisato N, Sakurai T, Furuyama S, Sugiya H. Comparison of the characteristics of human gingival fibroblasts and periodontal ligament cells. J Periodontol. 1995;66:1025–31.

28. Cross D, El-Angbawi A, McLaughlin P, et al. Developments in autotransplantation of teeth. Surgeon. 2013;11:49–55.

29. Imazato S, Fukunishi K. Potential efficacy of GTR and autogenous bone graft for autotransplantation to recipient sites with osseous defects: evaluation by re-entry procedure. Dent Traumatol. 2004;20:42–7.

30. Aoyama S, Yoshizawa M, Niimi K, Sugai T, Kitamura N, Saito C. Prognostic factors for autotransplantation of teeth with complete root formation. Oral Surg Oral Med Oral Pathol Oral Radiol. 2012;114:S216–28.

31. Mahal NK, Singh N, Thomas AM, Kakkar N. Effect of three different storage media on survival of periodontal ligament cells using collagenase-dispase assay. Int Endod J. 2013;46:365–70.

32. Ghasempour M, Moghadamnia AA, Abedian Z, Amir MP, Feizi F, Gharekhani S. In vitro viability of human periodontal ligament cells in green tea extract. J Conserv Dent. 2015;18:47–50.

33. Khademi AA, Saei S, Mohajeri MR, et al. A new storage medium for an avulsed tooth. J Contemp Dent Pract. 2008;9:025–32.

34. Osmanovic A, Halilovic S, Kurtovic-Kozaric A, Hadziabdic N. Evaluation of periodontal ligament cell viability in different storage media based on human PDL cell culture experiments—a systematic review. Dent Traumatol. 2018;34:384–93.

35. Skoglund A, Hasselgren G, Tronstad L. Oxidoreductase activity in the pulp of replanted and autotransplanted teeth in young dogs. Oral Surg Oral Med Oral Pathol. 1981;52:205–9.

36. Skoglund A, Tronstad L, Wallenius K. A microangiographic study of vascular changes in replanted and autotransplanted teeth of young dogs. Oral Surg Oral Med Oral Pathol. 1978;45:17–28.

37. Andreasen JO, Paulsen HU, Yu Z, Bayer T, Schwartz O. A long-term study of 370 autotransplanted premolars. Part II. Tooth survival and pulp heal-

ing subsequent to transplantation. Eur J Orthod. 1990;12:14–24.

38. Siers ML, Willemsen WL, Gulabivala K. Monitoring pulp vitality after transplantation of teeth with mature roots: a case report. Int Endod J. 2002;35:289–94.

39. Abd-Elmeguid A, ElSalhy M, Yu DC. Pulp canal obliteration after replantation of avulsed immature teeth: a systematic review. Dent Traumatol. 2015;31:437–41.

40. Murray PE, Garcia-Godoy F, Hargreaves KM. Regenerative endodontics: a review of current status and a call for action. J Endod. 2007;33:377–90.

41. Bae JH, Choi YH, Cho BH, Kim YK, Kim SG. Autotransplantation of teeth with complete root formation: a case series. J Endod. 2010;36:1422–6.

42. Chung WC, Tu YK, Lin YH, Lu HK. Outcomes of autotransplanted teeth with complete root formation: a systematic review and meta-analysis. J Clin Periodontol. 2014;41:412–23.

43. Jang Y, Choi YJ, Lee SJ, Roh BD, Park SH, Kim E. Prognostic factors for clinical outcomes in autotransplantation of teeth with complete root formation: survival analysis for up to 12 years. J Endod. 2016;42:198–205.

44. Marques-Ferreira M, Rabaça-Botelho MF, Carvalho L, Oliveiros B, Palmeirao-Carrilho EV. Autogenous tooth transplantation: evaluation of pulp tissue regeneration. Med Oral Patol Oral Cir Bucal. 2011;16:e984–9.

45. Gaviño Orduña JF, Caviedes-Bucheli J, Manzanares Céspedes MC, et al. Use of platelet-rich plasma in endodontic procedures in adults: regeneration or repair? A report of 3 cases with 5 years of follow-up. J Endod. 2017;43:1294–301.

46. Iohara K, Imabayashi K, Ishizaka R, et al. Complete pulp regeneration after pulpectomy by transplantation of CD105+ stem cells with stromal cell-derived factor-1. Tissue Eng Part A. 2011;17:1911–20.

47. Laureys WG, Cuvelier CA, Dermaut LR, De Pauw GA. The critical apical diameter to obtain regeneration of the pulp tissue after tooth transplantation, replantation, or regenerative endodontic treatment. J Endod. 2013;39:759–63.

48. Fang Y, Wang X, Zhu J, Su C, Yang Y, Meng L. Influence of apical diameter on the outcome of regenerative endodontic treatment in teeth with pulp necrosis: a review. J Endod. 2018;44:414–31.

49. Schatz JP, Joho JP. Long-term clinical and radiologic evaluation of autotransplanted teeth. Int J Oral Maxillofac Surg. 1992;21:271–5.

50. Moorrees CF, Fanning EA, Hunt EE Jr. Age variation of formation stages for ten permanent teeth. J Dent Res. 1963;42:1490–502.

51. Demirjian A, Goldstein H, Tanner JM. A new system of dental age assessment. Hum Biol. 1973;45:211–27.

52. van Westerveld KJH, Verweij JP, Fiocco M, Mensink G, van Merkesteyn JPR. Root elongation after autotransplantation in 58 transplanted premolars: the radiographic width of the apex as a predictor. J Oral Maxillofac Surg. 2019;77:1351–7.

53. Andreasen JO. Experimental dental traumatology: development of a model for external root resorption. Endod Dent Traumatol. 1987;3:269–87.

54. Andersson L, Blomlöf L, Lindskog S, Feiglin B, Hammarström L. Tooth ankylosis. Clinical, radiographic and histological assessments. Int J Oral Surg. 1984;13:423–31.

55. Andersson L, Bodin I, Sörensen S. Progression of root resorption following replantation of human teeth after extended extraoral storage. Endod Dent Traumatol. 1989;5:38–47.

56. Malmgren B. Ridge preservation/decoronation. J Endod. 2013;39:S67–72.

57. Abbott PV. Prevention and management of external inflammatory resorption following trauma to teeth. Aust Dent J. 2016;61(Suppl 1):82–94.

58. Yu CY, Abbott PV. Responses of the pulp, periradicular and soft tissues following trauma to the permanent teeth. Aust Dent J. 2016;61(Suppl 1):39–58.

59. Gegauff AG. Effect of crown lengthening and ferrule placement on static load failure of cemented cast post-cores and crowns. J Prosthet Dent. 2000;84:169–79.

60. Stankiewicz NR, Wilson PR. The ferrule effect: a literature review. Int Endod J. 2002;35:575–81.

61. Juloski J, Radovic I, Goracci C, Vulicevic ZR, Ferrari M. Ferrule effect: a literature review. J Endod. 2012;38:11–9.

62. Khanberg KE. Intraalveolar transplantation of teeth with crown-root fractures. J Oral Maxillofac Surg. 1985;43:38–42.

63. Levine RA. Forced eruption in the esthetic zone. Compend Contin Educ Dent. 1997;18:795–803.

64. Davarpanah M, Jansen CE, Vidjak FM, Etienne D, Kebir M, Martinez H. Restorative and periodontal considerations of short clinical crowns. Int J Periodontics Restorative Dent. 1998;18:424–33.

65. Kohavi D, Stern N. Crown lengthening procedure. Part II. Treatment planning and surgical considerations. Compend Contin Educ Dent. 1983;4:413–9.

66. Smidt A, Gleitman J, Dekel MS. Forced eruption of a solitary nonrestorable tooth using mini-implants as anchorage: rationale and technique. Int J Prosthodont. 2009;22:441–6.

67. Das B, Muthu MS. Surgical extrusion as a treatment option for crown-root fracture in permanent anterior teeth: a systematic review. Dent Traumatol. 2013;29:423–31.

68. Tegsjö U, Valerius-Olsson H, Olgart K. Intra-alveolar transplantation of teeth with cervical root fractures. Swed Dent J. 1978;2:73–82.

69. Khanberg KE. Intra-alveolar transplantation. I. A 10-year follow-up of a method for surgical extrusion of root fractured teeth. Swed Dent J. 1996;20:165–72.

70. Kim CS, Choi SH, Chai JK, Kim CK, Cho KS. Surgical extrusion technique for clinical crown

lengthening: report of three cases. Int J Periodontics Restorative Dent. 2004;24:412–21.

71. Oikarinen KS, Stoltze K, Andreasen JO. Influence of conventional forceps extraction and extraction with an extrusion instrument on cementoblast loss and external root resorption of replanted monkey incisors. J Periodontol Res. 1996;31:337–44.

72. Hong B, Bulsara Y, Gorecki P, Dietrich T. Minimally invasive vertical versus conventional tooth extraction: an interrupted time series study. J Am Dent Assoc. 2018;149:688–95.

73. Muska E, Walter C, Knight A, et al. Atraumatic vertical tooth extraction: a proof of principle clinical study of a novel system. Oral Surg Oral Med Oral Pathol Oral Radiol. 2013;116:e303–10.

74. Kelly RD, Addison O, Tomson PL, Krastl G, Dietrich T. Atraumatic surgical extrusion to improve tooth restorability: a clinical report. J Prosthet Dent. 2016;115:649–53.

75. Dietrich T, Krug R, Krastl G, Tomson PL. Restoring the unrestorable! Developing coronal tooth tissue with a minimally invasive surgical extrusion technique. Br Dent J. 2019;226:789–93.

76. Kahler B, Hu JY, Marriot-Smith CS, Heithersay GS. Splinting of teeth following trauma: a review and a new splinting recommendation. Aust Dent J. 2016;61(Suppl 1):59–73.

77. Andersson L, Andreasen JO, Day P, et al. International association of dental traumatology guidelines for the management of traumatic dental injuries: 2. Avulsion of permanent teeth. Dent Traumatol. 2012;28:88–96.

78. Lengheden A, Jansson L. Ph effects on experimental wound healing of human fibroblast in vitro. Eur J Oral Sci. 1995;103:148–55.

79. Hinckfuss SE, Messer LB. An evidence-based assessment of the clinical guidelines for replanted avulsed teeth. Part II: prescription of systemic antibiotics. Dent Traumatol. 2009;25:158–64.

80. Grossman LI. Intentional replantation of teeth. J Am Dent Assoc. 1966;72:1111–8.

81. Dryden JA, Arens DE. Intentional replantation—a viable alternative for selected cases. Dent Clin N Am. 1994;38:325–53.

82. Garrido I, Abella F, Ordinola-Zapata R, Duran-Sindreu F, Roig M. Combined endodontic therapy and intentional replantation for the treatment of palatogingival groove. J Endod. 2016;42:324–8.

83. Becker BD. Intentional replantation techniques: a critical review. J Endod. 2018;44:14–21.

84. Torabinejad M, Dinsbach NA, Turman M, Handysides R, Bahjri K, White SN. Survival of intentionally replanted teeth and implant-supported single crowns: a systematic review. J Endod. 2015;41:992–8.

85. Mainkar A. A systematic review of the survival of teeth intentionally replanted with a modern technique and cost-effectiveness compared with single-tooth implants. J Endod. 2017;43:1963–8.

86. Bender IB, Rossman LE. Intentional replantation of endodontically treated teeth. Oral Surg Oral Med Oral Pathol. 1993;76:623–30.

87. Nosonowitz DM, Stanley HR. Intentional replantation to prevent predictable endodontic failures. Oral Surg Oral Med Oral Pathol. 1984;57:423–32.

88. Andreasen JO, Hjorting-Hansen E. Reimplantation of teeth. Radiographic and clinical study of 110 human teeth reimplanted after accidental loss (part I). Acta Odontol Scand. 1966;24:263–86.

89. Chércoles-Ruiz A, Sánchez-Torres A, Gay-Escoda C. Endodontics, endodontic retreatment, and apical surgery versus tooth extraction and implant placement: a systematic review. J Endod. 2017;43:679–86.

90. Cotter MR, Panzarino J. Intentional replantation: a case report. J Endod. 2006;32:579–82.

91. Choi YH, Bae JH, Kim YK, Kim HY, Kim SK, Cho BH. Clinical outcome of intentional replantation with preoperative orthodontic extrusion: a retrospective study. Int Endod J. 2014;47:1168–76.

92. Sugaya T, Tomita M, Motoki Y, Miyaji H, Kawamami M. Influence of enamel matrix derivative on healing of root surfaces after bonding treatment and intentional replantation of vertically fractured roots. Dent Traumatol. 2016;32:397–401.

93. Nizam N, Kaval ME, Gürlek Ö, Atila A, Çalışkan MK. Intentional replantation of adhesively reattached vertically fractured maxillary single-rooted teeth. Int Endod J. 2016;49:227–36.

94. Solakoglu Ö, Filippi A. Transreplantation: an alternative for periodontally hopeless teeth. Quintessence Int. 2017;48:287–93.

95. Saida H, Fukuba S, Miron R, Shirakata Y. Efficacy of flapless intentional replantation with enamel matrix derivative in the treatment of hopeless teeth associated with endodontic-periodontal lesions: a 2-year prospective case series. Quintessence Int. 2018;49:699–707.

96. Espona J, Roig E, Durán-Sindreu F, Abella F, Machado M, Roig M. Invasive cervical resorption: clinical management in the anterior zone. J Endod. 2018;44:1749–54.

97. Kany FM. Single-tooth osteotomy for intentional replantation. J Endod. 2002;28:408–10.

98. Kim S, Kratchman S. Modern endodontic surgery concepts and practice: a review. J Endod. 2006;32:601–23.

99. Zachrisson BU, Stenvik A, Haanaes HR. Management of missing maxillary anterior teeth with emphasis on autotransplantation. Am J Orthod Dentofac Orthop. 2004;126:284–8.

100. Schatz JP, Joho JP. Indications of autotransplantation of teeth in orthodontic problem cases. Am J Orthod Dentofac Orthop. 1994;106:351–7.

101. Slagter KW, Meijer HJ, Bakker NA, et al. Feasibility of immediate placement of singletooth implants in the aesthetic zone: a 1-year randomized controlled trial. J Clin Periodontol. 2015;42:773–82.

102. Torabinejad M, Dinsbach NA, Turman M, et al. Survival of intentionally replanted teeth and implant-supported single crowns: a systematic review. J Endod. 2015;41:992–8.

103. Albrektsson T, Donos N, Working Group 1. Implant survival and complications. The Third EAO consensus conference 2012. Clin Oral Implants Res. 2012;23(Suppl 6):63–5.

104. Pjetursson BE, Karoussis I, Bürgin W, Brägger U, Lang NP. Patients' satisfaction following implant therapy. A 10 year prospective cohort study. Clin Oral Implants Res. 2005;16:185–93.

105. Fardal Ø, Grytten J. A comparison of teeth and implants during maintenance therapy in terms of the number of disease-free years and costs—an in vivo internal control study. J Clin Periodontol. 2013;40:645–51.

106. Cardona JL, Caldera MM, Vera J. Autotransplantation of a premolar: a long-term follow-up report of a clinical case. J Endod. 2012;38:1149–52.

107. Intra JB, Roldi A, Brandao RC, et al. Autogenous premolar transplantation into artificial socket in maxillary lateral incisor site. J Endod. 2014;40:1885–90.

108. Vignoletti F, Matesanz P, Rodrigo D, Figuero E, Martin C, Sanz M. Surgical protocols for ridge preservation after tooth extraction. A systematic review. Clin Oral Implants Res. 2012;23(Suppl 5):22–38.

109. Rohof ECM, Kerdijk W, Jansma J, Livas C, Ren Y. Autotransplantation of teeth with incomplete root formation: a systematic review and meta-analysis. Clin Oral Investig. 2018;22:1613–24.

110. Anitua E, Mendinueva-Urkia M, Galan-Bringas S, Murias-Freijo A, Alkhraisat MH. Tooth autotransplantation as a pillar for 3D regeneration of the alveolar process after severe traumatic injury: a case report. Dent Traumatol. 2017;33:414–9.

111. Veneziani M. Posterior indirect adhesive restorations: updated indications and the morphology driven preparation technique. Int J Esthet Dent. 2017;12:204–30.

112. Gonnissen H, Politis C, Schepers S, Lambrichts I, Vrielinck L, Sun Y, Schuermans J. Long-term success and survival rates of autogenously transplanted canines. Oral Surg Oral Med Oral Pathol Oral Radiol Endod. 2010;110:570–8.

113. Watanabe Y, Mohri T, Takeyama M, Yamaki M, Okiji T, Saito C, Saito I. Long-term observation of autotransplanted teeth with complete root formation in orthodontic patients. Am J Orthod Dentofac Orthop. 2010;138:720–6.

114. Mendoza-Mendoza A, Solano-Reina E, Iglesias-Linares A, Garcia-Godoy F, Abalos C. Retrospective long-term evaluation of autotransplantation of premolars to the central incisor region. Int Endod J. 2012;45:88–97.

115. Kindelan SA, Day PF, Kindelan JD, Spencer JR, Duggal MS. Dental trauma: an overview of its influence on the management of orthodontic treatment. Part 1. J Orthod. 2008;35:68–78.

116. Day PF, Kindelan SA, Spencer JR, Kindelan JD, Duggal MS. Dental trauma: part 2. Managing poor prognosis anterior teeth—treatment options for the subsequent space in a growing patient. J Orthod. 2008;35:143–55.

117. Paulsen HU, Andreasen JO, Schwartz O. Pulp and periodontal healing, root development and root resorption subsequent to transplantation and orthodontic rotation: a long-term study of autotransplanted premolars. Am J Orthod Dentofac Orthop. 1995;108:630–40.

118. Mensink G, van Merkesteyn R. Autotransplantation of premolars. Br Dent J. 2010;208:109–11.

Printed in the United States
by Baker & Taylor Publisher Services